Risk Management for Health/Fitness Professionals

Legal Issues and Strategies

Risk Management for Health/Fitness Professionals
Legal Issues and Strategies

JoAnn M. Eickhoff-Shemek, PhD, FACSM, FAWHP

Professor & Coordinator, Exercise Science
School of Physical Education & Exercise Science
University of South Florida
Tampa, Florida

David L. Herbert, JD

Member, David L. Herbert & Associates, LLC
Attorneys & Counselors at Law
The Renaissance Centre
Canton, Ohio

Daniel P. Connaughton, EdD

Associate Professor
University of Florida
Department of Tourism, Recreation & Sport Management
Gainesville, Florida

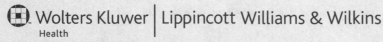 Wolters Kluwer | Lippincott Williams & Wilkins
Health

Philadelphia · Baltimore · New York · London
Buenos Aires · Hong Kong · Sydney · Tokyo

Acquisitions Editor: Emily Lupash
Development Editor: Jennifer P. Ajello
Marketing Manager: Christen D. Murphy
Production Editor: Paula C. Williams
Designer: Doug Smock
Compositor: International Typesetting and Composition
Printer: Data Reproductions Corporation

Library of Congress Cataloging-in-Publication Data

Eickhoff-Shemek, JoAnn M.
   Risk management for health/fitness professionals : legal issues and strategies / JoAnn Eickhoff-Shemek,
David L. Herbert, Daniel P. Connaughton.
        p. ; cm.
   Includes bibliographical references and index.
   ISBN-13: 978-0-7817-8364-4 (alk. paper)
   ISBN-10: 0-7817-8364-X (alk. paper)
   1. Exercise personnel—Malpractice—United States.   2. Physical fitness centers—Law
and legislation—United States.   I. Herbert, David L.   II. Connaughton, Daniel, 1963–
III. Title.
   [DNLM: 1. Fitness Centers—legislation & jurisprudence—United States.   2. Malpractice—legislation &
jurisprudence—United States.   3. Physical Education and Training—legislation & jurisprudence—United
States.   4. Risk Management—legislation & jurisprudence—United States.   QT 33 AA1 E34 2009]
   KF2915.E953E33 2009
   344.7304'11—dc22   2008018516

DISCLAIMER

Care has been taken to confirm the accuracy of the information present and to describe generally accepted practices. However, the authors, editors, and publisher are not responsible for errors or omissions or for any consequences from application of the information in this book and make no warranty, expressed or implied, with respect to the currency, completeness, or accuracy of the contents of the publication. Application of this information in a particular situation remains the professional responsibility of the practitioner; the clinical treatments described and recommended may not be considered absolute and universal recommendations.

The authors, editors, and publisher have exerted every effort to ensure that drug selection and dosage set forth in this text are in accordance with the current recommendations and practice at the time of publication. However, in view of ongoing research, changes in government regulations, and the constant flow of information relating to drug therapy and drug reactions, the reader is urged to check the package insert for each drug for any change in indications and dosage and for added warnings and precautions. This is particularly important when the recommended agent is a new or infrequently employed drug.

Some drugs and medical devices presented in this publication have Food and Drug Administration (FDA) clearance for limited use in restricted research settings. It is the responsibility of the health care provider to ascertain the FDA status of each drug or device planned for use in their clinical practice.

To purchase additional copies of this book, call our customer service department at (800) 638-3030 or fax orders to (301) 223-2320. International customers should call (301) 223-2300.

Visit Lippincott Williams & Wilkins on the Internet: http://www.lww.com. Lippincott Williams & Wilkins customer service representatives are available from 8:30 am to 6:00 pm, EST.

I dedicate this book to my husband, Patrick Shemek. I am very grateful for his love, support, sense of humor, and amazing patience through the completion of this book and many other academic endeavors. I also dedicate this book to my parents, Ralph and Hilda Eickhoff, now in their late 80s, who continue to enjoy an active retirement. I appreciate everything they have taught me but especially the importance of serving others. In addition, I would like to thank my coauthors and colleagues, David Herbert and Dan Connaughton. It was a distinct pleasure and honor to work with such gifted scholars. Lastly, I dedicate this book to the exercise science students who enrolled in my graduate risk management course over the last 10 years. Not only did they express a real need for a textbook like this one, but they contributed to the book in numerous ways.

JoAnn M. Eickhoff-Shemek

My work on this text is dedicated to someone who has had a profound and lasting impact on both my life and professional endeavors and to whom I am very grateful and appreciative: William G. Herbert, PhD, my brother and exercise physiologist extraordinaire.

David L. Herbert

I would like to thank my parents for their love and support. I would also like to acknowledge my dedicated coauthors for their tireless efforts, friendship, and assistance.

Daniel P. Connaughton

About the Authors

JOANN M. EICKHOFF-SHEMEK

Dr. Eickhoff-Shemek is a professor and the coordinator of the undergraduate exercise science program at the University of South Florida in Tampa. She has authored numerous peer-reviewed journal articles and book chapters addressing legal liability and risk management issues in the health/fitness field. At her former institution, the University of Nebraska at Omaha (UNOmaha), she developed and coordinated a master's degree program in health and fitness management (HFM) and taught a risk management course designed for HFM and exercise science graduate students. While at UNOmaha, she received the College of Education's Outstanding Teaching Award. Dr. Eickhoff-Shemek has been elected or appointed to serve in many national leadership positions for over 25 years, and since 2000, she has served as the legal columnist and an associate editor for *ACSM's Health & Fitness Journal*. Dr. Eickhoff-Shemek is a certified ACSM Health/Fitness Director and ACSM Exercise Test Technologist and a fellow of ACSM and the former AWHP. Before becoming a full-time academician in 1994, she worked as a health/fitness manager in various settings for nearly 18 years.

DAVID L. HERBERT

David L. Herbert is a senior member of the law firm of David L. Herbert & Associates, LLC, Attorneys and Counselors at Law, Canton, Ohio. He is a graduate of Kent State University and The University of Akron, School of Law. Mr. Herbert is a former assistant prosecuting attorney and was previously on the faculty of Kent State University. He is the author of more than 40 books/book chapters and approximately 600 articles on legal topics dealing with health and fitness facilities, sports medicine, negligence, malpractice, and similar legal topics. He has been a writer and column author for *Fitness Management* magazine for nearly 20 years and has published articles there as well as in *ACSM's Health & Fitness Journal, American Fitness, The Trial Lawyers Journal*, law reviews, and numerous other publications. Mr. Herbert was formerly an editor for *The Physician and Sportsmedicine* journal. He is coeditor of *The Exercise Standards and Malpractice Reporter, The Sports Medicine Standards and Malpractice Reporter*, and *The Sports, Parks & Recreation Law Reporter*, all published by PRC Publishing, Inc. of Canton, Ohio. He has assisted the ACSM, NSCA, AFAA, and other organizations in the development of their various standards and guidelines over the last 25 years. He has been a presenter for annual meetings of the ACSM, NATA, ASCM, AHA, AOASM and numerous other organizations and has made a variety of presentations for programs at Akron General Hospital, SummaCare, Aultman Hospital, St. Thomas Hospital, The Cleveland Clinic, and many other hospitals and similar groups. He is a trustee of the National Board of Fitness Examiners (NBFE).

DANIEL P. CONNAUGHTON

Dr. Dan Connaughton is an associate professor at the University of Florida (UF) where he conducts research and teaches sport law and risk management. He received a bachelor's degree in exercise and sport sciences, and a master's degree in recreational studies from UF, a master's degree in physical education from Bridgewater State College, and a doctorate in sport management from Florida State University. An author of numerous peer-reviewed articles and book chapters, and the recipient of several teaching and scholar awards, Dr. Connaughton is a fellow with the Research Consortium of AAHPERD. He is also a licensed emergency medical technician and holds numerous professional certifications, including ACSM Health/Fitness Instructor and NSCA Certified Strength and Conditioning Specialist. He has several years of experience in the health/fitness field as a fitness instructor, fitness director, and program director. Dr. Connaughton frequently serves as a consultant and expert witness in health/fitness and sport-related litigation.

Preface

Risk Management for Health/Fitness Professionals: Legal Issues and Strategies is specifically designed to provide education and information to fitness, exercise, allied healthcare/ wellness and health promotion students, practitioners, and managers. The book has been written with an awareness of the following facts:

- Health/fitness facilities typically offer access to free weights, stationary bicycles, climbers/steppers, plate-loaded exercise devices, treadmills, rowers, and programs/services including group exercise and personal fitness training for various populations.
- Health/fitness facility membership and use is continuing to grow, although the U.S. population is aging. More facility users are older than ever before. Canadian facilities are experiencing similar growth patterns.
- Current estimates indicate that almost 40 million U.S. citizens are members of nearly 27,000 health clubs. The health club industry currently has revenues exceeding $14 billion. These data do not reflect the proliferation of many other health/fitness facilities, such as in corporate, community, university/college, hospital/clinical, government, and retirement settings. For example, more than 2,600 YMCAs in the United States serve over 20 million people each year.
- Although estimates for Canada are somewhat more difficult to quantify, there are over 10,000 health/fitness facilities in that country, and approximately half of all Canadians report they are physically active.
- Health/fitness professionals design and direct exercise programs in the United States and Canada in a variety of settings. Participation in exercise programs can create risks for many types of personal injuries. Therefore, a major responsibility of health/fitness professionals is to provide reasonably safe conditions for the participants they serve.
- A variety of medical emergencies occur in health/fitness facilities each year, including life-threatening events such as sudden cardiac arrests. When such incidents occur, injured parties often file negligence claims or lawsuits against health/fitness personnel and facilities to recover monetary damages. As a result, insurance companies sometimes pay out large sums of money when these liability claims are asserted or established in court settlements, judgments, or even for defense costs, all of which might be prevented through sound risk management practices as described in this book.
- Health/fitness safety standards and guidelines have been published in the United States principally through professional organizations. Applicable Canadian standards and guidelines have also been developed.
- Although most health/fitness professionals believe that compliance with the law and published safety standards and guidelines is important, research has shown that many professionals are not familiar with the law and these published statements, and therefore they are not complying with such laws and statements.
- The lack of familiarity with the law as well as published standards and guidelines can and does lead to the delivery of some programs/services below the so-called legal standard of care. This exposes participants to untoward risks of

injury and even death, while exposing professionals and facilities to the risk of claim and suit because of this lack of knowledge and familiarity with standards statements.

- Research indicates that most undergraduate and graduate programs in exercise science (or related areas) do not offer or require a risk management/legal liability course for their students. Although academic programs (undergraduate exercise science and personal fitness training and graduate clinical and applied exercise physiology) can become nationally accredited and recognized for meeting quality standards, it is important that accreditation standards include adequate course work in risk management and the law.
- The demand for personal fitness trainers is at an all-time high. Various professional organizations, including the International Health, Racquet and Sportsclub Association (IHRSA), the National Board of Fitness Examiners (NBFE), and other similar organizations are presently raising educational requirements and training standards for these professionals through their recommendations and activities.
- Specific education and training of health/fitness students and professionals is needed through a textbook that provides risk management concepts, information as to published standards and guidelines, and an understanding of various legal concepts and potential problems in the delivery of programs/services that can be eliminated or at least managed through the application of risk management principles and concepts.

ORGANIZATION

The 14 chapters of this book are divided into three different parts. Each part focuses on an important area for review and learning.

Part I begins with an introduction into the area for study and includes a broad but necessary review of various principles of law and risk management and a review of the legal system including civil and criminal law issues. Topics of major concern focus on concepts of negligence and the elements that must be established in legal proceedings based on such concepts, as well as common defenses (e.g., assumption of risk, release/waiver, and informed consent) to negligence claims and lawsuits.

Part II focuses on specific topics to which legal and risk management principles will be applied and includes the following:

- Employment issues with a focus on the distinction between employees and independent contractors, legal principles related to employer–employee relationships, and the importance of protecting health/fitness personnel and facilities through liability insurance.
- Hiring, training, and ongoing education of personnel in core competencies and emerging issues of concern such as an understanding and appreciation of applicable laws and risk management.
- The use of pre-activity health screening processes and a discussion of circumstances under which program participants need medical clearance prior to commencing activity.
- Health/fitness assessments and the prescription or recommendation for participant activity and the need for the setting of activity parameters.
- Proper instruction and supervision of participants in diverse service settings including a discussion of issues dealing with the provision of service by personal fitness trainers and group exercise leaders.
- The selection, installation, inspection, and maintenance of exercise equipment as well as the provision of proper instruction/supervision and posting of equipment safety and warning signs or labels.

- Facility risks including adherence to the Americans with Disabilities Act (ADA) and proper maintenance of premises inside and outside of the health/fitness facility, as well as important risk management strategies for off-premises activities and sponsored events.
- Compliance with the Bloodborne Pathogens Standard established by the Occupational Safety and Health Administration (OSHA) that includes the development of a written Exposure Control Plan.
- Medical emergency procedures including the development of a written emergency action plan (EAP) concentrating on the importance of properly carrying out the facility's EAP by qualified and well-trained staff members.

Applicable laws and actual case examples from claims and litigation are provided for each of the areas just described to stimulate discussion. Summaries of important standards and guidelines published by professional organizations (see Publication Notice and Authors' Note) are included, followed by recommended risk management strategies that can assist health/fitness professionals in the exercise of professional judgment to provide a reasonably safe environment for their participants. Implementing these risk management strategies may result in fewer medical emergencies and less subsequent litigation.

Part III focuses on the implementation and evaluation of a comprehensive risk management plan that includes the development of a Risk Management Policies and Procedures Manual (RMPPM) and staff training. Additional selected topics and related risk management strategies are also presented, such as copyright laws, unsupervised health/fitness facilities, employer-sponsored programs, and steps to take if ever named in a lawsuit, as well as how to select a lawyer. Finally, a summary of the book is presented using a newly developed Risk Management Pyramid that provides at a glance seven lines of defense that health/fitness professionals can implement to protect themselves and the organizations they represent.

ADDITIONAL RESOURCES

Risk Management for Health/Fitness Professionals: Legal Issues and Strategies includes additional resources for students and instructors, available on the book's companion website at http://thePoint.lww.com/Eickhoff.

- Downloadable blank forms from the text.
- Searchable Full Text Online.

Purchasers of the text can access these resources by going to the *Risk Management for Health/Fitness Professionals: Legal Issues and Strategies* website at http://thePoint.lww.com. See the inside front cover of this text for more details, including the passcode you will need to gain access to the website.

SUMMARY

This textbook was written to fill a decided void in the educational materials covering this topic. Given recent survey findings, this textbook should provide important information to a profession that needs a much better understanding of the applicable risks and their attendant consequences. This book also provides clear guidance on how applicable risks may be managed. In addition, the LWW website, http://thePoint.lww.com/Eickhoff, provides an electronic version of the many forms and documents contained in this book so that health/fitness professionals, and their risk management advisory committees can easily review them.

The information contained in this book should not be construed as legal or medical advice. Health/fitness professionals need to consult with competent local attorneys and other qualified experts for specific guidance. Please see the Publication Notice below.

JoAnn M. Eickhoff-Shemek, PhD, FACSM, FAWHP
Professor and Coordinator, Exercise Science
School of Physical Education & Exercise Science
University of South Florida
4202 East Fowler Avenue, PED214
Tampa, FL 33620-8600
Phone: (813) 974-4676
Fax: (813) 974-4979
E-mail: eickhoff@tempest.coedu.usf.edu

David L. Herbert, JD
David L. Herbert & Associates, LLC
Attorneys and Counselors at Law
4580 Stephen Circle NW, Suite 300
Canton, OH 44718
Phone: (330)499-1016
Fax: (330) 499-0790
E-mail: herblegal@aol.com or dlherbert@herblaw.com

Daniel P. Connaughton, EdD
Associate Professor
Department of Tourism, Recreation and Sport Management
University of Florida
P.O. Box 118208
Gainesville, FL 32611
Phone: (352) 392-4042 ext. 1296
Fax: (352) 392-7588
E-mail: danc@hhp.ufl.edu

PUBLICATION NOTICE

This publication is written and published to provide accurate and authoritative information relevant to the subject matter presented. It is published and sold with the understanding that the authors and publisher are not engaged in rendering legal, medical, or other professional services by reason of their authorship or publication of this work. If legal, medical, or other expert assistance is required, the services of competent professional persons should be obtained by those in need of such services. Moreover, in the field of health and fitness, the services of such competent professionals must be obtained.

Adapted from the Declaration of Principles of the American Bar Association and a committee of publishers and associations.

Reviewers

Sonja Anderson-Struzzo, NASM CPT,
 IDEA Elite, PFT
Fitness Center Director
Brentwood Country Club
Los Angeles, CA

Lisa Eldracher, MS
Fitness Professional
Woodbridge, CT

Bill Finnearty, MS
Department of Allied Health
Hocking College
Nelsonville, OH

Brian Leutholtz, PhD
Program Director-Exercise Science
Department of Health, Human Performance
 and Recreation
Baylor University
Waco, TX

Chad London, PhD
Associate Dean
Faculty of Health and Community Studies
Mount Royal College
Calgary, AB

Thomas Richards, JD
Public Policy Manager
International Health, Racquet, and Sportsclub
 Association (IHRSA)
Boston, MA

Janet Schumacher, MS
Area Manager, Program Director
Corporate Fitness and Wellness
San Jose, CA

Robert Steele, MS
Department Chair
Athletic Training Education Program
National American University
Rapid City, SD

Kristin Ugrob, BA
Fitness Director
Magdalena Ecke Family YMCA
Encinitas, CA

Acknowledgments

M any people have contributed to the preparation and completion of this text including the following staff members at Lippincott Williams & Wilkins (LWW): Jennifer Ajello (Development Editor), Emily Lupash (Acquisitions Editor), Paula Williams (Production Editor), and Christen Murphy (Marketing Manager), as well as Arushi Chawla of International Typesetting and Composition who served as our Project Manager. We would also like to thank LWW staff member Peter Darcy and former LWW staff member Karen Ruppert for their support and assistance in the early stages of the development of this book. In addition, we are grateful for the reviewers of this book who offered valuable suggestions to improve this book. They include Sonja Anderson-Struzzo, Lisa Eldracher, Bill Finnearty, Brian Leutholtz, Chad London, Thomas Richards, Janet Schumacher, Robert Steele, and Kristin Ugrob.

The authors would also like to thank those who provided permissions for the use of materials developed by a variety of professional organizations which has enabled the authors to incorporate standard statements within this work. These professional organizations include the American College of Sports Medicine (ACSM), Aerobics and Fitness Association of America (AFAA), American Heart Association (AHA), International Health, Racquet & Sportsclub Association (IHRSA), Medical Fitness Association (MFA), National Strength and Conditioning Association (NSCA), Ontario Association of Sport and Exercise Sciences (OASES), and Young Men's Christian Association (YMCA) of the USA. We would also like to thank the following organizations—the American Law Institute, American Society for Testing and Materials, Association Insurance Group, Canadian Society for Exercise Physiology, Creative Agency Group, Cybex International Inc., FranklinCovey, Human Kinetics, Kendall/Hunt Publishing, Lippincott Williams & Wilkins, National Heart Lung and Blood Institute, PRC Publishing, Inc., and Thomson Learning Global Rights Group, as well as the following individuals—Kris Berg, Aaron Craig, Jon Denley, Ken Reinig, and Susan Selde who have provided permissions for the use of their materials.

Authors' Note

Throughout this publication are a variety of citations and commentary about standards, guidelines, parameters of practice, and similar statements authored by a number of associations involved in the health and fitness profession. These standards, guidelines, and similar recommendations are subject not only to modification as time goes by but to interpretation and application to particular facts. As a consequence, the information presented in this publication needs to be evaluated through the application of individual professional judgment before adaptation to any particular program or practice. Furthermore, in light of the fact that such statements evolve as time progresses, these statements must be reviewed and interpreted periodically to determine the applicability of such statements to particular programs and practices.

JoAnn M. Eickhoff-Shemek, PhD
David L. Herbert, JD
Daniel P. Connaughton, EdD

Contents

PART I

INTRODUCTION

CHAPTER 1

Introduction to Risk Management

LEARNING OBJECTIVES After reading this chapter, health/fitness students and professionals will be able to:

1. Define "risks" and describe the types of risks that can lead to medical emergencies in health/fitness facilities.

2. Describe the types of personal injury claims that occur in health/fitness facilities and the effect they have had on the profession.

3. Describe studies that have reported the number of injuries associated with physical activity and sport activities.

4. Describe why health/fitness professionals typically have little knowledge about the law and risk management.

5. Define risk management and related terms.

6. Describe the four steps comprising the risk management planning process.

7. Understand the role of the risk management advisory committee.

8. Understand the various types of health/fitness professionals and their risk management responsibilities.

9. Describe the types of health/fitness facilities and settings.

10. Identify three major benefits of risk management.

This chapter is divided into four major sections: (a) Risks Presented to the Health/Fitness Profession, (b) Risk Management Defined, (c) Health/Fitness Professionals and Their Risk Management Responsibilities, and (d) Benefits of Risk Management. The first section introduces the topic of "risks" and the types of risks that occur in health/fitness facilities that often lead to litigation. The second section defines risk management and presents the four risk management steps used in this book. The third section focuses on the various types of health/fitness professionals and the role they each have regarding risk management, and the fourth section describes the major benefits of risk management.

RISKS PRESENTED TO THE HEALTH/FITNESS PROFESSION

This section defines "risk" and presents the two major types of risks (health risks and injury risks) that can lead to medical emergencies occurring in health/fitness facilities. When medical emergencies occur, legal claims and lawsuits often follow. In the last three decades, litigation has increased in the health/fitness field as it has generally in our society. Possible reasons to explain why there has been an increase in litigation in the health/fitness field are described.

WHAT ARE RISKS?

Many physiological and psychological benefits are obtained from participation in regular physical activity and exercise[1] (see Table 1-1). However, risks are also associated with physical activity and exercise. Appenzeller[2] defines **risk** as an element of danger. Two categories of risks exist in the health/fitness field: **Health risks** are medical conditions and/or risk factors that can lead to problems such as cardiac arrest, stroke, or an insulin reaction; and **injury risks** are conditions or situations that can lead to problems such as back injury, fractured bone, or cut/abrasion that causes bleeding. Both types of risks can result in medical emergencies occurring in health/fitness facilities.

The major goals of risk management are to prevent medical emergencies from occurring in the first place and to respond properly to them (e.g., appropriate first aid) when they do occur. Other goals of risk management, as we discuss later, are of a secondary but important nature to offset or manage risks through other strategies.

TABLE 1-1 Top 25 Reasons to Exercise

1. Strengthens heart muscle
2. Decreases the incidence of heart attack
3. Reduces risks for heart disease (e.g., reduces bad low-density lipoprotein [LDL] cholesterol and increases good high-density lipoprotein [HDL] cholesterol)
4. Improves circulation and oxygen/nutrient transport throughout the body
5. Helps lose weight and keep it off
6. Improves breathing efficiency
7. Strengthens and tones muscles and improves appearance
8. Helps prevent back problems and back pain
9. Improves posture
10. Strengthens bones and helps reduce risk of osteoporosis
11. Strengthens the tissues around the joints and reduces joint discomfort and arthritis if appropriate exercise is selected and properly performed
12. Decreases risk for several types of cancer
13. Improves immune function, which decreases risk for infectious diseases
14. Maintains physical and mental functions throughout the second half of life
15. Increases self-confidence and self-esteem
16. Boosts energy and increases productivity
17. Improves sleep
18. Helps create a positive attitude about life
19. Reduces anxiety and depression
20. Increases resistance to fatigue
21. May lengthen lifespan
22. Reduces blood pressure
23. Decreases the incidence of type 2 diabetes
24. Reduces stress
25. Improves cognitive function

Reprinted with permission from Eickhoff-Shemek JM, Berg KE. *Physical Fitness: Guidelines for Success.* 2003.[1]

Risk management as we investigate it not only involves identification of risks and taking steps to eliminate or reduce those risks, but it involves efforts to transfer those risks that cannot be eliminated or reduced through various mechanisms such as through the use of waivers or liability insurance.

There are several causes of medical emergencies that occur in health/fitness facilities. Some medical emergencies are a result of **inherent risks,** meaning they are inseparable from the activity and can happen as a result of participation. Almost everyone reading this book has probably experienced this type of injury when participating in physical activity or sports. These types of injuries are no one's fault, for example, spraining one's ankle while playing basketball.

Medical emergencies can also be related to **negligence:** the fault of the participant (e.g., misusing a piece of exercise equipment) or the fault of facility personnel (e.g., failing to inspect exercise equipment or deficiencies in providing safe instruction). Negligence is introduced in Chapter 2 but discussed throughout the book. The case law examples in this book present the many types of negligence claims and lawsuits that participants have brought against health/fitness professionals and facilities. A more serious form of negligence termed, *gross negligence,* can also lead to medical emergencies and is discussed in more detail in Chapter 2.

In addition, medical emergencies can also be caused by product liability, for example, defects or deficiencies in exercise equipment in which the manufacturer of the equipment would be liable for the participant's injury. In addition, medical emergencies can be caused by problems in the physical plant (e.g., improper floor surfaces).

MEDICAL EMERGENCIES CAN LEAD TO LITIGATION

Medical emergencies can be minor (e.g., injured ankle) or major (e.g., life threatening such as a cardiac arrest). Both minor and major medical emergencies can result in costly claims and lawsuits against health/fitness facilities. For example, the Association Insurance Group, Inc. conducted a study in which they analyzed the type and the number of liability claims that occurred over a 12-year period (1995–2007) for their health/fitness facility clients (personal communication, K. Reinig, President, Association Insurance Group, Inc., September 19, 2007) (Table 1-2). During this period, they received reports of 6,144 incidents of which 2,395 turned into actual claims. The highest number of claims came from member malfunction, premises liability (trip and falls), equipment malfunction, and treadmills. Member malfunction is a category of claims where members hurt themselves while working out; for example, they strain a muscle, drop a weight on their foot, or smash their fingers re-racking weights. Equipment malfunction claims included items such as cable failure on selectorized machines, exercise balls that burst, equipment that falls over because it is not installed properly, or seats that fall off spin bikes. Most of these claims were due to poor maintenance of the equipment. Professional liability claims reflect incidents involving improper instruction from employees, instructors, and trainers.

As shown in Table 1-2, liability claims can be quite costly (personal communication, K. Reinig, President, Association Insurance Group, Inc., September 19, 2007). For example, the equipment malfunction claims (N = 339), which resulted in an average claim value of $17,063, totaled $5,784,357 over the 12-year period. It is important to realize that insurance companies often "settle" cases out of court (i.e., the insurance company and the injured party agree on an amount to be paid to the injured party to resolve a claim without trial) because it is usually more cost effective to do so than going to trial and resolves the uncertainties associated with litigation. It is also important to recognize that many of the claims paid out by the Association Insurance Group, Inc. could be have been significantly reduced if health/fitness professionals would have incorporated the many risk management strategies presented throughout this book.

TABLE 1-2	Health Club Liability Claims Analysis over a 12-Year Period (January 1995–July 2007)	
Type of Claim	Number of Claims	Average Claim Value*
Sauna	28	$5,641
Tanning	31	$5,845
Child Care	142	$6,165
Aerobic Classes	121	$8,149
Member Malfunction	388	$8,902
Treadmill	233	$8,933
Slip and Fall—Wet Areas	252	$12,478
Spinning Bike	60	$12,682
Professional Liability	70	$13,631
Basketball/Racquetball	44	$13,982
Equipment Malfunction	339	$17,063
Property Damage Liability	106	$17,588
Premises Liability—Trip and Falls	350	$18,554
Day Spa Services	5	$21,516
Outside Premises—Trips and Falls	91	$22,112
Swimming Pool	48	$23,549
Steam Room	27	$23,747
Tennis	37	$26,080
Sexual Harassment & Discrimination	21	$26,958
Drowning	2	$135,100

Total Number of Claims: 2,395
Average Claim Value: $21,434
$14,678 without the two drowning incidents

* Claim value includes defense costs, expenses, and reserves.
Reprinted with permission, Courtesy of Association Insurance Group, Inc.

Today, when individuals experience a personal injury, they are not hesitant to file a claim or lawsuit. Personal injury claims and lawsuits have increased significantly in the last 30 years.[3] This increase in litigation is often referred to as the "litigation epidemic." The health/fitness field is not immune to these increases. and unfortunately, claims and lawsuits related to negligence are predicted to continue to increase in the health/fitness field.[4]

The increased number of claims and lawsuits (and associated costs) has forced insurance companies to increase their liability insurance premiums, sometimes significantly. For example, a health club in New York recently reported that their annual premium went from $12,000 to $59,000.[5] Interestingly however, some insurance companies are now providing financial incentives to some facilities by reducing premiums if the organization has an active risk management plan[2] or has agreed to engage in what is otherwise considered sound risk management practices. For example, one college in the northeastern United States was rewarded a 10% reduction in their liability insurance premiums (a $35,000 savings in one year) by organizing a campus-wide risk management plan.[2]

A comprehensive risk management plan should result in reducing the number of legal claims and lawsuits that any insurance company theoretically will have to pay out or defend, which keeps their costs down and, in turn, can lower (or contain) the cost of the premium paid by the health/fitness facility. Like auto insurance, a good "record" in this regard can help prevent potential increases in premiums. The possible savings on liability insurance premiums because of participation in risk management activities should motivate upper managers of health/fitness facilities to initiate the development of a comprehensive risk management plan. Liability insurance premiums paid by individual health/fitness professionals (discussed in Chapter 5) can also be contained with a good track record.

POSSIBLE REASONS FOR INCREASED LITIGATION IN THE HEALTH/FITNESS FIELD

As previously stated, the number of negligence claims and lawsuits has increased in the health/fitness field in recent years. This section explains some possible reasons why this has occurred, such as the high number of injuries in physical fitness and sport activities and the lack of education in the law and risk management among health/fitness professionals.

High Number of Injuries

In addition to some individuals' tendencies to file a claim or lawsuit, litigation may also be increasing in the health/fitness field because of the high number of injuries associated with physical activity and sports. The National Center for Injury Prevention and Control, a department within the Centers for Disease Control and Prevention, reported in July 2003 that 7 million Americans receive medical attention for sports and recreation-related injuries each year.[6] About a third (30.7%) of these injuries occurred at a sport or recreation facility. The highest reported injury rates were for children 5 to 14 years of age and for persons 15 to 24 years of age. Those 25 years or older were also frequently injured in activities such as racquet sports, biking, golfing, bowling, jogging, and exercising.

Another study that involved a 20-year retrospective review of weight training injuries that were treated in U.S. hospital emergency departments (based on National Electronic Injury Surveillance System data from the U.S. Consumer Product Safety Commission) estimated that 980,173 persons were treated for weight training injuries.[7] The study authors stated that there was a 35% increase in injuries treated in the emergency department over the 20-year period, and about 1 in 4 of these occurred from the misuse or abuse of weight training equipment. The most common venue of injury was the home (40.2%) followed by a sports or recreation site (17.8%).

The U.S. Consumer Product Safety Commission (CPSC) has also published sports and recreation-related injury reports for children (*Prevent Injuries to Children from Exercise Equipment*), baby boomers (*Baby Boomers and Sports Injuries*), and older adults (*Sports-Related Injuries to Persons 65 Years of Age and Older*) that are available at the CPSC website.[8] The CPSC estimates that each year about 8,700 children younger than 5 years are injured with exercise equipment (e.g., stationary bicycles, treadmills, and stair climbers), and an additional 16,500 injuries occur to children 5 to 14 years of age. About 20% of the exercise equipment-related injuries resulted in fractures and even amputations. Sports-related injuries to baby boomers (35 to 54 years of age) increased 33% from 1991 to 1998 (i.e., 276,000 to 365,000 hospital emergency room–treated injuries). For persons 65 years of age and older, there was a 54% increase in hospital emergency room–treated injuries (34,000 to 53,000) in a 7-year period (1990–1996). The findings in these studies indicate that a high number of injuries do occur in physical fitness and sport activities and the number of injuries is increasing, which may be one explanation for the increase in litigation that has occurred.

Lack of Education in the Law and Risk Management

Another possible reason for an increase in litigation in the health/fitness field is that health/fitness professionals have not received adequate education in relevant legal and risk management topics in order to avoid or manage relevant risk occurrences. Poor adherence to basic safety procedures (e.g., having and practicing an emergency action plan and conducting pre–health activity screening) and laws, for example, the Bloodborne Pathogens Standard of the Occupational Safety and Health Administration (OSHA), the Americans with Disabilities Act (ADA), and state statutes may demonstrate that a lack of education in the law and risk management exists among health/fitness professionals as well as poor academic preparation in this content area.

Poor Adherence to Basic Safety Procedures   One study[9] investigated 110 health/fitness facilities in Massachusetts and found that 45% had never practiced emergency drills, 39% did not routinely (or never) screened new members, and 31% had less than half of their fitness staff with a bachelor's degree in the field. Another study[10] of 65 health/fitness facilities in Ohio found, among other problems, that 53% of them had no written emergency response plan. These types of safety procedures (e.g., pre-activity health screening, emergency action plans, etc.) are often reflected in standards of practice published by professional organizations in the form of standards, guidelines, and position papers. Poor adherence to these published standards of practice can have legal implications for health/fitness professionals and facilities. Adhering to them can help protect from legal claims and lawsuits, but poor adherence to them can lead to increased legal liability, as discussed in more detail in Chapter 3.

A national study published in 2002[11,12] determined adherence levels to the six standards published in *ACSM's Health/Fitness Facility Standards and Guidelines* (2nd ed.).[13] This study of 437 highly qualified professionals found that in defined facilities, more than 50% of the respondents possessed a master's degree, were ACSM Health/Fitness Instructor (HFI) certified and in either upper management or middle management positions, and had 10 or more years professional experience in the field. The results of this study showed that 79% of the facilities had a written emergency plan, but only 61% had taken steps to ensure that the entire staff knew how to carry it out. In addition, only 66% of the facilities required adult members to complete a pre-activity health screening device. This study also compared adherence to standards among six different types of fitness facilities: private, for-profit; community, nonprofit; clinical/hospital; government; corporate/worksite; and college/university. Generally, the study found that clinical/hospital and corporate/worksite settings were more compliant to the ACSM's emergency and pre-activity procedures than the other four settings, as well as with applicable laws such as OSHA's Bloodborne Pathogen Standard and the ADA.

Another study[14] conducted recently by the attorney general's office in New York involved surveying health clubs to determine whether or not they were in compliance with two state statutes. The first requires cardiopulmonary resuscitation (CPR) equipment and signage indicating the availability and location of the CPR equipment in public places; and the other requires health clubs with more than 500 members to have an automated external defibrillator (AED) and an employee (or authorized volunteer) present who holds valid certifications in CPR and AED during business hours. Of the 231 respondents, 78 of the clubs (34%) were in compliance with both state statutes. However, 153 clubs (66%) were not compliant with one or the other or both.

Poor Academic Preparation   Education about the law and risk management should be included in academic programs that prepare health/fitness professionals for the field. However, it appears that this content area is not being adequately addressed. One study[15] investigated law and legal liability content in 98 sports medicine and exercise science academic programs. At the graduate level, 32% of the programs included legal and liability content through an entire course, 26% within an existing course, and 42% did not include this content in the curriculum at all. At the undergraduate level, these percentages were 16, 62, and 22, respectively. For those graduate academic programs that did offer an entire course, the course was most often a sport law course, which meets the educational needs for those pursuing sport-related fields, but not necessarily the specific needs of those pursuing the health/fitness field. In addition, students in exercise science (or related) specializations were required to take this course in only 5 of the 98 programs studied.

Of the graduate programs that covered legal content within an existing course, 80% covered the law/legal liability content area in six or less contact hours of instruction. Although helpful, this may not be an adequate amount of instruction. Most alarming was the high percentage (42%) of graduate programs that did not cover this content at all. Individuals who pursue master degrees often want to qualify for higher-level management positions. Given the fact that upper managers are ultimately responsible for risk management (discussed later), it would make sense that individuals preparing for these positions have an entire course in this content area. Clearly these data indicate that academic programs are not adequately covering the law and legal liability content for their exercise science (or related) majors.

Published competencies often influence the development of certain course work in academic programs as well as content covered on certification examinations. However, competencies are often limited in the area of law and risk management.

For example, of the many knowledge, skills, and abilities (KSAs) listed for the ACSM HFI certification examination, the following three are included under the Safety, Injury Prevention, and Emergency Procedures category that cover legal content:

1.10.10 Knowledge of the health/fitness instructor's responsibilities, limitations, and the legal implications of carrying out emergency procedures.

1.10.13 Knowledge of the components of an equipment maintenance/repair program and how it may be used to evaluate the condition of exercise equipment to reduce the potential risk of injury.

1.10.14 Knowledge of the legal implications of documented safety procedures, the use of incident documents, and ongoing safety training.[16]

Although these KSAs address important legal and risk management concepts, they are limited in their scope.

Limited emphasis on legal issues can also impact the curriculum of academic programs in exercise science and related areas. For example, in order for an academic program to become ACSM endorsed[17] or accredited through the Commission on Accreditation of Allied Health Education Programs (CAAHEP), the courses need to cover the HFI KSAs. Exposure to legal and risk management content in published competencies, as well as in academia needs to be increased in order to help health/fitness students and professionals appreciate the importance of developing knowledge and skills in these areas.

RISK MANAGEMENT DEFINED

The term *management* can be defined as "the process of planning, organizing, leading, and controlling an organization's or other entity's resources to fulfill its objectives cost-effectively."[18] An organization may have several objectives, such as growth, profit, and service. To prevent a slowing in growth, reduction in profits, or just general interruption of operations, an organization must prevent four types of accidental losses:[19] property losses (e.g., property damage caused by fire/theft), net income losses (e.g., an increase in expenses or a reduction in revenue as result of an accident), **liability losses** (e.g., claims or lawsuits owing to negligence), and personnel losses (e.g., premature death of an employee). Preventing the third type of accidental losses (liability losses) is the risk management focus of this book as applied to health/fitness activities and operations.

In a broad context to address all four types of accidental losses, Head and Horn define risk management as "the process of making and implementing decisions that will minimize the adverse effects of accidental and business losses on an organization."[20] For the purpose of this book, **risk management** is defined as a proactive administrative process that will help minimize liability losses for health/fitness professionals and the organizations they represent.

Head and Horn also describe risk management as a decision-making process that includes the following five sequential steps:

1. Identify and analyze loss exposure.
2. Examine alternative risk management techniques.

3. Select risk management techniques.
4. Implement techniques.
5. Monitor results.[19]

These five steps can be collapsed into four steps using terms that are familiar to health/fitness professionals: assessment, development, implementation, and evaluation. For example, at an individual level, when health/fitness professionals help a participant begin an exercise program, they often first *assess* the participant's health risks and fitness levels. The data collected in the assessment are then used to *develop* an exercise prescription tailored for that participant. In conjunction with health/fitness professionals, the participant then *implements* his or her exercise program. After a certain period of time, the health/fitness professional e*valuates* the progress the participant has made toward personal health/fitness goals.

At the program planning level, these four steps are used to plan health/fitness programs.[21] For example, when planning a new program, the health/fitness needs and interests of the population to be served are assessed. The results of this assessment are then used to direct the development of the program. The program staff members then implement and evaluate the program. Assessment, development, implementation, and evaluation phases are also used in strategic management planning in health/fitness facilities.[22] Therefore, because these four steps and terms are commonly used in the health/fitness field, it made sense to incorporate them in the risk management approach used in this book as follows:

Step 1—Assessment of Legal Liability Exposures
Step 2—Development of Risk Management Strategies
Step 3—Implementation of the Risk Management Plan
Step 4—Evaluation of the Risk Management Plan.

In their step 1, Head and Horn[19] refer to "loss exposure." An exposure is any situation that can create the possibility of an accidental or inadvertent loss or the occurrence of an untoward event. This book addresses **legal liability exposures** that exist in the health/fitness field. A legal liability exposure is any situation that creates a probability of a medical emergency occurring (e.g., failure to conduct pre-activity health screening, proper instruction/supervision, and regular inspections of exercise equipment) or increases the severity of a medical emergency when one occurs (e.g., failing to carry out appropriate emergency care). Legal liability exposures are also created when health/fitness facilities do not adhere to federal, state, and local laws, as well as published standards of practice that are applicable to the field. To prevent liability losses (and the subsequent financial losses that can result), health/fitness professionals must first understand and appreciate the many legal liability exposures they face. Therefore, step 1 involves the assessment of legal liability exposures.

STEP **1** ASSESSMENT OF LEGAL LIABILITY EXPOSURES

Various approaches exist for health/fitness professionals to assess legal liability exposures. First, it is important to become familiar with the laws that apply to the health/fitness field. For example, legal cases that have occurred involving health/fitness facilities are interesting to review not only because case law decisions may set **precedent** —a rule that future similar cases will have to follow—but also because they demonstrate the many types of claims that plaintiffs (injured parties) can bring against a facility. In addition, statutory and administrative laws such as ADA and the OSHA Bloodborne Pathogens Standard, respectively, are laws that health/fitness professionals must understand and comply with.

Once the applicable laws are determined, standards of practice published by health/fitness professional organizations (e.g., standards, guidelines, and position papers) and independent organizations, for example, Consumer Product Safety Commission (CPSC),

American Society of Testing and Materials (ASTM), and equipment manufacturers, need to be examined. Health/fitness professionals should incorporate published standards of practices into their daily operations because they can be used in the presentation of evidence about standard of care (legal duty) in negligence claims and lawsuits, as discussed in Chapter 3. Adherence to published standards of practice decreases legal liability exposures, whereas the failure to adhere to them increases legal liability exposures. Although the assessment step in this book focuses on identifying applicable laws and published standards of practice, health/fitness professionals should also consider the following when determining their legal liability exposures:

1. Review accident/injury reports to become familiar with the types of medical emergencies that have occurred at the health/fitness facility (e.g., a high number of similar injuries may indicate a particular legal liability exposure that exists in that facility).
2. Conduct a facility inspection to determine if there are any situations that are unique to the health/fitness facility (e.g., an area where participants have to step up or down that is not easily visible and that may lead to untoward events and then potential claims and lawsuits).
3. Evaluate the demographics of the population that is served—their ages, genders, and health histories—because older participants and those who are classified as moderate or high risk (discussed in Chapter 6) create additional legal liability exposures.
4. Consult with local experts who would be familiar with any local laws (e.g., state, county, and city) that would apply to facility operations.

Of course it is impossible to identify all legal liability exposures that exist, but by following the approaches outlined here, health/fitness professionals can feel confident that they are on the right track with their risk management efforts. Once the assessment of legal liability exposures is completed, the next step is to develop risk management strategies.

STEP **2** DEVELOPMENT OF RISK MANAGEMENT STRATEGIES

Risk management strategies as described by Head and Horn[19] and applied in a health/fitness context are referred to as **loss prevention,** that is, strategies that eliminate or reduce the frequency of medical emergencies occurring; **loss reduction,** that is, strategies that lower the severity of liability loss when medical emergencies occur such as staff members providing appropriate emergency care; and **contractual transfer of risks,** that is: (a) waivers signed by participants where they contractually agree not to sue the health/fitness facility for its own negligence, and (b) liability insurance purchased where by the insurance provider agrees to pay for any damages (financial losses) within the limits of the insurance policy. This book focuses on loss prevention strategies that are presented in Chapters 5 through 10, but it also addresses loss reduction strategies that are discussed in Chapter 11, as well as strategies involving the contractual transfer of risks, described in Chapters 4 and 5.

Many of these risk management strategies necessitate the development and implementation of various documents. For example, a loss prevention strategy such as conducting pre-activity health screening involves the use of a pre-activity health screening device. A loss reduction strategy such as providing emergency care entails completing an incident/injury report after a medical emergency occurs. A strategy that involves a contractual transfer of risks such as a waiver of liability would entail having participants signing a waiver document of some type. Many examples of these types of documents are presented throughout this book. Not only is it important to use these documents to help demonstrate adherence to the law and/or the standard of care, it is wise to have a second set of these documents (written and/or electronic) stored at another location. **Duplication**[19] of documents serves as a backup procedure in case the primary documents are ever lost or destroyed, for example, in a fire.

STEP 3 IMPLEMENTATION OF THE RISK MANAGEMENT PLAN

This step involves the development of a Risk Management Policy and Procedures Manual (RMPPM), in which all of the risk management strategies are presented in an organized manner. For example, the written procedures and documents related to pre-activity health screening are all included in logical sequence in one section of the RMPPM entitled Pre-Activity Health Screening. Staff training using the RMPPM is essential. Staff training is an ongoing function of health/fitness facilities for their professionals. It must be done when a new staff member is hired and periodically throughout the year for all staff members so they are reminded of their risk management responsibilities and kept up to date on new developments and changes in the risk management plan. Evaluation of the risk management plan is the fourth and final step in the risk management process.

STEP 4 EVALUATION OF THE RISK MANAGEMENT PLAN

Evaluation of the risk management plan is both formative and summative. **Formative evaluation** is conducted throughout the year on an ongoing as-needed basis. For example, after injury, formative evaluation involves answering questions such as (a) what was the cause, (b) was it preventable, and (c) was the Emergency Action Plan (EAP) carried out properly? The information gathered should then be used to correct any problems right away. If the EAP was not carried out properly by the staff, an inservice training would be necessary to review the EAP. **Summative evaluation** is a formal annual review of the entire Risk Management Plan and RMPPM. It will be important to make any revisions if the law and/or any published standards of practice have changed. Figure 1-1 depicts the major components for each of the four risk management steps.

OUR APPROACH TO THE FOUR RISK MANAGEMENT STEPS

Chapters 5 through 11 focus on the major responsibilities and functions of health/ fitness professionals while carrying out various programs and services. Many legal liability exposures exist with regard to these responsibilities and functions that need to be addressed in the daily operations of any health/fitness facility. Each of these chapters contains two major sections addressing the first two risk management steps: (a) assessment of legal liability exposures, and (b) development of risk management strategies. The first section describes the laws and published standards of practice that apply for that chapter's topic. The second section focuses on the development of risk management strategies that directly reflect the law and published standards of practice. The goal is first to learn the applicable laws and published standards of practice, and then to understand how to put them into practice by developing risk management strategies.

Many examples of risk management strategies are described that can then be adapted to meet the specific needs of any health/fitness facility. Many of the sample forms and documents that appear throughout the book are available electronically on the Lippincott Williams & Wilkins website, http://thePoint.lww.com/Eickhoff, so they can be reviewed. However, in the case of certain sample documents such as waivers and informed consents, it is essential that competent legal counsel review these in the jurisdiction where they will be used *prior* to implementing them. Toward the end of Chapters 5 through 11 is a "Put into Practice Checklist" that includes the major risk management strategies that should be developed. Health/fitness professionals can use this checklist to self-assess their progress for each of the risk management strategies: developed, partially developed, or not developed.

Steps 3 (Implementation of the Risk Management Plan) and 4 (Evaluation of the Risk Management Plan) are presented in Chapter 12. See Figure 1-2 for the Risk Management icon that will appear throughout Chapters 5 to 12. As each step is described, it is highlighted to help you identify which risk management step is being discussed.

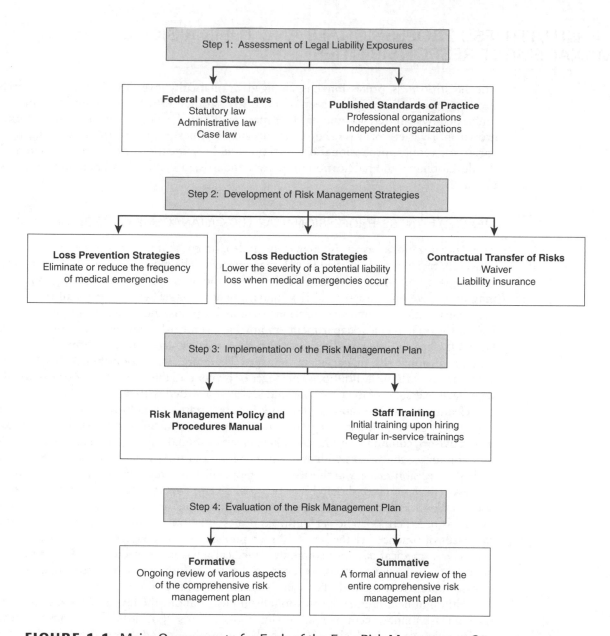

FIGURE 1-1 Major Components for Each of the Four Risk Management Steps

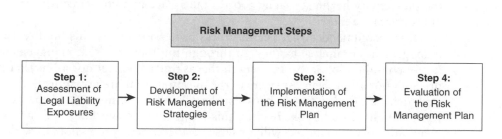

FIGURE 1-2 Icon: Risk Management Steps

HEALTH/FITNESS PROFESSIONALS AND THEIR RISK MANAGEMENT RESPONSIBILITIES

The health/fitness profession has changed dramatically over the last two or three decades. Not only has there been a concerted national effort to promote the importance of physical activity among all Americans, but the profession has evolved and grown in a variety of ways. For example, health/fitness facilities are now found in a variety of venues, professional organizations and certifications have proliferated, and the development and publication of many standards, guidelines, and position papers is ongoing.

HEALTH/FITNESS PROFESSIONAL AS RISK MANAGEMENT PROFESSIONAL

Many organizations have a risk management department that is managed by professionals educated, trained, and certified in risk management. The existence and structure of any such department usually depends on the size of the organization. A small organization may only have one professional risk management manager who oversees all risk management functions. Large organizations such as hospitals and major corporations may have a risk management department employing several risk management professionals. Generally, health/fitness facilities do not have a risk management department or a full-time professional risk management manager. Therefore, the responsibility of risk management lies with the health/fitness manager or owner and the health/fitness professionals who have oversight of the programs and services provided within the facility.

Health/fitness professionals who work for organizations that have a risk management department should include a representative from this department on their **risk management advisory committee**. All health/fitness facilities should have a risk management advisory committee that works with and assists the health/fitness managers and professionals with the decision-making authority throughout all four steps of the risk management process. This committee should be made up of diverse experts (e.g., legal, medical, insurance, and exercise science) who can provide specific input and perspective in their respective areas of expertise. Some health/fitness professional organizations that have published standards of practice (see the list of 10 such publications in Chapter 3) recommend facilities have a medical advisory committee, medical advisor, or medical liaison. However, none of them recommend, as we do here, having an advisory committee made up of diverse experts to assist with the facility's risk management efforts.

Although health/fitness professionals will learn about the law and how to apply it through risk management by reading this book, it can still be difficult at times to know exactly what to do in all situations. The law is not black and white (there can be a lot of gray), and the interpretation of published standards of practice may not always be clear, thus creating the need for a risk management advisory committee and often the advice of a lawyer that can help health/fitness professionals with the sometimes difficult decisions. For example, all health/fitness facilities should conduct pre-activity health screening on all participants prior to their participation. However, for facilities with very large groups of prospective participants like colleges and universities, how should the pre-activity health screening process take place in a cost-effective yet prudent and appropriate manner?

It is recommended that health/fitness professionals use this book with their risk management committee as they go through the four-step risk management process. It will contain a lot of the answers to the risk management questions that may come up—but not all of them. Answers to the questions that are not addressed in this book can then be decided jointly between the advisory committee and the health/fitness professionals. In addition, reading this book prior to working with a risk management advisory committee will provide health/fitness professionals with necessary legal and risk management knowledge to communicate intelligently with the experts on their advisory committee and make the risk management process efficient.

TYPES OF HEALTH/FITNESS PROFESSIONALS

The health/fitness profession is not government regulated as are many related professions (e.g., athletic training, physical therapy) that require a state license prior to practicing in that profession. However, some states have proposed legislation for licensure for health/fitness professionals, and in the future this may become a reality. The health/fitness profession has primarily been self-governed through professional certifications and accreditation of academic programs and certification examinations. See Chapter 5 for more discussion on these credentialing issues. Therefore, professional organizations have defined the role and/or scope of practice of health/fitness professionals by providing descriptions of their major functions/responsibilities. For example, ACSM has defined the scope of practice for a certified Health/Fitness Instructor as follows:

The ACSM Health/Fitness Instructor® (HFI) is a degreed health and fitness professional qualified for career pursuits in the university, corporate, commercial, hospital, and community settings. The HFI has knowledge and skills in management and administration and training and supervising entry level personnel. The HFI is skilled in conducting risk stratification, conducting physical fitness assessments and interpreting results, constructing appropriate exercise prescriptions in motivating apparently healthy individuals with medically controlled diseases to adopt and maintain healthy lifestyle behaviors.[23]

The HFI certification requires an associate's or bachelor's degree in a health-related field from a regionally accredited college or university, and current adult CPR certification that has a practical skills examination component (e.g., American Heart Association or American Red Cross).[23]

Although either an associate's or bachelor's degree is required for the HFI certification, most health/fitness professionals possess a bachelor's degree. This is probably because there are more academic programs that offer a bachelor's degree in the field than an associate's degree, and many employers in the field require a bachelor's degree for entry-level professional positions.

A person who possesses the HFI certification (or other similar entry-level professional certifications that require a degree in exercise science or a related area such as the National Strength and Conditioning Association's Certified Strength and Conditioning Specialist) would obviously be considered a health/fitness professional. However, for the purposes of this book, health/fitness professionals also include those individuals who do not necessarily have an associate's or bachelor's degree in the field or related field, but perhaps possess health/fitness certification(s) (e.g., personal training, group exercise leadership). These individuals have risk management responsibilities, as do entry-level and advanced-level professionals in the field, and therefore they also need adequate background in the law and risk management. Those professionals in advanced-level positions (managers/owners, executive directors) have the ultimate responsibility for risk management in their health/fitness facilities. See Figure 1-3 for a sample organizational chart for a typical health/fitness facility and a brief description of the key risk management responsibilities that the various types of professionals have. Note that staff members who are not considered health/fitness professionals (e.g., front desk staff, child care, and maintenance staff members) also have risk management responsibilities.

TYPES OF HEALTH/FITNESS FACILITIES AND SETTINGS

At a basic level, health/fitness facilities may be initially defined as places where physical activities are performed by individuals with or without supervision for recreational or other defined purposes such as fitness. The American College of Sports Medicine (ACSM) and the American Heart Association (AHA) have classified fitness facilities into the following five levels:[24]

Level 1—Unsupervised Exercise Room
Level 2—Single Exercise Leader

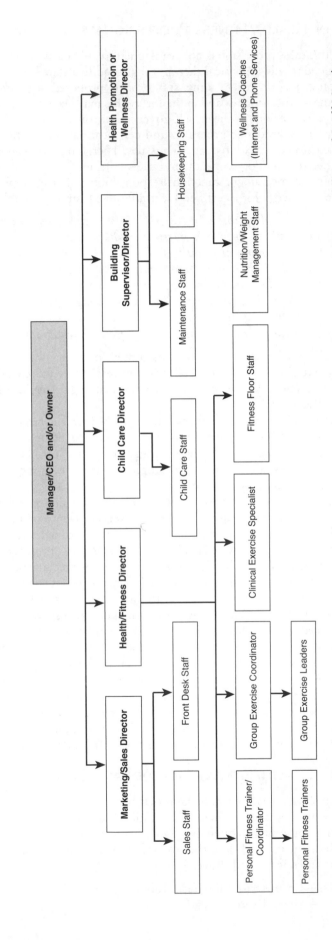

FIGURE 1-3 Sample Organizational Chart for a Typical Health/Fitness Facility and Key Risk Management Responsibilities of Staff Members

Key Risk Management Responsibilities of Staff Members

Manager: Has overall responsibility for the facility's risk management plan; primary liaison with risk management advisory committee; ensures that staff members with risk management responsibilities are trained, supervised, and evaluated so that the risk management plan is carried out properly; ensures staff members are qualified prior to employment

Directors: Working with the manager, directors are responsible for the development of the risk management plan in their respective areas; train, supervise, and evaluate their staff members to help ensure they are properly carrying out the risk management plan; ensure their staff members are qualified prior to employment

Personal Fitness Coordinator: Working with the health/fitness director, is responsible for the development of the risk management plan involving the personal fitness training program; trains, supervises, and evaluates personal fitness trainers to help ensure they are properly carrying out the risk management plans; ensures their personal fitness trainers are qualified prior to employment

Personal Fitness Trainers: Carry out risk management policies and procedures related to client safety (e.g., proper pre-activity health screening, instruction, and supervision)

Group Exercise Coordinator: Working with the health/fitness director, is responsible for the development of the risk management plan involving the group exercise program; trains, supervises, and evaluates group exercise leaders to help ensure they are properly carrying out the risk management plan; ensures their group exercise leaders are qualified prior to employment

Group Exercise Leaders: Carry out risk management policies and procedures related to participant safety (e.g., proper instruction and supervision)

Clinical Exercise Specialist: If the health/fitness director does not have adequate knowledge, skills, and abilities in clinical exercise, then a clinical exercise specialist should be hired who would work with all health/fitness staff members to help ensure that risk management strategies are properly carried out (e.g., programs and services for participants who have medical risks and/or certain medical conditions are "safely" designed and meet the current standard of care)

Fitness Floor Staff: Carry out risk management policies and procedures properly (e.g., supervise participants to help ensure they are adhering to the facility's safety policies/procedures and utilizing the exercise equipment properly); report/document incidents that occur (e.g., equipment breaking down, participant nonadherence to safety policies/procedures or misuse of equipment)

Nutrition/Weight Management Staff: Carry out risk management policies and procedures properly related to nutrition and weight management programs including proper scope of practice (e.g., provide "general" nonmedical nutrition information to participants—only licensed (as required by many state statutes) professionals such as registered dietitians can provide "individualized" nutritional/dietary advice

Wellness Coaches: Carry out risk management policies and procedures properly related to wellness coaching services provided over the Internet and by phone (e.g., contractual terms including the limitations involved in these services are clearly communicated); practice within proper scope (e.g., educational and motivational strategies only)

Sales Staff: Carry out risk management policies and procedures properly related to sales (e.g., sections within membership contracts such as a waiver of liability are communicated properly)

Front Desk Staff: Carry out risk management polices and procedures properly (e.g., certain aspects of the pre-activity health screening process and the medical emergency action plan)

Child Care staff: Carry out risk management policies and procedures properly related to child care programs and services

Maintenance and Housekeeping Staff: Carry out risk management policies and procedures properly related to the maintenance and cleaning of the facility

FIGURE 1-3 *(Continued)*

Level 3—Fitness Center for Healthy Clients
Level 4—Fitness Center Serving Clinical Populations
Level 5—Medically Supervised Clinical Program

Unsupervised exercise rooms are often found in places such as apartment complexes and hotels. Facilities that involve single exercise leaders could be private studios designed for personal fitness training or group exercise programs. Health/fitness facilities that serve healthy clients and clinical populations (levels 3 and 4) describe the clientele that most health/fitness facilities serve today. However, note that these same populations also patronize the "single exercise leader" facilities (level 2). Given the prevalence of chronic diseases in the United States, it would be rare for health/fitness facilities to serve only healthy individuals, that is, low-risk individuals with no medical risk factors or medical conditions. In addition, physicians often recommend that their patients who have medical risk factors and/or diagnosed medical conditions join a health/fitness facility because of the significant role that regular physical activity plays in the prevention and control of chronic diseases.

Based on the preceding description, the information in this book primarily applies to health/fitness facilities that are classified as levels 2 through 4. Most health/fitness professionals work in these types of facilities. We have prepared a section in Chapter 13 (Selected Topics, Part II) to address risk management strategies for unsupervised health/fitness facilities (level 1). Health/fitness professionals who work in medically supervised clinical programs (level 5), such as cardiac rehabilitation programs, should also learn about applicable laws and the many risk management strategies set forth in this book. However, specific published standards of practice designed for medically supervised clinical programs, such as those published by the American Association of Cardiovascular and Pulmonary Rehabilitation (AACVPR), are not included here. As stated earlier, there has been a significant increase in the types of settings over the last two or three decades where health/fitness professionals work. No longer do they work only in private health clubs and YMCAs. These settings include the following:

- Corporate
  - Employer-sponsored health/fitness programs
- College/University
  - Campus recreation for students and employees
  - Strength and conditioning for athletes
- Commercial (for profit)
  - Health clubs
  - Country clubs/resorts
  - Personal fitness training and group exercise studios
  - Sports performance centers for youth, adults, and professional athletes
- Community (nonprofit)
  - YMCAs/YWCAs
  - Jewish Community Centers (JCCs)
  - Public schools
- Government
  - Military branches
  - Firefighters/police
  - City/county parks and recreation
- Hospitals/Medical Clinics
  - Community health/fitness
  - Cardiac and pulmonary rehab*
  - Orthopedic rehab*
- Retirement Centers
- Home Gyms
  - Personal fitness trainer's home
  - Client's home

BENEFITS OF RISK MANAGEMENT

Although the major benefit of risk management is the reduction of legal liability exposures that will result in decreased liability losses (and subsequent financial losses), a comprehensive risk management plan also enhances the quality of the programs and

---

* These types of programs often hire clinical exercise specialists, but they also hire health/fitness specialists.

services provided to participants and increases the overall operational efficiency of the many daily procedures that take place within a health/fitness facility.

Health/fitness programs and services that are both *safe* and *effective* are considered high quality. Risk management focuses on providing a reasonably safe environment for participants (e.g., the exercise equipment is inspected on a daily basis to help ensure proper function, and group exercise leaders and personal trainers teach properly using principles of safe exercise).

A comprehensive risk management plan also increases the efficiency of daily operations. Health/fitness professionals have the responsibility to ensure that all staff members are carrying out their daily responsibilities properly. When they don't, this not only creates a lot of stress for other health/fitness professionals, but it also results in inefficient use of their time to solve problems or to put out "operational" fires. Many of these daily problems can be prevented through staff training. Once staff members are trained using the RMPPM, it will likely result in fewer operational problems. More staff time can be spent on program development and expansion than on dealing with or solving problems.

These benefits of risk management not only protect the financial assets of a health/ fitness facility (fewer liability losses), but they can also increase its financial assets. Enhanced quality can result in an increase and greater retention of the number of participants. Increased operational efficiency can help ensure that the staff's time is used wisely, thus getting the most out of one the largest expenses of health/fitness facilities: staff costs.

SUMMARY

This chapter presented the types of risks that exist in health/fitness facilities and explained how these risks can lead to medical emergencies, which subsequently often result in legal claims and lawsuits against health/fitness professionals and the organizations they represent. Litigation has increased in the health/fitness field as it has generally in our society. Reasons to possibly explain the so-called litigation epidemic that exists in the health/fitness field were offered and described, including the high number of injuries and a lack of education among health/fitness professionals about the law and risk management.

This chapter also defined risk management and related terms as well as presented the four steps involved in the risk management process used in this book. It also described the function of a risk management advisory committee and how health/fitness professionals should work with this committee in the risk management decision-making process. The risk management responsibilities of various health/fitness professionals were described, as well as the types of health/fitness professionals and facilities that will benefit from this book. Lastly, reduction of legal liability exposures was listed as the major benefit of risk management along with enhanced quality of programs/services and increased operational efficiency.

RISK MANAGEMENT ASSIGNMENTS

1. Develop a list of the types of medical emergencies that could occur in a health/fitness facility—both those related to health risks and injury risks. Or, review the incident report forms for the last five years at your facility and classify the incidents as resulting from either health risks or injury risks.

_____

_____

_____

_____

2. Utilizing the results of research studies presented in this chapter, prepare a PowerPoint presentation describing the possible reasons for litigation increasing in the health/fitness field.

_____

_____

_____

_____

3. Prepare a written description of risk management including key terms and the four major risk management steps, as well the major benefits of risk management that can be inserted in the front of a Risk Management Policy and Procedures Manual (RMPPM) as an introduction or preface.

_____

_____

_____

_____

4. Describe the types of health/fitness professionals in relationship to their risk management responsibilities and the role of the risk management advisory committee.

_____

_____

_____

_____

KEY TERMS

Contractual transfer of risks
Duplication
Formative evaluation
Health risks
Inherent risks
Injury risks

Legal liability exposure
Liability losses
Loss prevention
Loss reduction
Negligence
Precedent

Risk
Risk management
Risk management advisory
   committee
Summative evaluation

REFERENCES

1. Eickhoff-Shemek JM, Berg KE. *Physical Fitness: Guidelines for Success.* 2003. Available by contacting lead author at: eickhoff@tempest.coedu.usf.edu, Tampa, FL.
2. Appenzeller H, ed. *Risk Management in Sport. Issues and Strategies.* 2nd ed. Durham, NC: Carolina Academic Press, 2005.
3. Hronek BB, Spengler JO, Baker TA. *Legal Liability in Recreation and Sport.* Champaign, Ill: Sagamore, 2007.
4. Herbert D. New Year's predictions for the health and fitness industry for the year 2003—A look into the future. *Exercise Standards and Malpractice Reporter.* 2003;17:12–13.
5. Cotten D. Minimizing legal liability for exercise programs. Presentation given at the 8th Annual ACSM Health & Fitness Summit & Exposition, Orlando, Fla, April 2004.
6. Herbert D. Seven million Americans treated for sports and recreation-related injuries each year. *Exercise Standards and Malpractice Reporter.* 2003;17:92–93.

7. Jones CS, Christensen C, Young M. Weight training injury trends. A 20-year survey. *Phys SportsMed.* 2000;28(7):61–72.

8. U.S. Consumer Product Safety Commission. Available at: http://www.cpsc.gov. Accessed August 24, 2007.

9. McInnis KJ, Hayakawa S, Balady GJ. Cardiovascular screening and emergency procedures at health clubs and fitness centers. *Am J Cardio1.* 1997;80:23–25.

10. McInnis KJ, Herbert WG, Herbert DL. Low compliance with national standards for cardiovascular emergency preparedness at health clubs. *Chest.* 2001;120:283–288.

11. Eickhoff-Shemek J, Deja K. Are health/fitness facilities complying with ACSM standards? Part I. *ACSM's Health Fitness J.* 2002;6(2):16–21.

12. Eickhoff-Shemek J, Deja K. Are health/fitness facilities complying with ACSM standards? Part II. *ACSM's Health Fitness J.* 2002;6(3):19–24.

13. Tharrett SJ, Peterson JA, eds. *ACSM's Health/Fitness Facility Standards and Guidelines.* 2nd ed. Champaign, Ill: Human Kinetics; 1997.

14. Report on the Attorney General's survey of health clubs concerning the presence of automated external defibrillators and CPR equipment. *Exercise Standards and Malpractice Reporter.* 2006;20:92–93.

15. Eickhoff-Shemek JM, Evans JA. An investigation of law and legal liability content in master academic program in sports medicine and exercise science. *J Leg Aspects Sport.* 2000;10:172–179.

16. Whaley MH, ed. *ACSM's Guidelines for Exercise Testing and Prescription.* 7th ed. Philadelphia: Lippincott Williams & Wilkins; 2006:330.

17. American College of Sports Medicine. ACSM certification and registry programs—The university connection. Available at: http://www.acsm.org/Content/NavigationMenu/Certification/UniversityConnectionEndorsementProgram/UC_Main1.htm. Accessed August 29, 2007.

18. Head GL, Horn S. *Essentials of Risk Management,* vol 1, 3rd ed. Malvern, Pa: Insurance Institute of America; 1997:4.

19. Head GL, Horn S. *Essentials of Risk Management,* vol 1, 3rd ed. Malvern, Pa: Insurance Institute of America; 1997.

20. Head GL, Horn S. *Essentials of Risk Management,* vol 1, 3rd ed. Malvern, Pa: Insurance Institute of America; 1997:5.

21. Green LW, Kreuter MW. *Health Program Planning: An Educational and Ecological Approach.* 4th ed. Boston: McGraw-Hill Higher Education; 2005.

22. Grantham WC, Patton RW, York TD, et al. *Health Fitness Management.* Champaign, Ill: Human Kinetics; 1998.

23. American College of Sports Medicine. *ACSM Health/Fitness Instructor® Scope of Practice,* Available at: http://www.acsm.org/Content/NavigationMenu/Certification/ACSMCertifications/ACSMHealthFitnessInstructo/Health_Fitness_Instr.htm#scope_of_practice, n.d. Accessed October 24, 2007.

24. American College of Sports Medicine and American Heart Association Joint Position Statement: Recommendations for cardiovascular, screening, staffing, and emergency policies at health/fitness facilities. *Med Sci Sports Exerc.* 1998;30:1009–1018.

CHAPTER 2

Introduction to the Law and Legal System

LEARNING OBJECTIVES After reading this chapter, health/fitness students and professionals will be able to:

1. Understand the sources of U.S. law.
2. Identify how U.S. law is classified.
3. Understand the U.S. court system.
4. Understand basic legal terminology.
5. Explain the steps in a civil trial.
6. Describe the basic types of tort law.
7. Understand the concept and elements of negligence.
8. Describe several defenses to negligence.
9. Describe various types of strict liability.
10. Understand the basic elements of a contract.
11. Understand various types of contracts typically found in the health/fitness field.

This chapter provides health/fitness students and professionals with an introduction to the U.S. legal system as well as to two areas of law (torts and contracts) that greatly impact the health/fitness field. Having a general understanding of the legal system as well as tort and contract law will serve as a foundation for the other chapters in this text, as well as assist you in managing associated risks.

SOURCES OF LAW

Sources of U.S. law can be categorized as primary or secondary. Primary sources are the law and are created by the three main branches of the government. Secondary sources analyze, describe, comment, or summarize legal issues and topics. Both types are further described later.

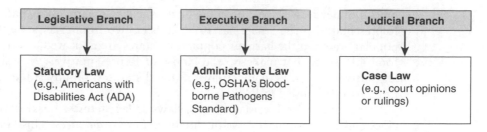

FIGURE 2-1 Branches of Government (Both Federal and State Levels) and Primary Sources of Law

PRIMARY SOURCES

U.S. laws are typically categorized according to their source as either constitutional law, statutory law, case law, or administrative law. These sources are known as **primary sources.** The three main branches of our government, the executive, judicial, and legislative, all create primary law (see Figure 2-1). Each of the branches is discussed in the following sections.

Constitutional Law

The federal government and every state have documents, termed *constitutions,* whose chief purpose is to create the government and define its functions and responsibilities in relationship to the people of the United States and of the respective citizens of each state. The U.S. Constitution, which became operative in 1789, is the supreme law of the land.[1,2] Any law that conflicts with it is void.

The U.S. Constitution has three primary functions. First, it creates the national government with its three branches (legislative, executive, and judicial). It creates the Congress (legislative branch) and dictates what laws it may pass. Furthermore, it creates the office of the president (executive branch) and the responsibilities that accompany it. The U.S. Constitution also creates the federal courts (judicial branch) and describes what cases they may decide.[2]

Second, the U.S. Constitution guarantees that the individual states retain all power not given to the federal government. Therefore, state governments play a pivotal role in all of our lives. Major issues of criminal law, tort law, and property law, as well as many other areas, are primarily regulated by the individual states.[2]

Third, the U.S. Constitution ensures many basic rights and privileges for the American people. Many of these rights are found in the amendments to the Constitution, including the Bill of Rights, which are contained in the first ten amendments. For example, the First Amendment provides the rights of free speech and press, and the free exercise of religion. Several of these other amendments pertain to the rights of criminal defendants in our legal system. Additional amendments ensure that the government treats all people equally. By establishing a limited government and guaranteeing basic rights for all citizens, the U.S. Constitution has become one of the most important documents ever written.[2] The full text of the U.S. Constitution can be found at http://www.house.gov/house/Educate.shtml.

Besides the U.S. Constitution, every state has a constitution that establishes its own government. They are typically patterned after the federal constitution and incorporate comparable provisions. Whenever a question of state law is an issue, that individual state's constitution is the supreme law. Thus two separate systems of government affect every one of us. These include the federal government, which has power over the whole country, and the state governments, which have powers that the U.S. Constitution did not grant the federal government.[2,3]

Statutory Law (Legislative Branch)

A second important source of U.S. law is **statutory law.** Generally speaking, statutory law is the body of law that has been enacted through our legislative process. The legislative branch of our federal government (Congress) has two parts, the Senate and the House of Representatives. The Senate has 100 members, two from every state that are elected by popular vote. On the basis of population, states are allocated a certain number of the total 435 seats that make up the House of Representatives. A basic function of the legislative branch is to enact laws. Federal statutes, on any subject, can be found at http://uscode.house.gov/.

State and federal legislators make laws called **statutes.** Local governments, such as cities and counties, make laws often termed *local ordinances.* This latter group includes such rules as building and licensing requirements, parking regulations, and leash laws. Together these statutes and ordinances are called the written law. The written law covers a wealth of subjects, such as civil rights, family law, housing, crime, and all matters in which the legislative branch has constitutional power to legislate. However, it is important to understand that statutory law is limited to matters of jurisdiction. For example, federal statutory law is limited to matters of federal jurisdiction; similar limitations hold for state statutes and local ordinances. When jurisdictions overlap (e.g., when two levels of governments have jurisdiction), conflicts occur. When that happens, the doctrine of supremacy applies, and federal law prevails over state law, as does state law over local law.[1]

Examples of federal statues that may apply to health/fitness professionals and programs are the Americans with Disabilities Act, the Age Discrimination in Employment Act, and the Volunteer Immunity Act. State statutes vary from state to state and may include laws that pertain to the use and operation of automated external defibrillators (AEDs), the unauthorized practice of medicine and other licensed professions, and various immunity provisions such as Recreational User statutes.

Administrative Law (Executive Branch)

Our government has assumed many functions through many departments, commissions, boards, and agencies. Numerous administrative agencies, specialized bodies created by legislation at all governmental levels, are granted lawmaking power to regulate specific activities. Administrative agencies exist at the federal, state, and local level. These agencies investigate problems within their respective jurisdictions, enact rules and regulations that have the force and effect of law, and resolve disputes, similar to court trials, to determine if their rules have been violated and, if so, what sanctions should be imposed.[1,2] Federal agencies such as the Food and Drug Administration (FDA), Internal Revenue Service (IRS), Federal Trade Commission (FTC), National Labor Relations Board (NLRB), and Occupational Health and Safety Administration (OSHA), as well as a myriad of state and local agencies, make and enforce numerous rules and regulations that impact the operations of health/fitness programs and facilities. The rules and regulations of these agencies are **administrative law.**

Case Law (Judicial Branch)

U.S. law is primarily based on English **common law,** a system in which laws were developed through the courts and case decisions. Common law is judge-made **case law.** Lawyers began to record decisions and urged judges to follow previously decided cases. As judges began to do so, the previously decided cases, termed *precedent,* took on greater importance. Finally, judges were obligated to follow precedent. Another term for precedent is *stare decisis,* which means "it stands decided." This means that if a particular factual dispute has been decided in court, and if the same factual dispute arises again, it must be resolved the same way as it was earlier. Precedence makes the law more efficient and predictable. However, not all litigation creates precedent. Most litigation ends in a resolution for the parties involved but no case precedent. Only in limited instances in which the judge writes the reasons why and how the dispute was resolved will precedent be created. If and when a judge writes these reasons, the result is termed a *written judicial opinion.* In most states, it is only at the appellate level that a judge writes a judicial opinion and creates law that others can access and use as guidance. However, most federal courts (trial as well as appellate level) write opinions. The published judicial opinions create precedent.[1-3]

Over many years, the common law developed into an extensive body of law. Many of the common law principles have been adopted by federal and state legislatures and thus have become statutory law. Nevertheless, the courts and their decisions play a crucial role in our legal system. Although most new law today is statutory, common law predominates in tort, contract, and agency law and is very important in employment, property, and other areas as well.

SECONDARY SOURCES

As previously stated, legal resources can be divided into primary and **secondary sources.** The primary sources, which we just reviewed, include court decisions (case law), federal and state constitutions, statutes, and administrative rules and regulations. Primary sources represent the actual law and therefore are the only legal sources that can be relied on to determine what the law requires. In contrast, secondary sources analyze, inform, or summarize various legal topics and issues. These publications are authored by private individuals, companies, and organizations.

Examples of secondary sources include books, treatises, legal encyclopedias and dictionaries, law review articles, and legal publications (e.g., *The Exercise Standards and Malpractice Reporter, Journal of Legal Aspects of Sport*). Although a court does not have to follow secondary authority, these sources can be very useful to the health/fitness professionals by providing insight into a specific legal issue or topic. They are also used to help a researcher gain access to primary sources because secondary sources frequently address issues that were raised by primary law, and they often refer to and cite primary sources.[3,4]

LOCATION OF PRIMARY AND SECONDARY SOURCES

Case law (court opinions) is published in sets of books known as *reporters.* At the federal level, all reported district court cases are published in the *Federal Supplement.* Federal circuit court decisions are reported in the *Federal Reporter.* U.S. Supreme Court cases are primarily reported in three major sets of reporters. These include the *United States Reports,* the *Supreme Court Reporter,* and the *United States Supreme Court Reports Lawyers' Edition.*[3,4]

Many states have official reporters for decisions from their courts, and some states have more than one reporter. Additionally, many state court opinions are published by the West Publishing Company in a set of reporters known as *regional reporters.* Every regional reporter prints opinions from courts in a geographical region. There are seven regional reporters, each printing the decisions for a number of states.[3,4]

Although these reporters are found in law libraries, case law can also be accessed via the Internet. Certain legal databases, such as *Westlaw* and *Lexis,* can only be accessed after paying a fee, and therefore are primarily only used by members of the legal profession, but the *Lexis/Nexis Academic Universe* database is often available to students at many academic institutions. This database allows researchers to obtain primary and secondary sources, and it offers keyword search engines for legal news, law reviews, statutes, and case law. Contact should be made to the local and/or school library to see if access is available to this powerful legal database.

SUBSTANTIVE LAW AND PROCEDURAL LAW

The U.S. law may be classified into several different categories. These include federal and state law, public and private law, civil and criminal law (described later), and **substantive law** and **procedural law.** Substantive law is the part of law that creates, defines, and regulates the rights, duties, and powers of parties.[5] Substantive law typically defines what the law is and creates the legal basis for any lawsuit.[1,2] Both of the two major categories of law, criminal and civil, are divided into substantive principles and procedural rules.

The two play very important roles in our legal system. For example, if the substantive law does not support a plaintiff's position, then the court has no basis for granting the plaintiff any legal remedy. Similarly, if a party does not follow the procedural rules, the court may not afford legal remedies even if they are allowed under substantive law.

Substantive laws exist for both criminal and civil actions, as do procedural rules. Substantive criminal law deals with crimes. Substantive civil law covers several different areas, including torts, contracts, and family law.

Procedural law, as compared to substantive law, are the rules that prescribe the steps for having a right or duty judicially enforced.[5] Procedural laws relate to the enforcement of the substantive rights. They set forth how a case should be handled once a dispute arises under substantive law. Procedural law includes all of the rules, or mechanisms, for processing civil and criminal cases through the federal and state courts.[1,2] For example, procedural law prescribes the dates and time limits when certain papers must be filed, what information legal papers must contain, how witnesses can be examined prior to trial, how the jury may be selected, when and where the trial will be held, and so on.

THE U.S. COURT SYSTEM

The U.S. court system is composed of various courts on both the state and federal levels, as well as specialized administrative courts. There are also special courts designed to hear only certain types of legal disputes (e.g., small claims courts). The various types and levels of courts are described next.

TYPES OF COURTS: CRIMINAL VERSUS CIVIL

U.S. law may also be classified into criminal and civil law. Both criminal and civil law attempt to induce people to act for the benefit of society. Nevertheless, they differ in their means of doing so. **Criminal law** is the body law that declares what conduct is criminal and dictates penalties for its commission. Most criminal laws are statutes, enacted by Congress or a state legislature. The statutory law of individual states regarding crimes is found in books often termed Penal Codes.[1-3]

In criminal court, which hears cases regarding the alleged commission of misdemeanors and felonies, the people (society) are represented by a governmental representative (district attorney). To convict a defendant in criminal court it must be shown that the person committed the crime beyond a reasonable doubt. A convicted criminal may be punished by a fine, community service, probation, imprisonment, or by a combination of these. If a fine is imposed, the money goes to the court, not to the victim of the crime. Although the courts have the inherent power to order restitution to a victim of a criminal act, for all general purposes, the victim of a crime leaves the courtroom empty handed. Health/fitness professionals may face criminal charges if they violate criminal statutes such as the unauthorized practice of medicine. Other examples of crimes include robbery, assault and battery, stalking, theft, and so on.

Civil law, in contrast, is the body of state and federal law that pertains to civil or private rights enforced by civil actions. Civil courts decide noncriminal matters, i.e., disputes between individuals, organizations, businesses, and governmental agencies. Two parties are involved in a civil lawsuit: a **plaintiff** (e.g., the injured participant in a health/fitness program who is bringing the lawsuit) and a **defendant,** the person or entity the plaintiff is suing (e.g., the health/fitness professional and/or organization that he or she represents). Typically, several defendants are named in a civil suit. A current trend is to name several parties as defendants regardless if they were directly involved in the alleged incident or not. For example, a lawsuit may not only name an aerobics instructor who allegedly performed the negligent act that led to the plaintiff's injury, but may also name the aerobic supervisor, fitness director, and the owners of the aerobic studio.

A plaintiff suing in civil court only has to show by a preponderance of evidence that the defendant is guilty (the term *liable* is used in civil court). The criminal law standard requires a much higher degree of certainty in the mind of the juror to find a defendant guilty (e.g., proof beyond a reasonable doubt). The civil standard only requires the jury to find more (51% or greater) evidence than not to hold a defendant liable.[1-3] Unlike criminal court, the plaintiff may leave the courtroom with a verdict that will require the defendant to compensate the plaintiff financially, right the alleged wrong, or both.

The overwhelming majority of lawsuits involving health/fitness practitioners and programs focus on civil claims. Thus, this book primarily focuses on civil law rather than criminal.

TRIAL COURTS

The U.S. court system, modeled after the English system, is hierarchical. The lowest level court, or entry level, typically a trial or district court, is followed by an intermediate appellate court, and ends with the highest court, typically a superior or supreme court. Trial courts carry out the initial proceedings in lawsuits. These proceedings have three discrete purposes: (a) to ascertain the facts of the dispute (what happened between the parties?), (b) to decide what rules of law should be applied to the facts, and (c) to administer those rules to the facts.[1]

Federal and state judges preside in these courts to settle legal disputes that are brought before them by parties. At the end of every trial, the judge, or a jury, renders judgment in favor of one or the other of the litigants. Typically, by applying existing law, these judgments are resolved at the entry-level court, and most are not appealed.

APPELLATE COURTS

Within a certain time following a trial court's final judgment, the losing party can appeal. An *appeal* is a formal request to a higher court to review the trial court's decision. These review courts are termed *appellate courts*. Comprised of three or more judges, these courts review trial court decisions for substantive and procedural correctness.

Appellate courts work from a court transcript of what was said and what evidence was presented in the lower court, such as photographs, business records, contracts, waivers, and agreements. These courts do not accept new evidence, listen to witnesses, make different or new determinations of fact, or use a jury. Rather, these courts receive written briefs prepared by attorneys that include legal arguments regarding how the law was mistakenly stated or applied to the facts presented to the trial court. The appellate court decides whether the trial court correctly applied rules of substantive and procedural law.[1,2]

If the appellate court determines the trial court incorrectly applied or interpreted the law, it may modify or reverse the lower court's decision, and either enter a new judgment or **remand** (send back) the case to the trial court for a new trial in compliance with the appellate court's instructions. However, just determining an error occurred at the trial court is not sufficient to overturn the trial court's decision. A minor error, or one that is not prejudicial to the interests of the appellant, is unlikely to affect the outcome of a case. An error found must be severe, demanding correction by the appellate court to escape a miscarriage of justice.[1,3]

If a case is heard on appeal, the appellate court typically writes and publishes a written opinion. In the opinion, the appellate court states the applicable rules of law as well as the rationale for reaching its decision. When reaching their decisions, appellate courts interpret and apply relevant statutory law along with appropriate common law derived from prior cases. Under the common law doctrine of *stare decisis*, also know as precedent, a lower court is bound to follow and apply decisions and interpretations of higher courts when similar cases arise. Occasionally, when there is no controlling statute

TABLE 2-1	The Federal and State Court Systems	
Federal (Rule on Federal Law Issues)	Type of Court	State (Example Florida) (Rule on State Law Issues)
U.S. Supreme Court	**Supreme Court** (Appellate Court)	Supreme Court of Florida
U.S. Courts of Appeals (United States has 13)	**Intermediate Courts of Appeal** (Appellate Courts)	District Courts of Appeals (Florida has 5)
U.S. District Courts (Florida has 3)	**General or Limited Jurisdiction Courts** (Trial Courts)	Circuit and County Courts in Florida

or precedent when ruling on a case, an appellate court may create a new rule or extend an existing principle to the case. Thus new law is created and is termed judge-made law, or case law. These court decisions become a part of our continually evolving common law system that must be followed by other courts when deciding future similar cases within their respective jurisdictions.[1-3]

STATE VERSUS FEDERAL COURTS

A typical state court system consists of both trial and appellate courts. Most states have three main levels: trial courts, intermediate appellate courts, and the highest court (typically termed the state supreme court). Although most states provide two levels of appeal, some have only one appellate court. Additionally, and unfortunately, names of state courts are not uniform. The names of courts in one state often apply to very different courts in another state. Information about state court systems can be found at the National Center for State Courts website, http://ncsconline.org.

Similar to the state court system, the federal court system consists of trial and appellate courts (see Table 2-1). The federal court system conducts trials involving federal matters, such as federal crimes and enforcement of federal laws. They also hear cases when parties are from different states and claimed damages are at least $75,000.

The federal trial courts are the U.S. District Courts. The United States is divided into 94 judicial districts, and there is at least one U.S. District Court in each state and territory. The two major federal appellate courts are the U.S. Courts of Appeals and the U.S. Supreme Court. The U.S. Courts of Appeals review the decisions of the U.S. District Courts. The U.S. is divided into 13 judicial circuits or geographical areas, each with one U.S. Court of Appeal. The top level of the federal court system is the U.S. Supreme Court. Nine justices sit on the U.S. Supreme Court. Most often this court acts as the court of final appeal for federal Courts of Appeals.[1-3] Additional information on federal courts may be obtained at the federal court website, http://www.uscourts.gov/.

THE PROCESS OF A CIVIL LAWSUIT

When a person decides to seek compensation through the civil court system, his or her attorney, if satisfied that the person has a cause of action (legal reason(s) for suing—referred to as reasonable or probable cause), often files a **complaint.** This formal document, which initiates a civil lawsuit, briefly states the facts the injured party (plaintiff) believes justify the claim and requests damages, or other relief, that the person is seeking from the defendant. Most often the complaint is served via a **summons,** commonly delivered by a court officer, which informs the defendant that a lawsuit has been filed and gives the person a prescribed amount of time to respond to the complaint.

Upon receiving the summons and complaint, a defendant typically retains the services of an attorney who will represent his or her interests. The defendant's attorney typically files an **answer,** which normally denies some or all of the allegations found in the complaint. The complaint and answer together are known as **pleadings.** Instead of an answer, the defendant's attorney may seek a dismissal of the complaint. This is known as a *motion to dismiss* and is used when the complaint is legally insufficient to justify an answer.

After the initial pleadings, the case proceeds to what is typically referred to as the **discovery phase.** The period, or process, of discovery encompasses the time period from the filing of the complaint to the beginning of the actual trial. This pretrial procedure is the time when both parties obtain facts and information about the case from each other, to assist in the preparation for trial. Very common discovery techniques are interrogatories, depositions, and requests to produce physical evidence. An **interrogatory** is a set of written questions sent by an attorney representing one party in the lawsuit to the other party involved in the suit. The questions must be answered under oath, within a certain time period, and may be used as evidence in trial. They should be answered only with the advice and guidance of an attorney. A **deposition** is an out-of-court oral examination of a witness taken before a trial. Attorneys from all parties are typically present at depositions where the witness answers questions, under oath, which are recorded by a court stenographer. Similar to interrogatories, deposition transcripts may also be used as evidence at trial. A **request to produce evidence** is a request by one party to another to produce, and allow for the inspection of, any designated physical evidence that they currently control or possess and is believed to be relevant to the lawsuit.[1-3] For instance, it is not uncommon for attorneys to request to examine specific documents such as accident/incident reports, preactivity health screening questionnaires, informed consents, waivers, and medical records, as well as to inspect equipment (e.g., resistance and/or cardiovascular equipment) that was used by the plaintiff at the time of the alleged incident.

If there are no disputes over the facts of the case that need to be resolved, it is possible that the case can be decided without having to go to trial. In a motion for **summary judgment,** the moving party, the one that requests summary judgment, argues there are not any significant questions of fact and that the applicable case law requires that they be awarded judgment. This motion may be made when a party believes discovery has shown there are no real disputes as to the facts. If the motion is granted, a trial does not occur.[1-3]

Typically, any party or the court can request a pretrial hearing or conference, which usually takes place after the discovery process is complete. The purpose of these informal conferences is to identify the matter(s) in dispute and to plan the course of the trial. At the pretrial hearing, a judge may motivate the parties to reach an out-of-court settlement. If a settlement cannot be reached, the case typically goes to trial.

In a civil court case, the plaintiff typically has the choice as to whether he or she wants the case to be heard by a jury or a judge. Through their respective attorneys, several steps occur. The plaintiff gives the opening statement, which may be followed by a statement from the defendant. These statements are designed to inform the **triers of fact** (either the judge or the jury) as to the nature of the case and what types of evidence will be presented during the trial. After opening statements, the plaintiff presents their case first. The plaintiff calls and examines their witnesses. The witnesses are then cross-examined by the defendant, often redirected by the plaintiff, and then typically recrossed by the defendant. The defendant then repeats this with their witnesses.

During trial, two types of witnesses may be called. **Fact witnesses** are called because they have specific information (perhaps something they saw, heard, or felt) regarding the alleged incident in question. In contrast, **expert witnesses** are called to educate the triers of fact by sharing their expertise and knowledge. Expert witness are often asked to testify through their opinions regarding the professional standards that apply to the incident in question and to the degree that the defendant adhered, or did not adhere, to those standards.

Once both sides have finished their questioning, final closing statements are made with the defendant proceeding first. After the final statements, the judge, in a jury trial, gives the jury instructions regarding their options in reaching a decision based on the applicable laws. Statutes, case law, and precedent are read and given to the jury. After deliberating, the jury renders a decision. In a trial without a jury, the judge can either recess the court while making a decision or render a decision just after closing statements.

Sometimes judgments by entry-level courts are appealed to a higher court. The party that lost the case makes a request to have the proceedings reviewed by a higher court, hoping that the lower court's decision will be reversed. The appellate court may affirm (agree with) the lower court's decision, reverse it (disagree with), remand it (send it back, with instructions, for a new trial), or modify the lower court's judgment in some manner.[1,2,6-8]

TORT LAW

A **tort** can be defined as conduct that amounts to a legal wrong that also causes harm on which the courts can impose civil liability. Some torts can also be crimes. However, tort law is not concerned with the separate issue of criminal responsibility. Rather, the defendant's potential for civil liability to the plaintiff for harmful wrongdoing and the victim's potential for compensation is the essence of tort law.[9]

The source of tort law is predominantly the common law. Judges rather than legislatures typically define torts and how compensation will be measured. However, a statute may deem certain conduct legally wrong and may allow recovery of damages for such conduct. In the vast majority of tort cases, a favorable judgment for the plaintiff results in an award of money as compensation for the harm caused by the conduct in question. The concepts and nuances of tort law are contained in the Restatement of Torts (Third).[10]

The Fault Basis of Tort Liability

Tort law has to do with an infringement (a civil wrong) by one person of the legally recognized rights of another. The infringement can be categorized according to three levels of fault, which include intentional conduct, negligence, and strict liability[9] (see Figure 2-2).

Intentional Torts

An **intentional tort** (wrong) involves an intent on behalf of the defendant to participate in behavior that the law regards as wrongful. Typically, the intentional tort defendant is consciously aware of the wrongdoing. Many crimes are also intentional torts because criminal acts are typically intended and often injure the victim. Therefore, the government may prosecute the criminal in criminal court for the public wrong to society, and

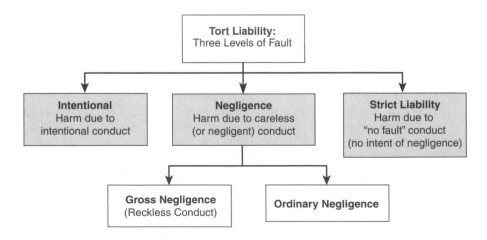

FIGURE 2-2 Fault Basis of Tort Liability

the individual victim may also sue the wrongdoer in civil court for the private wrong. Examples of intentional torts include battery, assault, false imprisonment, and intentional infliction of emotional harm.[1,3]

Battery is intentional bodily contact to a plaintiff in a way not justified by the plaintiff's apparent wishes, and the contact is harmful or against the plaintiff's will. The contact does not have to result in an injury. Any touching that violates ordinary social usages may be a battery unless the plaintiff has provided signs that it is acceptable. Violence or ill will is not mandatory.[1,3]

Assault is an act of putting someone in reasonable fear or apprehension of an immediate battery by means of an act amounting to an attempt or threat to commit a battery.[5] In other words, assault is the victim's subjective apprehension that he or she is about to be touched in an impermissible way that is a battery if it occurs.[9]

An example of an assault that occurred in the health/fitness setting is found in the case of *State v. Dennis Farias*.[11] The defendant, Dennis Farias, appealed his conviction after a jury found him guilty of one count of second-degree sexual assault. The sexual assault occurred at a health club where Farias groped and sexually pawed his victim while they were both seated in the health club's whirlpool tub. The case was remanded for a new trial.

In its simple form, false imprisonment occurs when the defendant confined or instigated the confinement of the plaintiff. *Confinement* means the plaintiff was constrained against his or her will. The confinement must be within a given area, large or small, by means of a physical barrier and/or physical force, or the threat of force. Locking someone in a room against his or her will is a classic example of false imprisonment. False imprisonment may be alleged when a business restrains an innocent shopper they wrongfully accused of shoplifting.[1,3]

Emotional harm is a highly unpleasant mental reaction (i.e., anxiety, anguish, grief, diminished enjoyment, humiliation, fright) that is the result of another person's intentional conduct. These harms are referred to as *mental distress* or *mental suffering* and can be actionable in court. However, the defendant's conduct must be extreme and outrageous, based on an intent to cause severe emotional harm or at least a reckless disregard of such harm, and a cause of direct harm to recover damages.[9] Recently, this intentional tort has often been linked with harassment in the workplace, either owing to sex, race, age, or sexual orientation.[3]

Several other intentional torts exist, including but not limited to defamation, invasion of privacy, and breach of fiduciary duty. *Defamation* is the act of harming the reputation of another by making a false statement to a third party. Before a statement is deemed defamatory, it must not only be untrue, but it must also be a statement of fact rather than opinion. Defamation in written form is *libel*, whereas defamation communicated orally is *slander*. Defamatory statements tend to harm a person's reputation, often by subjecting the person to public disgrace or ridicule, or by negatively affecting the person's business.[5] The crucial element is the effect on third parties, people in the community.[1]

Invasion of privacy is an unjustified exploitation of one's personality or intrusion into one's personal activity.[5] In other words, it is an intentional tort that offensively intrudes on the solitude of another or on their private affairs or concerns.[3] All U.S. citizens are entitled to protection from unreasonable invasions of privacy.

A fiduciary relationship is a special relationship in which a person in a position of trust puts their needs second to act for the benefit of another. The beneficiary places special confidence in the fiduciary who, thereby, is obligated to act in good faith and candor.[1,2] An attorney–client relationship is an example of a fiduciary relationship. An attorney who breaches this duty could face civil liability.

Once again, it is important to realize that a victim of an intentional tort could file a civil lawsuit against the person who committed the harmful act (the defendant), but the government could also prosecute the defendant in criminal court if the conduct violated a federal or state statute. For example, a massage therapist who sexually assaults a client could face criminal charges (e.g., battery charges made by the government) and a civil lawsuit (e.g., a negligence claim made by a client).

Negligence

The vast majority of lawsuits brought against health/fitness professionals allege negligence. According to Dougherty, Goldberger, and Carpenter,[7] negligence is essentially failing to do something that a reasonable, prudent person would have done under the same or similar circumstances, or doing something that a reasonable, prudent, and knowledgeable person would not have done. Negligence may therefore arise from an act of omission or commission.

The Elements of Negligence   Unlike intentional torts, described earlier, negligence is unintentional. For example, a person, or maybe an organization, does some act, neither intending nor expecting someone to get hurt, but someone is harmed. For a defendant to be held liable for negligence, the plaintiff must show four elements of negligence: a legal duty, breach of duty, causation, and damage or harm[12] (see Figure 2-3).

DUTY   **Duty** arises from a special relationship between the health/fitness professional and the client that requires the health/fitness professional to protect the client from exposure to unreasonable risks that may cause harm.[12] If the injured party was a health/fitness club member or cycling class participant, the legal duty of the fitness instructor or cycling instructor is virtually indisputable. Although a special relationship may exist, it must be shown that the defendant should have been able to predict the possibility of harm under the circumstances in question. In other words, the health/fitness professional should have realized that a health/fitness participant might suffer some type of harm. This is known as *foreseeability*.[7] If the defendant could have foreseen injury to the health/fitness participant, then he or she has a duty to the participant. However, if the defendant could not have foreseen the harm, there is typically no duty.

BREACH OF DUTY   The **breach of duty** (also referred to as the act) is the error, or omission, that harmed the plaintiff. The key issue is essentially whether or not the defendant failed to act reasonably under the specific circumstances involved. In basing its decision on this issue, a court will not only apply the "reasonable person" test, but

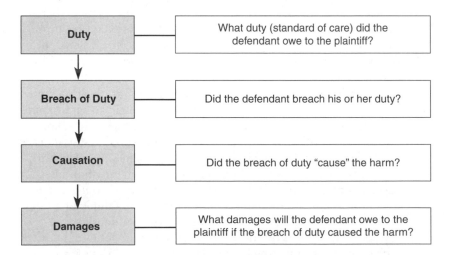

FIGURE 2-3 Four Essential Elements of Negligence: Plaintiff Has Burden of Proof

will also determine if the standard of care was met. A determination of negligent conduct is made by comparing the defendant's action, or inaction, against the conduct of a reasonable and prudent person under similar circumstances. In other words, the court considers what an average, reasonable person would have done in the same circumstances. However, a reasonable "person" means a person of the defendant's occupation.[2] For instance, a fitness instructor must instruct as a reasonable fitness instructor would instruct. Whether a defendant acted reasonably or not is a question for the judge or jury.

The **standard of care** required is that of a prudent person acting in like circumstances. Simply stated, standards describe the level of care that is owed to others to protect them from unreasonable harm.[13] In a broad sense, the standard of care may be set by case law, legislation, by organizations and associations, or by the profession. When published standards do not exist, the common practices of the profession are the norm. Because jurors cannot be expected to know the standards of various professions, expert witnesses attest to the accepted, desirable practices. Therefore, the standard of care provided must be that of the best professional practices.[12] To keep up with this ever-changing standard of care, it is necessary for health/fitness professionals to stay abreast of the developments and modifications to the standard of care. For additional information regarding standards of practice, see Chapter 3.

CAUSATION   Factual cause, or **causation,** refers to the fact that the breach of duty, the negligent act, was what caused the injury. Conduct is considered factual cause of harm when the harm would not have occurred absent the conduct in question.[10] In most cases this is apparent and determined by asking, "If not for the negligent conduct, would the injury have happened?" This is often referred to as the "but for" test. For example, suppose a fitness instructor prescribes a contraindicated exercise that injures a client. If the fitness instructor had not prescribed that contraindicated exercise, no injury would have occurred. However, cases are not always this simple. When analyzing situations, the "but for" test does not always work, so courts may use another type of analysis. The substantial factor test asks, "Was the defendant's negligence a substantial factor in causing the injury?" If the negligent act was a substantial factor in causing the injury, then the requirement of causation is satisfied. *Proximate cause* is a term frequently used, defined as "a cause that directly produces an event and without which the event would not have occurred."[14]

DAMAGES   Finally, the negligent act must have resulted in **damages** or losses to the plaintiff. If there is no injury, there is no cause of action for negligence. The injury can be a physical and/or emotional injury to a person or property damage. Compensatory damages, often referred to as actual damages, are awarded to cover actual injury or economic losses. They are intended to put the plaintiff in the same position the person was in prior to the injury. Examples of compensable damages include medical expenses, lost wages, and the repair or replacement of property. General damages, also referred to as non-economic losses, are intended to cover injuries when an exact dollar amount cannot be specified. General damages often include compensation for pain and suffering, but they may also consist of payment for a decreased life expectancy, loss of companionship of a loved one, and, in defamation cases, loss of reputation. Punitive damages, also referred to as exemplary damages, are awarded in addition to compensatory and general damages to punish the wrongdoer (defendant) for malicious, reckless, or willful conduct.[5,15] Punitive damages are rarely awarded for ordinary negligence (i.e., when someone is unintentionally injured).

In *Nimis v. Saint Paul Turners et al.,*[16] the plaintiff, Marion Nimis, was a member of the Saint Paul Turners health club when she was injured during a stretching demonstration. She sued, seeking damages for past and future medical expenses, pain and suffering, loss of earnings, and loss of consortium. **Consortium** is the benefits that one person, especially a spouse, is entitled to receive from another. These may include companionship, affection, cooperation, aid, and, between spouses, sexual relations.[5] Because Marion was not able to work for the family business as she had, she also sought lost profits.[16]

Gross Negligence   **Gross negligence** (sometimes also referred to as reckless conduct or willful/wanton conduct) is a conscious, voluntary act, or omission (failure to act), in reckless disregard of a legal duty and of the consequences to the plaintiff. It has been described as the failure to exercise even slight care. In such cases the plaintiff may recover punitive damages.[5] Additionally, several defenses to negligence may not apply to a defendant who was grossly negligent. For example, in most states, a waiver is not upheld if the defendant was grossly negligent. Other types of immunity may also be unavailable to a defendant who acted with gross negligence or with recklessness.[17] According to the Restatement of Torts (Third), "a person acts recklessly in engaging in conduct if: (a) the person knows of the risk of harm created by the conduct or knows facts that make the risk obvious to another in the person's situation, and (b) the precaution that would eliminate or reduce the risk involves burdens that are so slight relative to the magnitude of the risk as to render the person's failure to adopt the precaution a demonstration of the person's indifference to the risk."[18] (From the *Restatement of the Law Third. Restatement of the Law—Torts: Liability for Physical Harm.* Proposed Final Draft No. 1, § 2. Recklessness. April 6, 2005, Copyright (2005) by the American Law Institute. Reprinted with permission. All rights reserved.)

In summary, the success of a negligence claim depends on a plaintiff's ability to prove that the defendant owed a duty of care; that the defendant's act, or omission, was unreasonable in breaching that duty; that the plaintiff suffered damage; and that the defendant's act or inaction was the cause of the plaintiff's damage.[7]

Defenses Against Claims of Negligence   Just because a health/fitness business or professional is named as a defendant in a negligence lawsuit does not necessarily mean the person will be held liable. A defendant can use several defenses to counter claims of negligence. Perhaps the best defense is to show one of the four elements of a cause of action based on negligence does not exist: duty, breach of duty, causation, and injury. Other possible defenses include contributory negligence, comparative negligence, assumption of risk, expiration of the statute of limitation, various types of immunity, and the application of waivers.

CONTRIBUTORY NEGLIGENCE   **Contributory negligence** refers to negligence on the part of the person claiming damages (plaintiff). Under contributory negligence, if the plaintiff is even slightly negligent, he or she is barred from recovering any damages. In other words, if the plaintiff contributed to his or her own injuries, to any degree, the person cannot recover any damages from the plaintiff. If a plaintiff was 1% negligent, they could not recover from a defendant who was 99% negligent.

This harsh rule, which originated in England and was commonly applied in the U.S. during the 1800s, was attacked by critics as unreasonable. However, it survived into the 20th century and frequently blocked recovery of damages in motor vehicle accidents. Although this used to be the law in the United States, it remains in effect in only a few states.[1]

COMPARATIVE NEGLIGENCE   The vast majority of states have abandoned contributory negligence in favor of **comparative negligence.** Under comparative negligence, the plaintiff's negligence reduces but does not completely eliminate the defendant's liability for the plaintiff's injury. The damages are reduced in proportion to the amount of fault (negligence) attributable to the plaintiff. Liability for damages is allocated to the parties in proportion to the amount of fault that each contributed in causing the injury, as determined by the jury.[1] For example, if a defendant is 80% at fault and the plaintiff is 20% at fault, then the plaintiff recovers 80% of the damages.

Some states limit the concept of comparative negligence. Some states allow the plaintiff to always recover damages even if the defendant was only 1% at fault. This is known as a pure comparative negligence system. Other states have modified comparative negligence systems, under which the plaintiff can only recover if they are not as (50%) or more (51%) at fault than the defendant.[2,3]

ASSUMPTION OF RISK   **Primary assumption of risk** involves the plaintiff assuming well-known inherent risks to participating in the activity. For instance, when health/fitness participants know and understand the inherent risks involved in plyometric training and voluntarily participate, they assume those inherent risks and the health/fitness facility and staff are not liable, absence negligence on their parts, for injuries resulting from those inherent risks. However, three elements must exist to use this defense successfully: (a) the risk must be inherent to the activity, (b) the participant must voluntarily agree to participate, and (c) the participant must know, understand, and appreciate the inherent risks. A method often utilized in the health/fitness profession to assist in meeting these elements is the use of informed consents and agreements to participate.[17] When a health/fitness participant signs an informed consent, the assumption is express. In other words, they expressly assume the risk by signing an informed consent. Assumption of risk can also be implicit. Health/fitness participants may not expressly state that they assume the risk, but their conduct does so by implication. For additional information regarding assumption of risk and documents that help strengthen this defense, see Chapter 4.

PROCEDURAL DEFENSES   **Statutes of limitations** are legislative enactments that restrict the length of time an injured party has to formally file a lawsuit. The limitations vary from state to state and depend on the type of claim. Most states allow 2 to 3 years to file a tort claim; however, limitations vary from 1 to 4 years.[17] A 1- or 2-year time limit is typical for negligence torts; the time limit is usually 2 years for oral contracts and 4 years for written contracts.[1]

IMMUNITY   **Governmental immunity** originally barred liability claims against governmental entities; although not, typically, against their individual employees. However, the federal and state governments have passed varying degrees of tort claims legislation that permit injured parties to sue governmental entities under certain circumstances.[7] However, many put a cap on monetary damages for ordinary negligence. Another type of immunity—volunteer immunity—may protect volunteers while acting within the scope of their responsibilities for a nonprofit organization under the Volunteer Protection Act (VPA), a federal statute. However, the act only protects individual volunteers from liability for negligence, not the nonprofit organization.[17]

DEFENSES BASED ON CONTRACT LAW   Possible negligence defenses based on contract law include the use of waivers, facility lease agreements, and independent contractors. A waiver, or release of liability, is a contract in which the signer agrees to relinquish the right to recover damages from the health/fitness provider in the event that the health/fitness provider's (ordinary) negligence causes an injury to the signer. The validity of waivers varies greatly from state to state. Furthermore, waivers must be properly written and administered to be the upheld in court. For further information regarding waivers, see Chapter 4.

A facility lease agreement may be useful for health/fitness facility owners who allow other groups or businesses access to their facilities. For example, a local youth sports team may ask to use a health/fitness facility to conduct a practice, workout, or event. Waiver and facility lease agreements must be carefully written and should always be approved by an attorney prior to use. The use of independent contractors may also provide a defense from negligence claims. Typically, if a client is injured due to the negligence of an independent contractor, the liability for that injury is shifted from the health/fitness facility to the independent contractor.[18] However, facilities may be liable if they were negligent in hiring or supervising an independent contractor.

For example, a health/fitness facility owner may be liable for the actions of his/her aerobic instructor (an independent contractor) if he/she was hired without appropriate certification. For further information on independent contractors and negligent hiring, see Chapter 5.

DEFENSES THAT DON'T WORK   Many health/fitness professionals have never been sued, and some do not feel the need to manage risk. Others feel that managing risk is too time consuming, bad for business (making clients sign forms), takes too much staff time, is not required by law so why should they do it, or no matter what they do, they'll lose in court anyway. These excuses are clearly not valid in court, and are unwise to follow.

Another trap to which health/fitness professionals may succumb is not staying current with the accepted standard of care. From a legal standpoint, what was acceptable last year or a few years ago may not be today. The standard of care and accepted practices evolve and change as new scientific medical, professional knowledge develops. It is imperative to stay abreast with these changes, or a professional may suffer the negative legal consequences for failing to do so. Therefore, a defense such as "that is how we do things" or "that is how other health/fitness facilities do things" will not be an effective defense.[19] However, if the "current" standard of care has been applied, a stronger defense can be put forth.

Financial costs are never a valid excuse for not complying with the standard of care. If services cannot be provided that meet the standard of care because of budgetary constraints, those services should not be delivered.

There are known foreseeable risks associated with physical activity. Clients have a right to know, understand, and appreciate those risks that injure and/or even cause death, especially if they are paying for the privilege to participate in the activity. These risks should not be kept or hidden from clients.

Ultimately, it is the health/fitness professionals who must make these decisions. It is their business or employment that is at stake. However, health/fitness professionals should always remember that the bottom line to any standards issues is always predicated on a desire to make an activity safer or to protect a client from unnecessary harm.[18]

Strict Liability

Another type of tort is **strict liability**. Intentional torts and negligence are both based on the concept of fault. If someone does something wrong, intentionally or negligently, and causes injury, that person must pay for damages. However, strict liability is not based on fault but instead on public policy. In certain situations, the injured plaintiff does not need to prove intent or negligence; the defendant is liable even if not at fault. For instance, when people engage in certain types of conduct or activities and that conduct injures someone, that person or those people must compensate the injured party, even if there was no intentional wrongdoing or negligence.[1,3] The two main areas of business that incur strict liability are ultrahazardous activity and defective products.

Ultrahazardous Activities   Ultrahazardous activities include operating explosives, using dangerous chemicals, bringing harmful substances onto property, keeping dangerous animals, operating a nuclear reactor, and other similar activities in which the danger to the general public is very great. Defendants who engage in an ultrahazardous activity are virtually always liable for any harm they cause.[2]

Product Liability   If a product is negligently manufactured, distributed, or sold, the negligent party is liable for injuries as long as the product was being used in a foreseeable manner. Strict liability applies to the manufacturer, distributor, and seller. Even though the distributor and the seller had nothing to do with making the product, and may even be completely separate businesses from the manufacturer, they too can be liable.

Although liability only arises when the product is defective, the defect can originate in the design of the product, in the manufacturing of the product, or in the warnings that may come with the product. Certain states mandate that the defect make the product unreasonably dangerous. **Product liability** extends to the person who purchases the product, to one who uses it, or to a bystander injured by the product.

Prior to product liability being imposed, the injured parties must show they were using the product in a foreseeable manner. However, it is not required that it was used in the intended manner.[1,3] For example, a weight bench with stanchions is intended for bench-pressing. But it is foreseeable that someone may use it for other exercises. If the bench collapsed when someone was using it for shoulder presses, assuming all the other elements were present, strict liability would still apply. See Chapter 9 for additional information on liability issues associated with exercise equipment.

Workers' Compensation Workers' compensation is a form of strict liability imposed on the employer without fault. These statutes ensure that employees receive payment for injuries incurred at work. Prior to these statutes, injured employees could only recover damages if they sued their employer.

Workers' compensation statutes provide a fixed (by state statutes), reasonably certain recovery to the injured employee, no matter who was at fault for the injury. The injured worker is not required, or permitted, to sue to obtain damages. Although the amounts allowed for medical expenses and lost wages are typically less than an employee may recover in court, the injured employee trades the certainty of some award for the higher risk of going to trial. Claims are subject to review and approval by an administrative board that conducts an informal hearing. Injured employees are sometimes entitled to the assistance of legal counsel without cost to them.[1,2] For additional information on employment issues, see Chapter 5.

Vicarious Liability Under the common law doctrine of *respondeat superior,* an employer can be held liable to third parties for injuries caused by the negligence of their employees while they are acting within the scope of their employment. This doctrine imposes **vicarious liability** on an employer for the wrongful acts of their employees that occur when the employee is on the job. Vicarious liability is imposed even though the employer has not been careless. Because liability exists without the fault of the employer, this doctrine is similar to strict liability in tort.[1]

CONTRACT LAW

In simple terms, a **contract** is an agreement that can be enforceable in court. Typically, a contract is formed when two (or more) parties exchange binding promises. When making a promise, a party declares that they will, or will not, take a specified action sometime in the future. If that promise is not fulfilled, the contract has been breached (broken), and the party that failed to keep their promise must compensate the party to whom the promise was made. The nonperforming party is usually required to pay financial damages for the failure to perform the promise. In special situations a court may instead require actual performance of the promised act. However, in most cases when a contract is breached, the parties agree to some acceptable alternative without litigation and the payment of damages.[1]

Contract law varies among major types of businesses and from state to state. Many contracts are based on case law (court decisions), and specialized statutes exist for certain types of contracts (e.g., insurance policies, real estate transactions, employment contracts). Many contracts also involve the sale and/or purchase of goods, which are governed by the Uniform Commercial Code (UCC).[20] All states have adopted, at least in part, the UCC as part of their statutory law. Because the UCC does not attempt to answer all contract questions, common-law rules also provide answers to many contract questions.

Additionally, the Second Restatement of Contracts, although it does not have the force of law, is a highly persuasive summary that provides guidance and clarity of U.S. common law of contracts.[21]

FOUR ELEMENTS OF A CONTRACT

Four essential elements must be met for a valid contract to exist. If any of these elements are missing, a contract will not have been legally formed. These are the four elements:

1. *Agreement.* An agreement to form a contract includes an *offer* and an *acceptance.* One party must offer to enter into a legal agreement, and another party must accept the terms of the offer.
2. *Consideration.* Any promises made by the parties to the contract must be supported by legally sufficient and bargained for *consideration* (something of value received or promised, such as money, to convince a person to make a deal).
3. *Contractual capacity.* Both parties entering into the contract must have contractual capacity to do so; the law must recognize them as possessing characteristics that qualify them as competent parties.
4. *Legality.* The contract's purpose must be to accomplish some goal that is legal and not against public policy.[21–22]

TYPES/CLASSIFICATIONS OF CONTRACTS

Contracts may be *express,* when formed in spoken or written words, or they may be *implied* in fact, when manifested by conduct or body language (e.g., a hand waved at a football stadium vendor during a game followed by the passing of money and a return of a bag of peanuts). The majority of contracts combine express and implied terms. However, certain contracts must be in writing under what is termed the **Statute of Frauds,** such as contracts involving the sale of goods at $500 or more.[22]

In the majority of contracts, both parties exchange promises. This type of agreement is known as a *bilateral* contract; a promise made in exchange for another promise. For example, a fitness instructor promises to provide *XX* fitness-training sessions to a client in exchange for the client's promise to pay the instructor *XX* dollars. Bilateral contracts are the most common type of contract used in the health/fitness industry. In contrast, a promise in exchange of an act is known as a *unilateral* contract. In this case, one party makes a promise to induce some completed act by another party.[2] For example, a health/fitness facility offers their members a free 2-week membership extension for every new member they refer to the club. No member is legally obligated to refer members, nor is the facility obligated to extend memberships by 2 weeks unless the requested act is performed.

VOIDABLE AND UNENFORCEABLE CONTRACTS

A contract must comply with certain essential elements for it to be valid. If an essential element of a contract is missing, it is said to be a **voidable contract,** and either party may withdraw without liability. For example, a minor (less than 18 years of age) may usually void a contract even if freely and intentionally made because such a minor lacks the legal capacity to enter into a binding contract.

A contract is deemed an **unenforceable contract** if it violates a statute or is contrary to public policy. For instance, agreements that contemplate violating statutory laws such as tax laws, or the commission of torts such as fraud or defamation, may be declared illegal.[1,2]

A valid contract must be made with genuine assent. Assent is negated if either party acted under duress or because of undue influence. It will also be negated if it resulted from fraud or certain mistakes. *Duress* may occur when one party is unfairly persuaded or coerced by a wrongful act or threat from the other party. The threat of physical harm is an example. A victim of duress can usually choose to carry out the contract or cancel the entire contract without penalty.[1,2]

Undue influence, although peaceful and subtler than duress, has the same legal effect. Wrongful persuasion and persistent pressure may deprive a party from exercising sound judgment and free will. This may occur when one party is in a position of power or authority over the other and unfairly exploits the victim's trust and confidence when entering a contract.[1,2]

Misrepresentation is a false assertion of fact that entices a party to enter into a contract. The misrepresentation may be fraudulent and intentional or it may be a mistake and unintentional. If the misrepresentation is fraudulent, the victim has the option of considering the contract voidable. If the misrepresentation was innocent, the party who relied on the misrepresentation may cancel the contract with no penalty; however, this must be done promptly on learning the truth.[1,2]

When both parties have a false understanding about a fact that is an important element to the contract, there is a bilateral mistake that generally makes the contract voidable by either party. In other words, when both parties are mistaken about an important fact(s), either party may cancel the contract without liability. A unilateral mistake occurs when only one party is mistaken about a vital fact of the bargain. In these cases, if certain conditions occur the contract may be voidable.[1,2]

USES IN THE HEALTH/FITNESS FIELD

Although there are many examples where contract law is utilized in the health/fitness field, waivers, independent contractors, and purchasing/leasing equipment are three common applications. Prior to participation, health/fitness facilities may have their clients (or participants) sign a waiver, also called a prospective release. When clients sign a waiver, they agree to release the health/fitness facility for any liability associated with negligence on the part of the health/fitness facility or its employees. Within the waiver, the exculpatory clause is the specific language that releases the health/fitness facility from its own negligence. Additional information regarding waivers is found in Chapter 4. The use of independent contractors to carry out various programs and services is becoming more common in the health/fitness field. For example, independent contractors often provide massage therapy, teach group exercise classes, train clients, and maintain/clean the facility. Many corporate and hospital-based health/fitness facilities establish third-party contracts with management firms that manage the facility and program. In these situations, the staff are typically employees of the management firm and not of the hospital or corporation. Chapter 5 provides additional information regarding the use of independent contractors. Finally, many health/fitness programs use purchasing or leasing equipment contracts.

BREACH OF CONTRACT

A **breach of contract** is not typically a crime or a tort, except in unusual cases. If litigation becomes necessary, the breaching party may be obligated by a court to pay compensatory damages. These compensatory damages are designed to place the victim in essentially the same economic position that would have resulted from the performance of the contract. A damaged party's ability to recover damages for such a breach is limited by their duty to mitigate. In other words, they may not collect for damages that they allowed to accumulate or those that they may have reasonably avoided.[2,21]

If financial damages are inadequate, the court could require the specific performance of the contract. This is typically granted when the interest involves land or the sale of goods that are unique or rare (e.g., limited antique sports equipment). On the contrary, courts do not usually require a contract for personal services (e.g., personal training) to be specifically performed.[2,21]

SUMMARY

The U.S. legal system is operated by our government—federal, state, and local levels. The core of the American legal system is the courts, which include both the federal and state, and criminal and civil court systems. The federal courts, and most of the states, operate with a three-tier system: trial courts, appellate courts, and a Supreme Court. The purpose of the trial courts is to resolve factual disputes and then apply the appropriate law to facts determined at trial. The primary role of the appellate courts is to make sure the trial court was fair and the law was appropriately applied. The purpose of the Supreme Court is to resolve disputes that exist among the various appellate courts and to rule on issues of prime importance.

All health/fitness professionals should develop an appreciation of all areas of tort law, but negligence is of particular importance. To help reduce and prevent negligence liability, health/fitness professionals must understand how courts determine negligence and then take the necessary steps to meet the many legal duties they have in their daily practices. Finally, although verbal contracts can be enforced, contracts should be written because they will provide documentation of what the parties agreed on should a contractual dispute arise. Although health/fitness professionals can draft contracts using the many resources and examples available to them, it is strongly recommended that a qualified lawyer, knowledgeable in contract law in the relevant state, review all contracts before they are implemented.

RISK MANAGEMENT ASSIGNMENTS

1. Visit your local law library. Locate and read case law related to the health/fitness industry.

   _____

   _____

   _____

   _____

2. Perform an Internet search for legal information related to a current legal issue in the health/fitness field.

   _____

   _____

   _____

   _____

3. Identify several publications that are devoted to, or devote parts of the publication to, keeping health/fitness professionals current on legal issues.

   _____

   _____

   _____

   _____

4. Contact your local courthouse to inquire about observing a civil court case.

   _____

   _____

_____

_____

5. Obtain several different health/fitness-related contracts (e.g., membership, employ-ment, waivers). Compare and contrast the differences. What would you consider the strengths and weaknesses of each one to be?

_____

_____

_____

_____

6. Write down a hypothetical health/fitness facility–related example of negligence. Identify each of the elements of negligence. What could be possibly used as a defense?

_____

_____

_____

_____

7. Save as "favorites" on your computer the following websites to easily obtain addi-tional information about the law, legal definitions, and so on: www.law.cornell.edu, www.findlaw.com, www.lectlaw.com, and www.nolo.com.

_____

_____

_____

_____

KEY TERMS

Administrative law
Answer
Breach of contract
Breach of duty
Case law
Causation
Civil law
Common law
Comparative negligence
Complaint
Consortium
Contract
Contributory negligence
Criminal law
Damages
Defendant
Deposition

Discovery phase
Duty
Expert witnesses
Fact witnesses
Governmental immunity
Gross negligence
Intentional tort
Interrogatory
Plaintiff
Pleadings
Primary sources
Procedural law
Primary assumption of risk
Product liability
Remand
Request to produce evidence
Respondeat superior

Secondary sources
Standard of care
Stare decisis
Statutes
Statute of Frauds
Statutes of limitations
Statutory law
Strict liability
Substantive law
Summary judgment
Summons
Tort
Triers of fact
Unenforceable contract
Vicarious liability
Voidable contract

REFERENCES

1. Carper DL, Mietus NJ, West BW. *Understanding the Law.* 3rd Ed. Cincinnati: West Legal Studies in Business/Thomson, 2000.
2. Beatty JF, Samuelson SS. *Essentials of Business Law.* 2nd Ed. Mason, Ohio: West Legal Studies in Business/Thomson, 2005.
3. Hames JB, Ekern Y. *Introduction to Law.* Upper Saddle River, NJ: Prentice Hall, 1998.
4. Harris MA. *Legal Research: Fundamental Principles.* Upper Saddle River, NJ: Prentice Hall, 1997.
5. Garner BA, ed. *Black's Law Dictionary.* 7th Ed. St. Paul, Minn: West, 2000.
6. Friedenthal JH, Kane MK, Miller AR. *Civil Procedure.* 2nd Ed. Saint Paul, MN: West, 1993.
7. Dougherty NJ, Goldberger AS, Carpenter LJ. *Sport, Physical Activity, and the Law.* 3rd Ed. Champaign, Ill: Sagamore, 2007.
8. Wong GM. *Essentials of Amateur Sports Law.* 3rd Ed. Westport, Conn: Praeger, 2002.
9. Dobbs DB. *The Law of Torts.* St. Paul, Minn: West, 2000.
10. *Restatement of the Law Third. Restatement of the Law—Torts.* Philadelphia: American Law Institute, 2006.
11. *State v. Dennis Farias,* 796 A2d 1074 (R.I., 2002).
12. van der Smissen, B. *Legal Liability and Risk Management for Public and Private Entities.* Cincinnati: W.H. Anderson, 1990.
13. Napolitano F. What do lawn mower safety and Par-Q have in common? *ACSM's Health Fitness J.* 1997;1:38–39.
14. Garner BA, ed. *Black's Law Dictionary.* 7th Ed. St. Paul, Minn: West, 2000:174.
15. Nolo.com. Legal Glossary. 2007. Available at: http://www.nolo.com/glossary.cfm. Accessed September 1, 2007.
16. *Nimis v. Saint Paul Turners et al.,* 521 N.W.2d 54 (Minn. App., 1994).
17. Cotten DJ. Defenses against negligence. In: Cotten DJ, Wolohan JT, eds. *Law for Recreation and Sport Managers.* 4th Ed. Dubuque, Iowa: Kendall/Hunt, 2007.
18. Restatement of the Law Third. Restatement of the Law—Torts: Liability for Physical Harm. Proposed Final Draft No. 1, § 2. Recklessness. Philadelphia: American Law Institute, 2005:18.
19. Herbert DL. Struggling with legal issues in a non-legal environment. *Exercise Standards and Malpractice Reporter.* Canton, Ohio: Professional Reports Corporation, 1997.
20. Uniform Commercial Code (UCC) 2–206(1)(a). St. Paul, Minn: American Law Institute, 1987.
21. *Restatement of the Law—Contracts.* 2nd Ed. St. Paul, Minn: American Law Institute, 1981.
22. Clarkson, KW, Miller RL, Jentz GA, Cross FB. *West's Business Law.* 8th ed. St. Paul, Minn: West, 2001.

CHAPTER 3

Determination of Duty in Negligence Claims and Lawsuits

LEARNING OBJECTIVES After reading this chapter, health/fitness students and professionals will be able to:

1. Understand that judges, as opposed to juries, determine whether or not a legal duty exists, the breach of which is actionable.

2. Describe how courts determine duty in negligence cases.

3. Understand the elements involved when courts establish the reasonable person standard of care.

4. Explain why health/fitness professionals are held to a professional standard of care.

5. Describe the potential legal impact of published standards of practice in negligence cases using case law examples.

6. Understand the legal implications that exist because of inconsistencies among published standards of practice.

7. Describe duties that can arise from special relationships, such as person(s) on land and landowner/occupier as well as patient and health care provider.

8. Understand the attractive nuisance doctrine that applies to children trespassers.

9. Describe the standard of care related to children and related implications that arise for health/fitness facilities.

This chapter explains how courts determine whether or not duty exists, the breach of which is actionable in negligence claims and lawsuits. The focus is on the duties that arise out of relationships that are formed between health/fitness professionals and the participants they serve—those that are inherent and arise out of special relationships. This chapter also describes how standards of practice published by professional and independent organizations can be introduced into a court of law via expert testimony to determine legal duties in negligence cases. The information here is especially important for health/fitness professionals to understand because it provides the foundation for the information that follows in Chapters 5 through 11. Issues related to many inconsistencies that exist among published standards of practice in the health/fitness field are also discussed.

DETERMINATION OF DUTY: A BASIC OVERVIEW

As discussed in Chapter 2, in a negligence claim or lawsuit the plaintiff must first prove that the defendant owed him or her a certain duty determined by reference to a so-called standard of care. But how is this duty determined? First, it is important to understand that the court (or judge) determines duty, not juries. However, whether or not a defendant breached his or her duty as first found to exist by a judge will be determined by the jury (or by the judge if there is no jury). Courts determine duty in a variety of ways, but this chapter focuses on those that are most relevant for health/fitness professionals to understand and appreciate.

Betty van der Smissen[1] states that duty is formed from three primary origins: (a) relationship inherent in the situation, (b) voluntary assumption, and (c) mandated by statute. This chapter focuses on the various inherent relationships that are formed between health/fitness professionals and the participants they serve. These include the obvious relationships that occur between the health/fitness facility managers, owners, and staff members and the individuals—their clients/customers—that participate in the programs and services provided.

A legal duty can be created through a voluntary assumption of duty even when no relationship existed initially but is formed based on the action or conduct of an individual. The Restatement (Third) of Torts §42 states, "An actor who undertakes to render services to another that the actor knows or should know reduce the risk of physical harm to the other has a duty of reasonable care to the other in conducting the undertaking if: (a) the failure to exercise such care increases the risk of harm beyond that which existed without the undertaking, or (b) the person to whom the services are rendered or another relies on the actor's exercising reasonable care in the undertaking."[2] (From the *Restatement of the Law Third. Restatement of the Law—Torts: Liability for Physical Harm.* Proposed Final Draft No. 1, § 42. Duty based on understanding. April 6, 2005, Copyright (2005) by the American Law Institute. Reprinted with permission. All rights reserved.)

For example, in *Parks v. Gilligan,*[3] the defendant agreed gratuitously (like a volunteer) to spot for the plaintiff while he performed a bench-press exercise using dumbbells. As the plaintiff placed the dumbbells on the floor, his left index finger was crushed when his left hand came in contact with a weight on the floor. The plaintiff claimed the volunteer spotter had assumed a duty owed him and failed to carry out that duty (i.e., failed to ensure that the floor area where the exercise was taking place was free of weights or other objects that could cause an injury), and thus proximately caused the plaintiff's injury. The case resulted in a settlement when the defendants, the facility, and the volunteer spotter paid $15,000 and $5,000, respectively, to the plaintiff. This case demonstrates how those who voluntarily assume a duty can be potentially liable for an injury.

So even though no legal duty may exist to help another individual, once that duty is assumed voluntarily, a relationship is formed that results in a responsibility (or duty) to provide reasonable care. Health/fitness professionals who are working out at a facility on their own time do not have a *legal duty* to provide assistance to anyone (e.g., spotting, first aid) but perhaps a *moral duty* to do so. However, "while on the job," because of the various types of relationships inherently formed in such circumstances in health and fitness settings, health/fitness professionals have numerous duties that require them to be proactive to protect participants from foreseeable risks of harm. Chapters 5 through 11 describe many of these legal duties and the proactive risk management steps that can be taken to help ensure adherence to these legal duties.

A legal duty can also exist when a relationship is established by statute, for example, employment, supervisory requirements, or rendering first aid in certain situations.[1] For example, in Wisconsin, a statute there requires fitness centers to have a qualified supervisor (an employee who has satisfactorily completed a course or courses in basic first aid and basic cardiopulmonary resuscitation taught by an individual, organization, or institution of higher education approved by the department) present on the premises during all operating hours of the facility.[4] Several other states have also enacted statutes that require fitness facilities to have an automated external defibrillator (AED) as discussed in Chapter 11. Violation of statutes in these situations can result in **negligence** *per se,* a legal doctrine in which the plaintiff does not have to prove negligence as he or she would in an ordinary negligence case, but does have to show that the violation of the statute did *cause* the harm the statute was intended to prevent and the victim was in the class of persons that the statute was designed to protect.[5]

INHERENT RELATIONSHIPS: REASONABLE PERSON AND PROFESSIONAL STANDARD OF CARE

Inherent relationships are formed through the reasonable person standard of care and the professional standard of care. Distinct differences exist between these two standards of care. Generally, unsupervised health/fitness facilities (no staff or professional supervision) are held to the reasonable standard of care, and health/fitness facilities supervised by health/fitness professionals are held to the professional standard of care.

THE REASONABLE PERSON STANDARD OF CARE

Keeton et al.[6] state that the reasonable person standard, when used in reference to demonstrating negligence, requires one to act as a reasonable person or a person of ordinary/reasonable prudence. But how do the courts determine what is reasonable conduct? First, a reasonable person is one who has taken steps to avoid foreseeable, unreasonable risks of harm.[6] Foreseeable risks were discussed in Chapter 2 and the *Turner* case discussed later also explains how the concept of foreseeability is used in determining negligence. But what are unreasonable risks? Two factors are weighted: the defendant's burden of taking precautions, and the gravity (seriousness) and probability (frequency) of the risk the conduct creates. The defendant's burden of taking precautions is weighted against the gravity and probability elements resulting in a risk-benefit form of analysis to determine negligence using the reasonable person standard of care.[6] For example, if your car breaks down in the middle of a busy street, what would a reasonable person do? A reasonable person would put on their emergency flashers, put their hood up, and then call for a tow truck. None of these steps create an undue burden for the driver (e.g., cost a lot of money), in light of the magnitude of the risks (gravity and probability) that a stalled car on a busy street can create. The probability of an accident could be high and the gravity could also be high if the driver did not take reasonable steps to avoid any foreseeable, unreasonable risks of harm. Therefore, in this situation, the burden of the defendant to take precautions is low, whereas the magnitude of risk is high. In a situation in which a driver did not take these steps and an accident/injury occurred because of the situation the driver's omissions created, the driver could be found negligent using the reasonable person standard of care.

In this setting, an examination of the case of *Turner v. Rush Medical College*[7] should assist in focusing on the issue of foreseeable, unreasonable risks. The plaintiff, a 23-year-old medical student at Rush Medical College, was required to run 1 mile in 8 minutes as part of an experiment in his pathology class. During the run, the plaintiff allegedly suffered many serious and debilitating injuries requiring over 2 months of hospitalization at a cost of approximately $250,000. The plaintiff contended the defendant, Rush Medical College, breached its duty to exercise reasonable care by requiring the plaintiff, in what was classified as an experiment, to run a timed mile without obtaining the following information or providing the following safeguards:

1. Learning what forms of physical exercise the plaintiff did and, specifically, whether the plaintiff had ever run in a timed mile run (a type of pre-activity health screening issue).
2. Conducting a physical examination of the plaintiff to check on his respiration and blood pressure (also a type of pre-activity health screening issue).

3. Having medical personnel present to assist the plaintiff during and after the timed mile run (an emergency response planning issue).
4. Making oxygen available to the plaintiff if he needed the same during and after the timed mile run (also an emergency planning response issue).
5. Providing for water to be available to the plaintiff if needed during and after the timed mile run (a safety issue involving program delivery).

The trial court granted the defendant's motion to dismiss stating that "the complaint did not allege facts which established that the defendants owed plaintiff a duty."[8] The trial court ruled that "lack of foreseeability of harm and public policy considerations required dismissal of plaintiff's complaint as a matter of law."[8] On appeal, the court stated "that at the time of the defendant's conduct a reasonably prudent person would not have foreseen plaintiff's injury."[9] The defendant viewed the plaintiff as a healthy 23-year-old man. Regarding the public policy concerns, the court held that to impose a duty in like or similar cases would impose an expensive financial burden on schools (i.e., a duty to provide medical precautions). The appellate court upheld the trial court's decision of granting the motion to dismiss.

In this case, the court decided that the burden of taking precautions (such as those suggested by the plaintiff) was too great of a financial burden for Rush Medical College and the magnitude of risk was small (e.g., low probability of the plaintiff being harmed and severity of any harm that might occur). In other words, the burden of the defendant to take precautions outweighed the magnitude of the risk. Therefore pursuant to the ruling in this case, the defendant had no duty to take any precautions and therefore did not breach any duty and was not liable for the plaintiff's injury.

The *Turner* case is interesting because most professionals in the health/fitness field would disagree with the court's holding and reasoning and would agree with the dissenting judge's view when balancing the burden of taking precautions against the magnitude of the risks. The dissenting judge stated, "It is practically a matter of common knowledge that running an eight-minute mile may cause injury. . . . An injury from such an undertaking is certainly reasonably foreseeable."[10] Regarding the public policy concerns, the dissenting judge stated that "schools and facilities have a duty to exercise reasonable care in supervising track and field events . . . and a duty to provide medical care when needed."[11] This case would have probably been much different if a professional standard of care (discussed later) was applied versus the reasonable person standard of care.

Supporting the dissenting judge's opinion in *Turner*, similar cases have had a different outcome than what occurred in *Turner*. For example, in *Kleinknecht v. Gettysburg College*,[12] the trial court stated it was not "reasonably foreseeable" that Drew Kleinknecht, a 20-year-old lacrosse player for Gettysburg College, would suffer a cardiac arrest, and therefore it determined that the defendant college owed no duty toward him to provide emergency medical care. However, the appellate court did rule that the college had a duty toward Drew to provide emergency medical care while engaged in a school-sponsored activity. The college was held liable for Drew's death in this case.

THE PROFESSIONAL STANDARD OF CARE

The previous discussion addressed the reasonable person standard of care, which is a minimum standard that requires all of us to act as a reasonable person, a person of ordinary prudence, or a person of reasonable prudence. However, if a person has special knowledge, skill, or even intelligence superior to that of an ordinary person, the law demands of that person conduct that is consistent with it.[6] The Restatement of Law (Third) of Torts states that "If an actor has skills or knowledge that exceed those possessed by most others, these skills and knowledge are circumstances to be taken into account in determining whether the actor has behaved as a reasonably careful person."[13] Keeton et al. state that "experienced milk haulers, hockey coaches, expert skiers, construction inspectors, and doctors must all use care which is reasonable in light of their superior learning and experience and any special skills, knowledge or training they may personally have over and above what is normally possessed by persons in the field."[14] Professional persons or those whose work requires special skill are required not only to exercise reasonable care, but also to possess a standard minimum of special knowledge and ability.[6] Because the work of health/fitness professionals requires specialized knowledge, skills, and abilities, they can be held to a professional standard of care, which is a higher standard of care than the reasonable person standard of care.

Deviation from the professional standard of care can result in professional negligence. One of the most common types of professional negligence is medical malpractice. However, many other professionals other than physicians (and even skilled trade workers) have been involved in professional negligence claims and lawsuits. The following discussion on medical malpractice provides an example of how professional negligence is determined that has application to health/fitness professionals.

First, in these medical malpractice cases, to establish the standard of care (duty) and any deviation from it (breach of duty), the plaintiff must use expert medical testimony. The purpose of expert testimony is to educate the court about the standard of care owed to the plaintiff. Keeton et al.[6] state that juries composed of laypeople are normally incompetent to pass judgment on matters of medical science and therefore, there can be no finding of negligence in the absence of expert testimony. They also state that the ultimate result of all expert testimony is "that the standard of conduct becomes one of good medical practice, which is to say what is customary and usual in the profession."[15] However, courts have said that *customary practice* should be just one factor in determining what good medical practice is and it is not conclusive. See *Darling v. Charleston Community Memorial Hospital,*[16] in which the court stated that just because the evidence showed the physician followed the customary practice, it is not the sole test of malpractice.

Another factor, *locality,* in medical malpractice cases was used by courts to establish the standard of care, which involved comparing the physician with other physicians in the same location (e.g., a county doctor should not be held to the same standard as an urban doctor). However, courts today are modifying this to mean similar locations or abolishing it completely, saying there is a minimum standard of care to which all physicians should be held. See *McGuire v. DeFrancesco,*[17] in which the court ruled that the physician should have followed a nationwide standard versus a statewide standard.

As in medical malpractice cases, health/fitness professionals must understand that customary practice or locality probably will not determine the standard of care in their profession; rather they probably will be held to a minimum standard of care owed by all health/fitness professionals as presented by expert testimony. As described in Chapter 1, there are various levels of health/fitness professionals: (a) those without a degree in the field but perhaps possessing a certification in the field (e.g., personal trainers, group exercise leaders, fitness floor supervisors), (b) those with a bachelor's degree in the field in typical professional positions (e.g., supervisors, coordinators, directors, and some personal trainers), and (c) those with a bachelor's degree who also have advanced training/ education (e.g., in management or clinical exercise). Each of these professionals will be held to a standard of care that is commensurate with the knowledge, skill, and abilities exercised by others, given the same or similar position and circumstances.

It is also important to realize that if health/fitness professionals represent themselves as having a higher level of knowledge, skill, and abilities than they possess, or take on responsibilities beyond their level of education and training (e.g., a personal trainer who trains moderate- or high-risk clients but does not have the credentials to do so, or a personal trainer who does not have a degree in the field but represents herself as having the same knowledge, skills, and abilities as a personal trainer who does have a degree), the person probably will be held to the higher standard. Therefore, health/fitness professionals should always stay within their **scope of practice,** that is, practicing within the limitations of their education, training, experience, and certification. As mentioned earlier, expert witnesses educate the court as to the standard of care and whether or not, in their opinion, a professional's conduct was consistent with that standard of care. In their testimony, experts often reference published standards of practice as evidence of the standard of care.

Published Standards of Practice

Published standards of practice are developed by professional organizations (e.g., ACSM, NSCA) and independent agencies, such as the Consumer Products Safety Commission (CPSC) or the American Society for Testing and Materials (ASTM). Professional organizations have published standards of practice (e.g., standards, guidelines, and position statements) to provide benchmarks of **desirable operating practices**[18] for health/fitness facilities. Desirable operating practices include staff functions such as providing emergency care when an injury occurs, conducting pre-activity health screening, inspecting exercise equipment, and providing proper instruction. They also can reflect certain credentials (e.g., degree, certification, and experience) that staff members should possess. Here are some examples of published operating practices for health/fitness facilities that are presented throughout this book:

1. *ACSM's Health/Fitness Facility Standards and Guidelines,* 3rd edition (**ACSM's H/F Standards**)[19]
2. *ACSM's Guidelines for Exercise Testing and Prescription.* 7th edition (**ACSM's Guidelines**)[20]
3. ACSM and AHA (American Heart Association) joint position statement, "Recommendations for Cardiovascular Screening, Staffing, and Emergency Policies at Health/Fitness Facilities" (**ACSM/AHA Joint PP**)[21]
4. NSCA (National Strength and Conditioning Association) *Strength & Conditioning Professional Standards & Guidelines* (**NCSA Standards**)[22]
5. IHRSA (International Health, Racquet & Sportsclub Association) Club Membership Standards, in *IHRSA's Guide to Club Membership & Conduct.* 3rd edition (**IHRSA Standards**)[23]
6. *Canadian Fitness Safety Standards & Recommended Guidelines.* 3rd edition. Published by the Ontario Association of Sport and Exercise Sciences (OASES) in Ontario, Canada (**Canadian Standards**)[24]
7. *The Medical Fitness Model: Facility Standards and Guidelines,* published by the Medical Fitness Association (MFA) (**MFA Standards**)[25]
8. *Exercise Standards & Guidelines Reference Manual,* 4th edition, published by the Aerobics and Fitness Association of America (AFAA) (**AFAA Standards**)[26]
9. ACSM and AHA joint position statement, "Automated External Defibrillators in Health/Fitness Facilities" (**ACSM/AHA Joint PP-AEDs**)[27]
10. *Medical Advisory Committee Recommendations: A Resource Guide for YMCAs,* published by the YMCA of the USA (**YMCA Recommendations**)[28]

Please note the abbreviations in bold. This is how the standards of practice will be referred to throughout the book. They are often updated and revised (e.g., the MFA Standards were in the process of being revised at the time final drafts of this book were being completed).

In addition to standards of practice published by professional organizations, van der Smissen[18] also classified published standards as **technical physical specifications.** Technical physical specifications are published by independent agencies such as the CPSC and ASTM. For example, the CPSC has published standard specifications on equipment such as bicycle helmets, and on facilities such as spas, hot tubs, and whirlpools. The ASTM has published standard specifications for playground equipment and safety signage for fitness equipment/facilities.

Health/fitness professionals need to adhere to both of these types of published standards of practice: desirable operating procedures and technical physical specifications.

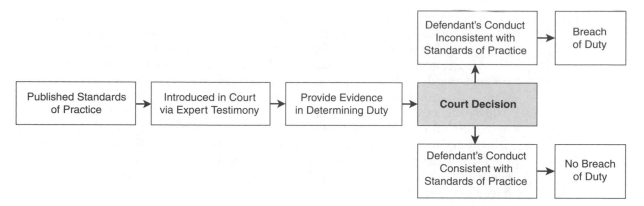

FIGURE 3-1 Example of the Potential Legal Impact of Published Standards of Practice (Reprinted with permission from Eickhoff-Shemek, J. and Kendall/Hunt Publishing Company. *Standards of practice.* In: *Law for Recreation and Sport Managers.*[29])

It is common for expert witnesses to introduce these published standards of practice as evidence of the standard of care. Adhering to these published standards of practice can serve as a shield for defendants (minimize liability associated with negligence) or as a sword for plaintiffs (increase liability associated with negligence) in situations in which defendants do not adhere to them. If it can be demonstrated that the defendant's conduct was consistent with the standards of practice, it will be difficult for the plaintiff to prove a breach of duty. However, if it can be shown that the defendant's conduct was inconsistent with the standards of practice, it can result in a breach of duty[29] (see Figure 3-1). As discussed in Chapter 1, selected laws and published standards of practice are presented in Chapters 5 through 11 so that health/fitness professionals can learn what these are and then how to apply them in their risk management plans.

Mandel v. Canyon Ranch, Inc.[30] and *Elledge v. Richland/Lexington School District Five*[31] are two cases that illustrate the importance of applying published standards of practice in a facility's risk management plan. In *Mandel,* published *operating practices* were introduced by an expert witness as evidence of duty, and in *Elledge,* the standard of care was determined from published *technical physical specifications*. Pertinent issues related to the proliferation and the inconsistencies that exist among published standards of practice are also discussed.

Mandel v. Canyon Ranch, Inc.[30]   In 1995, Robert Mandel purchased a spa package for his stay at Canyon Ranch, a health and fitness resort. While playing a game of wallyball with other guests, he collapsed onto the floor and died from an apparent cardiac arrest. The defendant's staff administered CPR and called paramedics immediately after the incident. Wendy Mandel, wife of the decedent, sued Canyon Ranch, claiming they had failed to appropriately handle the medical emergency because they did not use a heart defibrillation unit.

Expert witnesses for both parties testified in this case. The plaintiff's expert, a cardiologist, claimed the defendant Canyon Ranch breached its duty by failing to use a heart defibrillation unit when Mandel had an apparent cardiac arrest while playing wallyball. However, this expert witness did not introduce into evidence any published standards of practice that required or recommended health/fitness facilities to have and use a heart defibrillator unit.

The expert witness for the defendant Canyon Ranch, an exercise physiologist, testified that the conduct of the defendant in administering CPR and calling paramedics was consistent with standards of practice published in *ACSM's Health/Fitness Facility Standards and Guidelines,* 2nd edition, in effect at the time of this case.[32] This book contained six standards that "represent the standard of care that must be demonstrated by all health/fitness facilities toward their users."[33] Standard 1, which addressed emergency procedures, required health/fitness facilities to have personnel trained and certified in CPR but did not require facilities to have or use a heart defibrillation unit.

After considering all the evidence (including expert testimony from both the plaintiff and the defendant) in this case, the jury returned a verdict for the defendant Canyon Ranch. The expert testimony provided by the defendant indicating the defendant's conduct was consistent with the ASCM Standard 1 contributed, at least in part, to the jury's decision for the defendant. This case provides a good example of how published standards of practice can help protect a health/fitness facility from negligence, if the facility adheres to them. If Canyon Ranch had not carried out appropriate emergency procedures as required by ACSM Standard 1, the outcome of this case could have been quite different.

Elledge v. Richland/Lexington School District Five[31]   In 1994, Ginger Sierra, a 9-year-old fourth grader, was injured while playing on modified monkey bars on the school's playground. Three years earlier the school principal noticed children climbing on top of the bars rather than lying on the bench running underneath. The bars were originally designed to stand approximately 4.5 feet off the ground, and the children were to sit or lie on the bench underneath and pull themselves along the length of the bars. Believing that the original monkey bars were unsafe, the principal contracted with a playground equipment sales representative, who was not trained or licensed as an engineer, to modify the monkey bars. This modification resulted in removing the bench and lowering the bars, forming an inclined ladder ranging from 20 to 30 inches above the ground. Neither handrails nor a nonslip surface were added to the newly modified monkey bars.

While walking across the bars after a light rain, Ginger's foot slipped on a narrow bar resulting in a fall that trapped her right leg between the bars. She suffered a severe "spiral-type" fracture in her femur that resulted in damage to her femur's growth plate. Ginger's mother, Christine Elledge, sued the school district for injuries sustained by her daughter. Elledge claimed that the school district was negligent because it deviated from the accepted standard of care; that is, the modification of the monkey bars did not meet ASTM standards and CPSC guidelines for playground equipment. However, the trial court excluded Elledge's evidence that included video deposition testimony from an expert in playground equipment. This expert testimony would have clearly shown that the district did not adhere to industry standards as outlined by ASTM and CPSC. The trial court found for the defendant school district and Elledge appealed.

On appeal, Elledge asserted that the trial court erred in excluding evidence of ASTM standards and CPSC guidelines, arguing that such evidence was relevant to establish the appropriate standard of care. The appellate court agreed and reversed the trial court's ruling. Citing a variety of other cases to support its decision, the appellate court stated:

> *Safety standards promulgated by government or industry organizations in particular are relevant to the standard of care for negligence. . . . Courts have become increasingly appreciative of the value of national safety codes and other guidelines issued by governmental and voluntary associations to assist in applying the standard of care in negligence cases. . . . A safety code ordinarily represents a consensus of opinion carrying the approval of a significant segment of an industry, and it is not introduced as substantive law but most often as illustrative evidence of safety practices or rules generally prevailing in the industry that provides support for expert testimony concerning the proper standard of care.*[34]

The appellate court also stated the following as articulated by the New Jersey Supreme Court in *McComish v. DeSoi:*

[A] [safety] code is not introduced as substantive law, as proof of regulations or absolute standards having the force of law or scientific truth. It is offered in connection with expert testimony which identifies it as illustrative evidence of safety practices or rules generally prevailing in the industry, and as such it provides support for the opinion of the expert concerning the proper standard of care.[35]

This case was further appealed to the South Carolina Supreme Court. This court upheld the appellate court's decision, stating:

The general rule is that evidence of industry safety standards is admissible to establish the standard of care in a negligence case. The evidence of CPSC guidelines and ASTM standards which respondents sought to have admitted in the instant case is exactly the type of evidence contemplated by this general rule. The Court of Appeals correctly held the trial court committed reversible error in excluding the evidence.[36]

The *Mandel* and *Elledge* cases clearly demonstrate that courts allow published standards of practice (both desirable operating practices and technical physical specifications) as admissible evidence in determining the standard of care in negligence cases. This evidence, introduced by expert testimony, can provide powerful proof that the defendant either adhered or did not adhere to the standard of care. If the defendant adheres to published standards of practice, it can help protect the defendant from negligence, as demonstrated in *Mandel*. However, if the defendant does not adhere to published standards of practice, it can increase liability associated with negligence, as demonstrated in *Elledge*. Note: The preceding sections describing the *Mandel* and *Elledge* cases were reprinted with permission.[37]

Published Standards of Practice: Does Terminology Make a Difference?   The terminology that professional and independent organizations use to describe their published standards of practice can vary. For example, *ACSM's Health/Fitness Facility Standards and Guidelines,* 2nd edition,[32] contained six standards (requirements written as "must" statements) and over 500 guidelines (recommendations written as "should" statements) for health/fitness facilities. The six standards "represent the standard of care that must be demonstrated by all health/fitness facilities toward their users," whereas the "guidelines are not intended to be standards of practice or give rise to legal duties."[33] However, the ACSM/AHA joint position paper, *Recommendations for Cardiovascular Screening, Staffing, and Emergency Policies at Health/Fitness Facilities,*[21] includes both requirements (must statements) and recommendations (should statements), although the title specifically states "recommendations." In *ACSM's Guidelines for Exercise Testing and Prescription,*[20] it states that the "views and information . . . are provided as *guidelines* as opposed to *standards of practice.* This distinction is an important one, because specific legal connotations may be attached to such terminology."[38]

The National Strength and Conditioning Association (NSCA) defines standards and guidelines in a similar way to ACSM.[32] For example, *NSCA Strength & Conditioning Professional Standards and Guidelines*[22] contains 11 standards (written as must statements) and 12 guidelines (written as should statements). The NSCA publication defines a standard as "a required procedure that probably reflects a legal duty or obligation for the standard of care" and a guideline as "a recommended operating procedure formulated and developed to further enhance the quality of services provided."[39] The Medical Fitness Association (MFA) refers to standards as "minimum requirements that facilities must have in place to meet the definition of a 'Medical Fitness Center'" and "are not intended to be legal requirements," whereas guidelines "provide assistance/direction on how facilities can comply with the stated Standard."[40] The other published standards of practice selected to be included in this book either have not specifically defined the terms used (i.e., standards, guidelines, recommendations) or use them interchangeably.

Interestingly, in *ACSM's Health/Fitness Facility Standards and Guidelines,* 3rd edition,[19] the definitions of standards and guidelines have changed as follows:

1. *Standards are base performance criteria or minimum requirements that ACSM believes each health and fitness facility must meet to satisfy a facility's obligations to provide a relatively safe environment in which every physical activity or program is conducted in an appropriate manner. Furthermore, these standards are not intended to give rise to duty of care or to establish a standard of care; rather they are performance criteria derived from a consensus of ACSM leaders. The standards are qualitative in nature and are not intended to be restrictive or to supersede [sic] national, regional or local laws and regulations. Finally, as base performance criteria, they are steps designed to promote quality and to accommodate reasonable variations, based on local conditions and circumstances.*

2. *Guidelines are recommendations that ACSM believes health and fitness operators should consider using to improve the quality of the service they provide to users. Such guidelines are not standards, nor are they applicable in every situation or circumstance. Rather, they are illustrative tools that ACSM believes should be considered by health and fitness operators.*[41] (From American College of Sports Medicine, 2007, *ACSM's Health/Fitness Facility Standards and Guidelines,* 3rd edition, pages 4–5. © 2007 by American College of Sports Medicine. Reprinted with permission from Human Kinetics, Champaign, IL).

Other organizations such as the board of certification (BOC) for athletic trainers use the term "standards" in the title of their publication, *Standards of Professional Practice,* but the standard statements are written as "should" or "shall" statements. The American Association of Cardiovascular and Pulmonary Rehabilitation (AACVPR) in their *Guidelines for Cardiac Rehabilitation Programs* primarily uses "should" statements.

It is obvious that professional organizations and independent agencies define and use the terms standards and guidelines differently, but do courts distinguish these differences when establishing legal duty or the standard of care? In the *Elledge* case, although the ASTM published "standards" and the CPSC published "guidelines" both were introduced as evidence of the standard of care, the court made no distinction between standards and guidelines. The court did not exclude the CPSC guidelines, and it appeared that both standards and guidelines carried the same weight in determining the standard of care.

In another case, *Xu v. Gay,*[42] the court also did not exclude published guidelines when establishing the standard of care. In *Xu,* Ning Yan died from a severe head injury after falling off a treadmill. The treadmill only had 2.5 feet clearance behind it at the defendant's fitness facility. Dr. Marc Rabinoff, expert witness for the plaintiff, stated there should be a minimum of 5 feet behind treadmills to meet the industry's standard of care for the safety distance. He did not indicate the specific industry standards he was referring to, but he stated that they were voluntary not mandatory. The court made no distinction with regard to voluntary or mandatory standards when stating its ruling that the "defendant's ignorance of and failure to implement these standards . . . establishes a case of ordinary negligence."[43] Although the expert witness stated in his testimony that the industry standards were voluntary, the court still used them as evidence of the standard of care that the defendant owed to Yan.

Expert witnesses can introduce through their testimony into a court of law any evidence of published standards of practice they choose, regardless of how the professional or independent organizations have defined them. Responsible expert witnesses will make it clear to the court, as Rabinoff did in *Xu,* the distinction of mandatory versus voluntary as defined by the organization. However, not all expert witnesses will do so. Therefore, because courts may not even make the distinction between mandatory and voluntary standards of practice that are introduced as evidence of the standard of care (as demonstrated in *Xu*) when determining the standard of care, and because there is no guarantee that expert witnesses will distinguish mandatory from voluntary published standards of practice in their testimony, it is best for health/fitness professionals to adhere to all published standards and guidelines. In the event of inconsistency or conflict, they should follow those that are the most authoritative or safety oriented in their approach, regardless of how they are defined and/or stated by professional organizations or independent agencies.

Issues Related to the Proliferation of and Inconsistency Among Published Standards of Practice
Published standards of practice in the health/fitness profession, like those that had come before, primarily in the health field, were intended to standardize the delivery of service across the United States and Canada, while reducing claims and lawsuits based on negligence concepts where service delivery was claimed to be substandard. In a legal context, published standards of practice are "benchmark behaviors or actions that are universally exhibited by properly trained and experienced professionals."[44] From a professional perspective, such statements should be viewed "as the threshold or minimal acceptable level of service owed to a client, patient, or participant."[45]

Several issues are associated with the development and publication of standards of practice. First, the number of health/fitness professional organizations that have been formed in the last two or three decades has increased significantly. Many of these organizations have published standards of practice, as demonstrated by the 10 we selected to be included in this book. Because numerous published standards of practice now exist (labeled as standards, guidelines, recommendations, parameters of practice, baseline service delivery statements, optimal service standards, position papers, etc.), many inconsistencies have been created within them. As mentioned earlier, there is no consistency on how terms like *standards, guidelines,* and *recommendations* are defined. Sometimes, these inconsistencies even exist within the standards of practice published by the same organization, thus making it difficult for health/fitness professionals to understand and interpret them for their own health/fitness programs and facilities. This has led to loopholes in the adoption and application of published standards of practice in the delivery of programs and services.

One example of the inconsistencies that exist is best demonstrated by standards of practice published regarding AEDs. IHRSA has taken the position that AEDs are not yet part of the standard of care owed professionally or legally to health club participants.[46] However, in 2007, ACSM took the position that health/fitness facilities "must" have an AED, which thus became a requirement or a standard.[19] Where published standards of practice are inconsistent, "in the event of participant injury or death, such deficiencies may [thus] create confusion rather than clarity as to what should be the professional behavior expected in a specific exercise setting."[47]

Second, and as a significant result of the lack of consistency in the available published standards of practice, litigation results have been inconsistent. Moreover, such statements have been used as a sword to attack service delivery rather than a shield to protect from or against litigation. One of the primary reasons standards statements were developed in the first place was to minimize individualized expert witness opinions, which could differ from situation to situation and case to case and to let practitioners know in advance of service provision about the benchmarks of service delivery in their profession. If published standards of practice are deficient in the sense that they provide a standard of care below that which is as least perceived by the judiciary to be part of the required standard of care, the effectiveness of the standard statements will be diminished. A study by Harvard investigators regarding the use of standard statements indicated, among other observations, that many malpractice cases in which providers complied with published standards of practice might be settled or dismissed.[48] Time will tell if such statements in the health/fitness field live up to what would seem to be prudent, and if such statements were developed on a well-founded basis.

Given that the primary goal of such statements is to help minimize legal claims and lawsuits, it would only make sense that such statements reflect the many legal liability exposures that exist in the health/fitness field. This would require, for those who develop such statements, researching applicable law and then understanding how to incorporate the law properly into the published statements.

Third, the lack of clear, uniform, industrywide published standards of practice may have contributed to state governmental efforts to license health/fitness professionals, as well as studies that have shown poor adherence to safety standards and laws among health/fitness facilities, as presented in Chapter 1. To date, the health/fitness profession has been primarily self-governed through certification and accreditation efforts, but some states are now proposing legislative bills to license personal fitness trainers.[49-51] See Chapter 5 for more on this topic and the potential role of the National Board of Fitness Examiners (NBFE) with regard to these licensing efforts.

INHERENT RELATIONSHIPS: SPECIAL RELATIONSHIPS

In addition to the legal duties reflected in both the reasonable person standard of care and the professional standard of care, duties can also arise out of special relationships such as (a) a common carrier with its passengers, (b) an innkeeper and its guests, (c) a landlord and its tenants, and (d) an employer with its employees.[52] However, two additional special relationships are the focus of this next section: person(s) on land and land owner/occupier, and patient and health care provider, because of their particular application to the health/fitness field.

PERSON(S) ON LAND AND LAND OWNER/OCCUPIER

A special relationship is formed between a person(s) on land (e.g., a participant of a health/fitness facility) and a land owner/occupier (e.g., an owner/manager of a health/fitness facility). The law classifies persons that enter a health/fitness facility as *trespassers, licensees,* or *invitees.* Using *Duncan v. World Wide Health Studios,*[53] the differences in the legal duties that the health/fitness professionals have toward persons in each classification are described.

In *Duncan,* the plaintiff was seriously injured while using a leg press. On the day of the injury, the plaintiff was visiting the health club accompanied by a friend who was a regular member of the club. To determine whether the defendant health club was negligent, the court first examined the relationship between the plaintiff and the health club. The court stated that the standard of care owed to a person entering the land of an owner/occupier is determined by the circumstances surrounding his or her entry. The court in *Duncan* described the relationship between a land owner/occupier and a trespasser, licensee, and invitee as follows:

1. *A trespasser is one who enters the premises without the permission of the occupier or without a legal right to do so; and towards the trespasser no duty exists in most instances except to refrain from willfully or wantonly injuring him.*
2. *A licensee is one who enters the premises with the occupier's express or implied permission, but only for his own purposes which are unconnected with the occupant's interests; and to him in addition to the duty owed to a trespasser, is owed the duty of warning the licensee of latent dangers of the premises if actually known by the occupier.*
3. *An invitee is a person who goes on the premises with the express or implied invitation of the occupant . . . for their mutual advantage; and to him, the duty owed is that of reasonable and ordinary care, which includes the prior discovery of reasonably discoverable conditions of the premises that may be unreasonably dangerous, and correction thereof or a warning to the invitee of the danger.*[54]

An example of a **trespasser** would be a golfer entering the land of a homeowner to retrieve a lost ball without the permission of the homeowner. Although no duty exists other than not to injure the trespasser intentionally or willfully, land owners/occupiers do have duty to warn if they know of trespassers or if trespassing is frequent and it would be likely for trespassers to confront a dangerous activity/condition on their land. A special legal doctrine in reference to this concept called *attractive nuisance* applies to the child trespasser. In this situation, the duty or the standard of care of a land owner/occupier is higher compared with a typical adult trespasser. See the section later that describes a case involving a child who was hurt on a piece of exercise equipment in an apartment complex fitness center.

Examples of **licensees** are sales representatives entering a business to sell a product, or social guests in one's own home. Generally, there is no duty to warn of any dangerous condition unless the land owner/occupier knows that a dangerous condition exists, knows it is likely the licensee will confront the dangerous condition, and knows it is unlikely that the licensee will recognize the dangerous condition.

An example of an **invitee** would be a member, participant, or client of a health/fitness facility. Invitees are owed a higher standard of care than a trespasser or a licensee because a mutual benefit exists between an invitee and the land owner/occupier. For example, an owner of a health/fitness facility receives a monetary benefit from the fees that a member pays, and the member receives all the benefits that the membership provides. The land owners/occupiers owe a duty to act reasonably toward invitees regarding the activities/conditions on their land. This involves reasonable inspection of the property for dangers and to reasonably repair and/or warn of dangers.

After examining whether the plaintiff in *Duncan* was a trespasser, licensee, or an invitee, the court determined that the plaintiff was an invitee because he was "in the position of one who may confer a future benefit upon the defendant."[55] In other words, the plaintiff, who was a guest of the defendant health club on the day of the injury, would be considered a prospective purchaser of the health club's services and therefore classified as an invitee. The court stated that the defendant health club had a duty of ordinary and reasonable care toward invitees that included an obligation to inspect the premises, making them safe to visit. No evidence indicated that the health club had breached its duty to inspect the leg press machine the plaintiff was hurt on or that the leg press was dangerous in any way. The manager of the defendant health club testified that the leg press machine was functioning properly and the plaintiff's injury was related to his own misuse of it. Although the defendant health club clearly had a duty toward its members and guests (invitees) to inspect the leg press machine to ensure its safe use, the court found no breach of this duty and therefore concluded that the plaintiff's injury was not due to negligence on the part of the health club.

The Child Trespasser and Attractive Nuisance

The general rule for **attractive nuisance** is that if land owners/occupiers maintain a condition on their land that *attracts* children, and there are children around and the condition poses a possible danger, there is not only a duty to warn but also a duty to take reasonable steps to protect the child's safety. The Restatement (Second) of Torts, §339, states, "A possessor of land is subject to liability for physical harm to children trespassing thereon caused by an artificial condition upon the land if:

(a) *the place where the condition exists is one upon which the possessor knows or has reason to know that children are likely to trespass, and*

(b) *the condition is one of which the possessor knows or has reason to know and which he realizes or should realize will involve an unreasonable risk of death or serious bodily harm to such children, and*

(c) *the children because of their youth do not discover the condition or realize the risk involved in intermeddling with it or in coming within the area made dangerous by it, and*

(d) *the utility to the possessor of maintaining the condition and the burden of eliminating the danger are slight as compared with the risk to children involved, and*

(e) *the possessor fails to exercise reasonable care to eliminate the danger or otherwise to protect the children.*[56] (From the *Student Edition Restatement of the Law Second, Torts 2d, § 339. 1965.* Copyright (1965) by the American Law Institute. Reprinted with permission. All rights reserved.)

Smith v. AMLI Realty Co.[57] is an excellent case that demonstrates the attractive nuisance doctrine when applied to the health/fitness field. Nine-year-old Lucas Smith was visiting an apartment complex where his father lived. He was approached by another child, Dana Faulkenberg, who lived in the area and asked him to go to the apartment complex weight room so she could show him a trick she had learned. A Universal weight machine was in the room that had a "lat" exercise device a user could pull down by using the lat bar. By doing so, the weights would be raised. Dana took the pin to the lat exercise and set the weights at 70 pounds. Both children pulled the lat bar down so Dana could straddle it. As Lucas released the bar, it rose up in the air and Dana was hanging by her knees. After hanging in this position for a while, Dana asked Lucas to help her down. Lucas placed his hands under the suspended weight stack and lifted it up, causing the bar to go down. While he was doing this, Dana jumped off the bar, causing the 70 pounds to exert downward force pinning Lucas's left hand between the descending weights and the weights in the bottom stack. Lucas's fingers were seriously injured.

Smith's (Lucas's mother) lawsuit against AMLI Realty Co., owner of the apartment complex, was based on the attractive nuisance theory. In this type of negligence action, Smith had to show that the condition on AMLI's land (i.e., the weight machine in the apartment complex weight room) was *dangerous*. Whether or not a condition on the land of an owner/occupier is considered dangerous depends on the plaintiff's knowledge, understanding, and appreciation of the risk that the condition creates. The defendant claimed that the weight machine was not dangerous because Lucas had actual knowledge of the specific risk and understood and appreciated the risk. The trial court agreed with AMLI and dismissed the case. However, on appeal, the appellate court reversed the trial court's decision, stating that the weight machine was dangerous because "a child (of plaintiff's) age, knowledge, judgment, and experience would not have recognized the danger presented by attempting to hold the suspended weights while his friend endeavored to extricate herself from the bar."[58] The court stated that Lucas had knowledge and appreciation that 70 pounds could injure his hand, but it was not apparent to him that he could not hold up the weights once Dana jumped off the bar. Therefore, Lucas appreciated some but not all of the risks.

Another factor courts evaluate under an attractive nuisance theory claim is whether or not the land owner/occupier took *reasonable* steps to protect the child. To determine what the court would consider *reasonable,* the courts examine the burden of the defendant to eliminate the danger compared with the risk to children the danger can create—the same elements described earlier under the reasonable person standard of care. If the burden is light in comparison to the risk, the defendant could be found negligent under the attractive nuisance theory. In *Smith,* the court stated that the burden of defendant AMLI to eliminate the danger consisted of installing a lock and providing tenants with keys, which is arguably a very minor burden in comparison with the possibility of weights injuring children.

Children and Standard of Care

In *Smith,* Lucas, a 9-year-old boy, did not understand and appreciate all the risks involved when playing with the exercise equipment at the apartment complex. At what age do children fully understand and appreciate risks associated with any type of physical activity? Herbert provides the following:

Kids under the age of 7 +/− may not be capable legally of negligence (thus affecting their responsibility for their own actions and their liability toward others);

Kids 7 +/− to 14 +/− years of age may be rebuttably presumed to be incapable of negligence (thus affecting their responsibility for their own actions and their liability toward others);

Kids over 14 years of age are presumed to be capable of negligence.[59]

In *Campbell v. Morine*,[60] a 15-year-old boy was stuck and killed by a motorist on a rural road in the evening. He was jogging with a friend (also 15 years old) in the same direction as traffic. The decedent's mother brought a negligence lawsuit against the defendant motorist. The trial court found the defendant 65% negligent and the decedent 35% negligent, mainly because he failed to jog against oncoming traffic. On appeal, the defendant claimed that the decedent's conduct should have been based on an adult standard of care and not a child's standard of care. The defendant claimed that if the trial court would have used an adult standard of care in determining the amount of negligence, a larger proportion of negligence would have been attributed to the decedent. However, the court held that "even though a minor could be held to the same standard of care as an adult, he is not held to that standard, unless the trier of fact determines that his age, abilities, and experience require application of the adult standard of care."[61] A dissenting opinion in this case stated that the decedent should not have had the benefit of the minor's standard of care.

Recommendations: Person(s) on Land and Land Owner/Occupier

Because of the special relationship that exists between health/fitness facilities and its members, clients, and guests of such entities (who would be classified as invitees), it is essential that facilities do the following:

1. Inspect their premises and equipment regularly to determine if any condition(s) might be considered dangerous.
2. Document that the inspections have taken place, and file the documents in a secure place.
3. If a condition could be considered "dangerous" by an invitee, it is necessary to (a) correct the condition (e.g., repair or remove the condition), and/or (b) warn the invitee of the possible danger (e.g., post proper warning signage that an invitee will see and understand).

By implementing the steps just listed, owners/managers of health/fitness facilities can minimize their liability associated with the legal duties they have toward their invitees. Most often, the staff hired by the owner/manager of a health/fitness facility carries out these steps. Therefore, owners/managers should train their staff how to inspect the facility for any conditions that might be deemed dangerous (e.g., a piece of exercise equipment that is not functioning properly or a slippery floor surface). Staff members should take these responsibilities seriously and also use their common sense. If they see something that could be dangerous (or if a participant brings it to their attention), they should correct it and report it to management immediately. If the condition cannot be corrected right away, it will be important to adequately *warn* any invitee who may confront the potentially dangerous condition.

Health/fitness facilities can also take several steps to minimize liability associated with attractive nuisance. Children may think of exercise equipment as something fun to play on, as did the children in *Smith* who did not fully understand the potential dangers associated with the equipment. Health/fitness facilities that allow children in their facilities should establish and enforce supervision policies that will help prevent children from getting hurt. At no time should children be in a health/fitness facility without proper adult supervision. In facilities that do not have staff supervision, which is common in apartment complex and hotel exercise facilities, management should take reasonable steps that will prevent children from accessing the fitness facility. The preceding sections, (a) Person(s) on

Land and Land Owner/Occupier, (b) The Child Trespasser and Attractive Nuisance (except §339 of the Restatement of the Law Second, Torts 2d), and (c) Recommendations: Person(s) on Land and Land Owner/Occupier), were reprinted with permission.[62]

PATIENT AND HEALTH CARE PROVIDER

A physician–patient relationship is a special type of relationship called a **fiduciary relationship.** Fiduciary relationships are also formed between professionals and the persons they serve, such as a lawyer–client, agent–professional athlete, and perhaps personal trainer–client. Fiduciary relationships are created when one person trusts and relies on another (e.g., clients trust and rely on their personal trainer's fitness expertise). Fiduciary relationships involve additional duties on part of the professional, that is, good faith, trust, special confidence, and candor.[63] Because of the trust that is established, patients and clients will rely on the advice they receive.

In *Mikkelsen v. Haslam*,[64] the plaintiff was born with a congenitally dislocated right hip. After a total hip replacement surgery in 1974, the plaintiff contended that her physician told her she had no physical limitations and she could ski and play tennis. The defendant physician testified that he told the plaintiff not to run, twist, or lift. Five years after the surgery, the plaintiff felt she was ready to begin skiing and contacted her physician for clearance to do so. She, along with two of her coworkers who heard her conversations with the physician, testified that the physician endorsed the skiing. In 1979, the plaintiff went skiing 10 times with no problems. In 1980, she severely fractured her femur while skiing and the hip replacement was adversely affected and could not be repaired. She would need to use a wheelchair or crutches for the rest of her life.

The trial court provided an instruction to the jury that the plaintiff could have assumed the risks (contributory negligent) that would bar any recovery. The jury found the defendant negligent (medical experts testified that downhill skiing was contraindicated for patients with hip replacement), but the plaintiff was also negligent, and therefore the plaintiff was precluded from any recovery. (Note: This case was decided before the state of Utah adopted a comparative negligence rule.) On appeal, the plaintiff contended that "she could not, as a matter of law be contributorily negligent or have assumed the risk when she skied, if . . . [the defendant physician] advised her she could ski."[65] The appellate court held that "a physician has a duty to warn his patient of how to avoid injury following treatment" and that "the physician-patient relationship permits a patient to rely on a doctor's professional skill and advice."[66] The appellate court found that "it is not contributory negligence to follow the advice of a physician."[66] Therefore, the defenses of contributory negligence and assumption of risk did not apply, and the court returned the case to the trial court for a new trial.

Implications arise from *Mikkelsen* for health/fitness professionals such as personal fitness trainers because of the nature of the special relationships (potential fiduciary relationships) they may have with their clients. The advice, instruction, and any other information given to a client must be appropriate given each client's individual situation (e.g., health status, fitness level) to meet the standard of care. Failure to do so could result in negligence.

SUMMARY

Courts determine duty in a variety of ways in negligence cases. This chapter has focused on the duty that arises when relationships are formed (e.g., when health/fitness professionals provide programs and services there is little question that an inherent and obvious relationship is formed between them and the participants they serve). When these inherent relationships exist, health/fitness professionals have a legal duty *not* to expose their participants to foreseeable risks of harm. Therefore, it is necessary to learn what these potential legal duties are and the risk management steps that can be implemented to adhere to these legal duties, which is the major purpose of this book.

The standard of care that courts apply when determining duty vary depending on the situation. In most cases, especially for facilities supervised by health/fitness professionals, courts are likely to apply the professional standard of care. Expert witnesses provide testimony that educates the court as to whether or not the defendant's conduct was consistent with the proper standard of care. Courts allow expert witnesses to introduce, through their testimony, published standards of practice as evidence of the standard of care, as demonstrated in the *Mandel* and *Elledge* cases. Therefore, health/fitness professionals must be aware of these published standards of practice and implement them into their daily operations. However, one of the challenges for health/fitness professionals is that many inconsistencies exist among these published statements. For unsupervised health/fitness facilities (e.g., apartment complexes, hotels), it is likely in these cases that the court will apply the reasonable person standard of care as they did in the *Smith* case. This standard of care requires the management of such facilities to take precautions to avoid unreasonable, foreseeable risks of harm.

This chapter also described two additional types of special relationships and the duties that arise from such: (a) person(s) on land and land owner/occupier—the duties owed to trespassers, licensees, and invitees, and (b) patient and health care provider—duties that exist when a professional and a client form a relationship called a fiduciary relationship, perhaps between a personal trainer and a client. In addition, the standard of care that children are held to and the attractive nuisance doctrine that involves certain duties toward child trespassers were discussed, along with specific risk management steps that health/fitness professionals can take when providing programs and services to children.

RISK MANAGEMENT ASSIGNMENTS

1. Describe how the professional standard of care applies in your health/fitness facility.

   _____

   _____

   _____

   _____

2. Describe how the scope of practice may vary among the personal trainers in your facility.

   _____

   _____

   _____

   _____

3. Using case law examples, develop a PowerPoint presentation that you could use for staff training to help educate your employees on how standards of practice published by professional and independent organizations can reflect the standard of care and some of the challenges these published statements can create.

   _____

   _____

   _____

   _____

4. Describe the policies your facility should have in place with regard to any programs and services designed for children, especially those under the age of 14, as well as for all participants who would be classified as invitees.

_____

_____

_____

_____

5. Describe specific examples of the additional duties (e.g., good faith, trust, special confidence, and candor) that personal trainers have, given the possible fiduciary relationship formed between them and their clients.

_____

_____

_____

_____

KEY TERMS

Attractive nuisance	Invitee	Scope of practice
Desirable operating practices	Licensee	Technical physical specifications
Fiduciary relationship	Negligence _per se_	Trespasser

REFERENCES

1. van der Smissen, B. Elements of negligence. In: Cotten DJ, Wolohan JT, eds. _Law for Recreation and Sport Managers._ 3rd ed. Dubuque, Iowa: Kendall/Hunt; 2003.
2. Restatement of the Law (Third) of Torts: Liability for Physical Harm. Proposed Final Draft No. 1, § 42. Duty based on undertaking. Philadelphia: American Law Institute; April 6, 2005:809.
3. _Parks v. Gilligan,_ Analyzed in: Suit against volunteer spotter settled. _Exercise Standards and Malpractice Reporter._ 1998;12:41.
4. Fitness Center Staff Requirements. W.S.A. 100.178. West's Wisconsin Statutes Annotated, Thomson/West, 2007.
5. Restatement of the Law Third. Restatement of the Law Torts: Liability for Physical Harm. Proposed Final Draft No. 1, § 14. Statutory violations as negligence per se and § 38. Affirmative duty based on statutory provisions imposing obligations to protect another. Philadelphia: American Law Institute; April 6, 2005.
6. Keeton W, Dobbs D, Keeton R, Owen D. _Prosser and Keeton on the Law of Torts,_ 5th Ed. St. Paul, Minn: West, 1984.
7. _Turner v. Rush Medical College,_ 537 N.E.2d 890 (Ill. App. Ct. 1989).
8. _Turner v. Rush Medical College,_ 537 N.E.2d 890 (Ill. App. Ct. 1989), 894.
9. _Turner v. Rush Medical College,_ 537 N.E.2d 890 (Ill. App. Ct. 1989), 892.
10. _Turner v. Rush Medical College,_ 537 N.E.2d 890 (Ill. App. Ct. 1989), 895.
11. _Turner v. Rush Medical College,_ 537 N.E.2d 890 (Ill. App. Ct. 1989), 897.
12. _Kleinknecht v. Gettysburg College,_ 989 F.2d 1360 (U.S. App. LEXIS 6609, 1993).
13. Restatement of the Law Third. Restatement of the Law Torts: Liability for Physical Harm. Proposed Final Draft No. 1, § 12. Knowledge and skills. Philadelphia: American Law Institute, April 6, 2005.
14. Keeton W, Dobbs D, Keeton R, Owen D. _Prosser and Keeton on the Law of Torts._ 5th ed. St. Paul, Minn: West; 1984:185.

15. Keeton W, Dobbs D, Keeton R, Owen D. *Prosser and Keeton on the Law of Torts.* 5th ed. St. Paul, Minn: West; 1984:189.
16. *Darling v. Charleston Community Hospital,* 211 N.E.2d 253 (Ill. 1965).
17. *McGuire v. DeFrancesco,* 811 P.2d 340 (Ariz. Ct. App. 1990).
18. van der Smissen B. Standards and how they relate to duty and liability. Paper presented at the 13th annual conference for the Society for the Study of the Legal Aspects of Sport and Physical Activity, Albuquerque, NM, 2000.
19. Tharrett SJ, McInnis KJ, Peterson JA, eds. *ACSM's Health/Fitness Facility Standards and Guidelines.* 3rd ed. Champaign, Ill: Human Kinetics; 2007.
20. Whaley MH, ed. *ACSM's Guidelines for Exercise Testing and Prescription.* 7th ed. Philadelphia: Lippincott Williams & Wilkins; 2006.
21. American College of Sports Medicine and American Heart Association Joint Position Statement. Recommendations for cardiovascular screening, staffing, and emergency policies at health/fitness facilities. *Med Sci Sports Exerc.* 1998;30:1009–1018.
22. *NSCA Strength & Conditioning Professional Standards & Guidelines.* May 2001. Available at: http://www.nscalift.org/Publications/standards.shtml. *Colorado Springs:* National Strength and Conditioning Association (NSCA). Accessed September 2, 2007.
23. IHRSA Club Membership Standards. In: *IHRSA's Guide to Club Membership & Conduct.* 3rd ed. Boston: International Health, Racquet & Sportsclub Association (IHRSA); 2005.
24. *Canadian Fitness Safety Standards & Recommended Guidelines.* 3rd ed. 2004. Available at: http://www/oases.on.ca/safety/safetyStdsCurrent.htm. Ontario, Canada: Ontario Association of Sport and Exercise Sciences (OASES). Accessed September 2, 2007.
25. *The Medical Fitness Model: Facility Standards and Guidelines.* Richmond, Va: Medical Fitness Association (MFA); May 2006.
26. *Exercise Standards & Guidelines Reference Manual.* 4th ed. Sherman Oaks, Calif: Aerobics and Fitness Association of America (AFAA); 2005.
27. American College of Sports Medicine and American Heart Association Joint Position Statement. Automated external defibrillators in health/fitness facilities. *Med Sci Sports Exerc.* 2002;34:561–564.
28. *Medical Advisory Committee Recommendations: A Resource Guide for YMCAs.* Chicago: YMCA of the USA; February 2007.
29. Eickhoff-Shemek J. Standards of practice. In: Cotten DJ, Wolohan JT, eds. *Law for Recreation and Sport Managers.* 4th ed. Dubuque, Iowa: Kendall/Hunt; 2007.
30. *Mandel v. Canyon Ranch, Inc.,* Case no. 31277 (Super. Ct. of Ariz., Pima Co. 1998).
31. *Elledge v. Richland/Lexington School District Five,* LEXIS 108 (S.C. Ct. App. 2000).
32. Tharrett SJ, Peterson, JA, eds. *ACSM's Health/Fitness Facility Standards and Guidelines.* 2nd ed. Champaign, Ill: Human Kinetics; 1997.
33. Tharrett SJ, Peterson, JA, eds. *ACSM's Health/Fitness Facility Standards and Guidelines.* 2nd ed. Champaign, Ill: Human Kinetics; 1997:ix.
34. *Elledge v. Richland/Lexington School District Five,* LEXIS 108 (S.C. Ct. App. 2000), 477–478.
35. *McComish v. Desoi,* 42 N.J. 274 (N.J. 1964), 292.
36. *Elledge v. Richland/Lexington School District Five,* LEXIS 235 (S.C. 2002), 795.
37. Eickhoff-Shemek J. Do standards of practice reflect legal duties? *ACSM's Health & Fitness J.* 2001;5(5):23–25, 24–25.
38. *ACSM's Guidelines for Exercise Testing and Prescription.* 7th ed. Philadelphia: Lippincott Williams & Wilkins; 2006:x.
39. *NSCA Strength & Conditioning Professional Standards & Guidelines.* May 2001. Available at: http://www.nscalift.org/Publications/standards.shtml. Colorado Springs: National Strength and Conditioning Association (NSCA). Accessed September 2, 2007.
40. *The Medical Fitness Model: Facility Standards and Guidelines.* Richmond, Va: Medical Fitness Association (MFA); May 2006:7.
41. Tharrett SJ, McInnis KJ, Peterson JA, eds. *ACSM's Health/Fitness Facility Standards and Guidelines.* 3rd ed. Champaign, Ill: Human Kinetics; 2007:4–5.
42. *Xu v. Gay,* 668 N.W.2d 166 (Mich. App. 2003).
43. *Xu v. Gay,* 668 N.W.2d 166 (Mich. App. 2003), 171.
44. Herbert DL, Herbert WG. *Legal Aspects of Preventive, Rehabilitative and Recreational Programs.* 4th ed. Canton, Ohio: PRC; 2002:80–81.
45. Herbert DL, Herbert WG. *Legal Aspects of Preventive, Rehabilitative and Recreational Programs.* 4th ed. Canton, Ohio: PRC; 2002:205–206.

46. IHRSA. Automated external defibrillators (AEDs). A briefing paper. Available at: http://csdem080.citysoft.com/index.cfm/fuseaction/Page.viewPage/pageId/4341. Accessed June 30, 2006.

47. Herbert DL, Herbert WG. *Legal Aspects of Preventive, Rehabilitative and Recreational Programs.* 4th ed. Canton, Ohio: PRC; 2002:211.

48. Hyam AL, Brandenburg JA, Lipsitz SR, Shapiro DW, Brennan TA. Practice guidelines and malpractice litigation: A two-way street. *Ann Intern Med.* 1995;122(6):450–455.

49. Eickhoff-Shemek JM, Herbert DL. Is licensure in your future? Issues to consider—Part 1. *ACSM's Health & Fitness J.* 2007;11(5):35–37.

50. Eickhoff-Shemek JM, Herbert, DL. Is licensure in your future? Issues to consider—Part 2. *ACSM's Health & Fitness J.* 2008;12(1):36-38.

51. Eickhoff-Shemek JM, Herbert DL. Is licensure in your future? Issues to consider—Part 3. *ACSM's Health & Fitness J.* 2008;12(3):36-38.

52. Restatement of the Law (Third) of Torts: Liability for Physical Harm. Proposed Final Draft No. 1, § 40. Duty based on special relationship with another. Philadelphia: American Law Institute; April 6, 2005.

53. *Duncan v. World Wide Health Studios,* 232 S.2d 835 (La. Ct. App. 1970).

54. *Duncan v. World Wide Health Studios,* 232 S.2d 835 (La. Ct. App. 1970), 837.

55. *Duncan v. World Wide Health Studios,* 232 S.2d 835 (La. Ct. App. 1970), 838.

56. Student Edition Restatement of the Law Second, Torts 2d, § 339. Philadelphia: American Law Institute; 1965, 197.

57. *Smith v. AMLI Realty Co.,* 614 N.E.2d 618 (Ind. App. 1993).

58. *Smith v. AMLI Realty Co.,* 614 N.E.2d 618 (Ind. App. 1993), 622.

59. Herbert DL. What risk management concerns apply to clubs targeting kids as clients? *Exercise Standards and Malpractice Reporter.* 2005;19:10.

60. *Campbell v. Morine,* 585 N.E.2d 1198 (Ill. App. Ct., 1992).

61. *Campbell v. Morine,* 585 N.E.2d 1198 (Ill. App. Ct., 1992), 1202.

62. Eickhoff-Shemek J. Legal duties toward trespassers, licensees, and invitees. *ACSM's Health Fitness J.* 2002;6(3):30–32, 30–32.

63. Black H. *Black's Law Dictionary.* 6th ed. St. Paul, Minn: West; 1991.

64. *Mikkelsen v. Haslam,* 764 P.2d 1384 (Utah, 1988).

65. *Mikkelsen v. Haslam,* 764 P.2d 1384 (Utah, 1988), 1387.

66. *Mikkelsen v. Haslam,* 764 P.2d 1384 (Utah, 1988), 1388.

EDITORIAL NOTE: CAUTION!!!

Though many published standards of practice are described throughout this book, presented as either direct quotes or paraphrased summaries, by no means do they reflect the published standards of practice in their entirety. It is the responsibility of all health/fitness professionals and their risk management advisory committees to obtain these publications so they have access to the entire document and all of its contents when assessing legal liability exposures and developing risk management strategies. In addition, there may be other applicable published standards of practice that were not selected to be included in this book that also need to be considered. The main purpose of providing the published standards of practice selected for inclusion in this book was to make the reader aware of them and to focus on those that potentially reflect some of major legal liability exposures that exist in the health/fitness field.

CHAPTER 4

Defenses to Negligence Claims and Lawsuits: Assumption of Risk and Waivers

LEARNING OBJECTIVES After reading this chapter, health/fitness students and professionals will be able to:

1. Understand the legal doctrines of assumption of risk and waivers when used as defenses to personal injury/wrongful death actions arising out of health/fitness activities.

2. Understand the structure of assumption of risk and waiver documents and appreciate the factual and legal requirements for the use of these documents to support defenses to negligence claims and lawsuits.

3. Understand the difference between assumption of risk concepts when compared with waiver doctrines as defenses.

4. Realize the limitations associated with assumption of risk defenses when compared with waiver/release defenses.

5. Know that assumption of risk documents may be the only form of protective documents that may be available for use in health/fitness facilities in some jurisdictions.

6. Understand the use of prospectively executed waivers of liability, also referred to as releases, to bar and defend against negligence claims and lawsuits.

7. Appreciate the effectiveness of such documents in those jurisdictions where releases/waivers are recognized and legally effective.

8. Know the differences as well as the similarities between waivers/releases, assumption of risk documents, and informed consents.

9. Comprehend the limitations of release/waiver documents when used with minors and when applied to derivative claims and lawsuits filed by spouses or dependents of participants, at least in some jurisdictions.

10. Realize that these defensive documents need to be drafted by legal counsel familiar with the requirements applicable to these defenses in the jurisdiction where used.

11. Understand the need to establish guidelines, in conjunction with legal counsel, for the administration and use of these documents by staff members with participants.

As explained elsewhere in this text, risk management for health/fitness facilities involves a number of concepts. Risk management steps include the use of defensive measures that are designed to minimize claims and lawsuits while also providing legal defenses to those untoward events that cannot be totally eliminated. These defensive steps for managing risks include the use of assumption of risk concepts and documents as well as waiver/release documents where possible to help protect against untoward events that may occur within such facilities.

WHAT IS ASSUMPTION OF RISK?

Assumption of risk is a legal doctrine that can be used to assert a defense to a battery or personal injury/wrongful death action. Assumption of risk, among other things, simply involves a participant's voluntarily knowing, understanding, and agreeing to assume those ordinary and reasonable risks associated with certain activities. The doctrine is frequently used in the sports arena and with certain high-risk activities such as race car driving, parachute jumping, hang gliding, and similar activities. The doctrine is also applied to provide permission for contact with another participant, such as in football or boxing, or exposure to the possibilities of injury from certain other risks such as exercise activities.

Assumption of risk can be demonstrated by a participant's actions or words (implied assumption of risk), or even through his or her execution of a written document, which will then be referred to as an "express assumption of the risk." Examples of express assumption of the risk documents are included at the end of this chapter. These concepts and documents, if used, should be compared and contrasted with waivers/releases of liability executed in advance of an activity or, in other words, prospectively by the participants, examples of which are also located at the end of this chapter. In the health and fitness facility setting, these documents are often contained within membership agreements but may also be stand-alone documents.

As stated in *Hildreth v. Rogers*, "Three types of assumption of the risk defenses exist: (a) express or contractual assumption of the risk, (b) primary or "no duty" assumption of the risk, and (c) secondary or implied assumption of the risk."[1] **Express or contractual assumption of the risk** is an asserted defense to negligence that appears in a written or contractual form. **Primary or "no duty" assumption of the risk** is an asserted defense to negligence in which the defendant claims that no duty whatsoever was owed to the injured party. **Secondary or implied assumption of the risk** is an asserted defense to negligence in which the issue is whether or not a particular risk was assumed in a given activity where the participant knows that another has already acted in a negligent manner or will do so where established procedures, protocols, rules, or warnings are not followed. Although in years past an assumption of risk defense could be a complete bar to an injured party's right to recovery in a personal injury lawsuit, assumption of risk defenses may not now be a complete bar to recovery, but instead may serve to reduce any applicable recovery based on comparative negligence principles (see Chapter 2).

APPLICATION OF ASSUMPTION OF RISK: CASE LAW EXAMPLES WHERE THE ASSUMPTION OF RISK DEFENSE WAS NOT EFFECTIVE

The application of the express assumption of risk doctrine to health/fitness facilities may perhaps be best illustrated through an examination of a 2001 California case, *Santana v. Women's Workout and Weight Loss Centers, Inc.*[2] In this case, the plaintiff was injured while participating in a modified step aerobics class conducted at the defendant center. While participating in the activity that combined step aerobics and an overhead arm strength training exercise using a Dyna-Band, she fell when she stepped sideways onto a rectangular platform, fracturing her ankle. The injury required surgery to install pins in her leg for immobilization.

The evidence indicated that the instructor apparently led the class participants' use of the band in front of them and over their heads. According to the defendant, "Participants were instructed to keep their heads facing forward and not to look at their feet while doing the exercise but to look straight ahead at their reflections in a mirror for orientation."[3] Although the plaintiff was not inexperienced in "normal" step aerobics, the class was her first step experience that also involved the use of a Dyna-Band. After the incident, the plaintiff filed a negligence lawsuit alleging that the "peculiar design of the exercise was 'unnecessarily hazardous' in that the simultaneous performance of multiangled upward/downward steps and vigorous overhead arm exercises, combined with the forced inability to see one's feet in relation to the step platform, made normal balance unduly difficult and dangerous."[4]

Even though the plaintiff had executed a membership agreement that contained a waiver of liability provision on the back of the agreement, she filed suit against the facility for her injuries. The center, in turn, moved for summary judgment in its favor, contending that the membership agreement barred her action and asserted, among other defenses, assumption of the risk. The court reviewed the evidence in this regard and noted,

> *The back of the form contained two columns of 8-point type with paragraphs labeled in 12-point type. The last paragraph on the bottom is headed: "ASSUMPTION OF RISK RELEASE & INDEMNITY[.]" It states: 'The use of the Facilities naturally involve the risk of injury to you, whether you or someone else cause it. As such, you understand and voluntarily accept this risk and agree that FIT will not be liable for any injury, including without limitation, personal, bodily or mental injury, economic loss or any damage to you, your spouse, guests or relatives resulting from the negligence or other acts of FIT or anyone else using the Facilities. If there is any claim by anyone based on any injury, loss, or damaged [sic] described here, which involves you or your guest, you agree to (1) defend FIT against such claims and pay FIT for expenses relating to the claim and (2) indemnify FIT for all liabilities to you, your spouse, guests, relatives, or anyone else resulting from such claims."[4]*

On the basis of this and other language contained in the agreement, the trial court granted the defense motion. The plaintiff appealed. The appellate court ruled that the waiver was not effective, and as to the assumption of risk defense the appellate court explained,

> *[The] defendant owes no duty to protect against the risks inherent in the exercise of stepping on and off a platform, such as a sprained ankle. However, "defendants generally do have a duty to use due care not to increase the risks to a participant over and above those inherent in the sport." . . . In this case, defendants were not coparticipants in the sport or activity but were instead in control of it. They provided the instructor who decided what would be done and for how long. The instructor also gave direction on techniques. An instructor/student relationship is to be considered in determining the scope of defendant's duty. . . . Defendant also supplied necessary equipment, such as the platforms and Dyna-Bands. . . ." Under these circumstances, defendants owed a duty to plaintiff and the other participants not to increase the risks inherent in [step aerobics]. Thus, for example, they owed a duty not to supply faulty equipment."*
>
> *Defendant had no duty to eliminate the platforms entirely, which would transform the exercise from step aerobics into something else, and no duty to protect from injury arising from reasonably designed exercises. However, step aerobics does not inherently require exercises which are designed in such a*

way as to create an extreme risk of injury, such as, by combining movements that affect the balance and draw the participant's focus away from the platform while stepping on and off it or requiring the use of a mirror for orientation instead of looking where one's feet are going. Accordingly, premised on the duty not to utilize dangerously designed exercise, this case falls under the secondary assumption of risk category. Issues pertaining to plaintiff's comparative fault are for the trier of fact to decide. Plaintiff's expert's opinion regarding the design of the exercise is admissible at trial and creates a triable issue of material fact whether the exercise was designed in such a way as to create an extreme risk of injury.[5]

Based on the extract just cited, the trial court's decision was reversed and the case remanded for trial. As the appellate court's decision in this case illustrates, those who may prescribe, direct, lead, supervise, or promote certain physical activities will sometimes be prevented from asserting the defense of assumption of the risk where an activity goes "outside the bounds of reasonable conduct and outside the normal risks of play or behavior."[6]

Other cases dealing with the assumption of risk doctrine have also been determined in other jurisdictions. In the New York case of *Mathis v. New York Health Club, Inc.,*[7] the plaintiff was allegedly injured while using a weight training machine. The plaintiff filed a complaint naming both the health club and trainer who was supervising his training at the time of the injury as defendants. In response to these claims, the defendants moved for summary judgment and contended that the plaintiff assumed the risks that "materialized in his injury." The trial court denied the defendant's motion and the plaintiff appealed. On appeal, the appellate court stated,

Defendants have moved to dismiss the complaint, claiming in support of their motion that plaintiff voluntarily assumed the risks that materialized in his injury. While it is clear that plaintiff, who was not a novice to weight training, did assume those risks ordinarily entailed by properly supervised weight training, he cannot be said to have assumed risks in excess of those usually encountered in the activity, particularly unreasonably increased risks attributable to lapses in judgment by a trainer whose qualifications, plaintiff alleges, were not all they had been represented to be by defendant health club at the time plaintiff purchased the club's specialized training package. According to plaintiff, defendant trainer increased the weight on the training machine. Plaintiff had been using to 270 pounds and, despite plaintiff's repeatedly expressed doubts as to whether he could handle so much weight, urged plaintiff to continue with his repetitions. Given this scenario, factual issues are raised as to whether plaintiff's injury, which allegedly occurred in the course of the repetitions urged upon him by defendant trainer, was not the consequence of risks which, although inherent in weight training, were unreasonably augmented by culpable misjudgment as to plaintiff's capacity to bear so much weight.[8]

In another New York case, *Corrigan v. Musclemakers, Inc.,*[9] the plaintiff, a 49-year-old woman who had never patronized a health club or gym, joined a health club known as Gold's Gym. Three one-hour personal training sessions were included in the $400 annual membership fee. During her first personal training session, her personal trainer placed her on a treadmill. He set the treadmill at 3.5 miles per hour for 20 minutes and then left her unattended. In addition, the trainer did not instruct the plaintiff on how to use the machine (e.g., operate the control panel, stop the belt, or adjust the speed). Shortly into her walk on the treadmill, she began to drift back on the belt. She attempted to walk faster but was quickly thrown off the machine, sustaining a fractured ankle.

The plaintiff filed a negligence lawsuit against the defendant to seek recovery for her injury. However, the defendant facility moved for summary judgment claiming "that its duty to the plaintiff was lesser than that generally applicable to landowners . . . it needed only to ensure that the conditions of its facility were 'as safe as they appeared to be.' Defendant also claims that the plaintiff's voluntary participation in this 'athletic activity' warrants dismissal of the complaint under the doctrine of primary risk."[10] As in the *Mathis* case, previously described, the trial court denied the defendant's motion and the defendant appealed. The appellate court ruled that it was "unpersuaded" with the defendant's argument. In this regard, it stated,

> It is true that "[r]elieving an owner or operator of a sporting venue from lia-bility for inherent risks of engaging in a sport is justified when a consenting participant is aware of the risks; has an appreciation of the nature of the risks; and voluntarily assumes the risks." . . . Under such circumstances, "a premises owner continues to owe 'a duty to exercise care to make the con-ditions as safe as they appear to be. If the risks of the activity are fully com-prehended or perfectly obvious, [the] plaintiff has consented to them and [the] defendant has performed its duty'" . . . In our view, however, the fitness activ-ity undertaken by plaintiff was not a "sporting event" for which this lesser standard of care should be applied. Moreover, offering only the conclusory affidavit of its general manager, defendant did not establish as a matter of law that the risks associated with the use of the treadmill to plaintiff, a novice, were fully appreciated or perfectly obvious.
>
> In an attempt to establish that plaintiff voluntarily participated in an "ath-letic" activity and was aware of the inherent risks of using a treadmill, defen-dant makes repeated references to her status as a "former professional ice skater." Had plaintiff been injured while engaging in this type of activity, this fact might be relevant. What is relevant, is that plaintiff had never been on a treadmill, had not skated professionally for 16 years prior to this incident and had specifically informed the personal trainer that she was "very sedentary" and a newcomer to working out in a gym. It is undisputed that the personal trainer failed to ensure that plaintiff "understood the treadmill's operation before using it." Notably, the operator's manual for the machine states that this is a guideline for safe operation.
>
> Nor do we find, under the doctrine of primary assumption of risk, that plaintiff assumed the risks inherent in using this piece of equipment. "Primary assumption of the risk may be applied in cases where there is an elevated risk of danger, typically in sporting and recreational events" . . . We are unpersuaded that plaintiff's first time on the treadmill falls within the reach of this principle. . . . As noted, the risk of being ejected from this machine was not readily apparent. . . . Under these circumstances, a jury should assess whether plaintiff's injuries are the result of any breach of duty by defendant.[11]

It should be apparent from reviewing these cases that the assumption of risk defense is based on the facts and circumstances of each case. The defense as raised in response to personal injury/wrongful death lawsuits may often be difficult to prove. Questions of material fact related to this defense are very frequently left for a jury to determine. Therefore summary disposition of such cases is often difficult for defendants to achieve. Even when express—or written—assumption of risk defenses are asserted in defense of personal injury or wrongful death lawsuits, the delineation of risks contained within such documents may be insufficient to address risk issues successfully, and thus completely defend against these actions. It should also be pointed out, however, that sometimes no other similar defense may otherwise be available, such as those based on releases or waivers where the laws or statutes of particular states preclude the use of such protective documents. For example, in the state of New York, the use of waivers/releases in the health/fitness facility setting is pre-cluded by state statute.[12]

APPLICATION OF ASSUMPTION OF RISK: CASE LAW EXAMPLES WHERE THE ASSUMPTION OF RISK DEFENSE WAS EFFECTIVE

In a New York case, *Weithofer v. Unique Racquetball and Health Clubs, Inc.,*[13] the plaintiff slipped and injured himself while playing "walleyball" on an indoor court operated by the defendant health club. "According to the plaintiff, the court was damp and covered with water puddles. Despite this condition, the plaintiff chose to play anyway and injured himself during the game. Notably, the plaintiff had played on the same court, under similar conditions, several times in the past."[14] The defendant moved for summary judgment, which the trial court denied. On appeal of this decision, the appellate court noted,

> *The record demonstrates that the injury-producing defect was not concealed and that the plaintiff was fully aware of its existence prior to his voluntary participation in the game . . . As previously noted, the plaintiff stated that he had played on the very same court on prior occasions when similar conditions existed. Under these circumstances, the doctrine of assumption of the risk warrants the granting of judgment to the defendant.*[14]

In another case, *Rutnik v. Colonie Center Court Club, Inc.,*[15] the defendant was also successful in using the assumption of risk defense. In this case, a 47-year-old man who was an experienced racquetball player collapsed and died from a cardiac arrest while playing in a racquetball tournament at the defendant club. The defendant refuted the wrongful death action filed by the decedent's estate, claiming the decedent assumed the risks when he volunteered to participate in the tournament. The appellate court concurring with the defendant stated, "relieving an owner or operator of a sporting facility from liability for the inherent risk of engaging in sports is justified when the consenting participant is aware of the risk, has an appreciation of the nature of the risks and voluntarily assumes the risk."[16] Because the decedent had previously participated in similar tournaments and was an experienced racquetball player, the court indicated he must have known and appreciated the risk of cardiac arrest while playing racquetball.

Even though assumption of risk, particularly when used as a defense by health/fitness facilities to personal injury/wrongful death actions where no express or written document is secured may be somewhat difficult to assert successfully, the following case may seem by some in this field to go somewhat "overboard" in its application of the defense in this setting. In a somewhat significant 2006 California case, *Rostai v. Neste Enterprises,*[17] the court summarized its application of the assumption of risk doctrine to a health/fitness facility based on the particular facts of this case. In this regard it summarized the case as follows:

> *In this case we hold that the doctrine of primary assumption of risk is a complete defense to an action for damages based on the alleged negligence of a personal fitness trainer in failing to investigate the cardiac risk factors of a client as a result of which the client allegedly suffered a heart attack during his first training workout. Masood Rostai, plaintiff and appellant (hereafter plaintiff) sued Neste Enterprises, doing business as (dba), Gold's Gym (hereafter Gold's Gym), and Jared Shoultz, defendants and respondents (hereafter referred to either individually by name or collectively as defendants), for damages based on negligence. In his complaint, plaintiff alleged that he had entered into an agreement with defendants to provide him with a customized physical fitness program; defendants owed plaintiff a duty to investigate his health history, including his current physical condition and cardiac risk factors; on September 11, 2002, plaintiff participated in his first training session at Gold's Gym with defendant Shoultz; defendant Shoultz knew plaintiff was not physically fit and was overweight; defendant Shoultz was aggressive in his training of plaintiff; near the end of the 60-minute training session, after complaining several times*

to defendant Shoultz that he needed a break, plaintiff suffered a heart attack; and defendants' negligence was a proximate cause of plaintiff's injury.

In their answer to plaintiff's complaint, defendants asserted among other defenses that plaintiff's injury was the result of a risk inherent in strenuous physical activity; that defendants' neither increased that risk nor concealed any of the inherent risks; and therefore the doctrine of primary assumption of the risk bars plaintiff's claim. Defendants moved for summary judgment asserting the doctrine of primary assumption of the risk as the basis for their motion. Gold's Gym also asserted that it had no liability for the acts of defendant Shoultz because Shoultz is an independent contractor. Defendants prevailed on summary judgment and plaintiff appeals. We will affirm for reasons we now explain.[18]

Although the plaintiff contended that the doctrine of primary assumption of risk should apply only to "sports activities" and that "fitness training is not a sport," the court, on appeal of the trial court's grant of the defendant's motion for summary judgment, disagreed and used the doctrine to provide a complete defense to this action. In so ruling, the court, although admitting that no California case had previously dealt with the specific issue, "namely whether fitness training under the guidance of a personal trainer is an activity to which the doctrine of primary assumption of the risk applies," determined there were numerous cases in which the doctrine had been employed in sports-related cases and those involving students and instructors. Because the court determined that "fitness training under the guidance of a personal trainer is an activity in which a student learns from and is directed by an instructor," the court determined to rely on those cases in resolving the instant case.

Applying those principles from the other cases it cited, the court determined that "fitness training under the guidance of a personal trainer is . . . an activity," participation in which might be "chilled if the primary assumption of risk doctrine was not imposed so as to avoid assuming a duty which might chill vigorous participation in the implicated activity and thereby alter its fundamental nature." The court determined that "primary assumption of the risk is not limited to sports but applies to any physical activity that involves an element of risk or danger as an integral part of the activity."[19] In its application of the doctrine in this case, the court noted,

The obvious purpose of working out with a personal trainer is to improve physical fitness and appearance. In order to accomplish that goal, the participant must engage in strenuous physical activity. The risks inherent in that activity include physical distress in general and in particular . . . muscle strains, sprains, tears and pulls, not only of obvious muscles such as those in the legs and arms, but also of less obvious muscles such as the heart. Stress on the cardiovascular system as a result of the physical exertion that is an integral part of fitness training with a personal trainer is a risk inherent in the activity. Eliminating that risk would alter the fundamental nature of the activity.[19]

The court also further added,

Although plaintiff phrases his claim against defendant Shoultz in terms of failing to adequately assess plaintiff's physical condition and in particular his cardiac risk factors, the essence of plaintiff's claim is that Shoultz, in his capacity as plaintiff's personal fitness trainer, challenged plaintiff to perform beyond his level of physical ability and fitness. That challenge, however, is the very purpose of fitness training, and is precisely the reason one would pay for the services of a personal trainer. Like the coach in other sports or physical activities, the personal trainer's role in physical fitness training is not only to instruct the participant in proper exercise techniques but also to develop a training program that requires the participant to stretch his or her current abilities in order to become more physically fit. The trainer's function in the training process is, at bottom, to urge and challenge the participant to work muscles to their limits and to overcome physical and psychological barriers to doing so. Inherent in that process is the risk that the trainer will not accurately assess the participant's ability and the participant will be injured as a result.[20]

The court determined that the primary assumption of risk doctrine barred the plaintiff's suit because there was no duty imposed on the defendant to protect the plaintiff from those particular risks that the court identified and discussed. The court also determined that the plaintiff was required to "prove that the trainer acted either with intent to cause injury or that the trainer acted recklessly in that the conduct was 'totally outside the range of ordinary activity' . . . involved in [personal fitness training]." Because the appellate court determined that the plaintiff alleged only a claim of ordinary negligence, it could not prevail against the defendants based on the court's ruling. Although the court determined that "at most," the defending personal trainer did not accurately assess plaintiff's level of physical fitness and that the trainer "may have interpreted plaintiff's physical complaints, including his tiredness, shortness of breath, and profuse sweating, as the usual signs of physical exertion due to lack of conditioning rather than as symptoms of a heart attack," the court found no claim or evidence of recklessness, intent to injure, nor evidence of any increased risks in the activity itself. Because the claim against the facility was for vicarious liability owing to the acts of the trainer, the court similarly found no liability against the facility on either that basis or directly.

APPLICATION OF ASSUMPTION OF RISK DOCTRINE TO INFORMED CONSENTS

In those health/fitness facilities that provide staff-interpreted health/fitness assessments or other similar services—perhaps analogous to those that might otherwise be considered to be medical in nature—the informed consent process is used to disclose those risks associated with the procedures or activities to be undertaken. For example, prior to conducting health/fitness assessments, an informed consent should be properly administered. See Chapter 7 for a sample informed consent for this purpose. In this situation, the assumption of the risk "may be considered to be 'built in' to the informed consent process."[6]

In the case of *Smogor v. Enke*,[21] a participant with a prior history of a heart attack went to an emergency department of a hospital complaining of chest pain. Certain tests were performed or scheduled, including an exercise stress test to be performed the following day by one of the defendants, a cardiologist. The test was stopped in the last stage once the participant experienced chest pain. He died the following day, and suit was subsequently brought by his family. They contended that the cardiologist and a family physician defendant were negligent. As to the defendant cardiologist, they contended that he "failed to inform [the deceased patient] of risks of stress test or obtain . . . [the patient's] informed consent to undergo test." The informed consent document risk disclosure provision however, included the explicit disclosure of "risk of death." A jury returned a defense verdict, which, on appeal, was affirmed.

Assumption of risk documents are different in a legal sense than informed consent forms but have similar aspects. Such documents are also different than waiver/release forms as described later. Although the processes asserted with each document and the forms may seem at first brush to be similar, they are different. "A release discharges its recipient from liability . . . a consent [on the other hand] gives permission to act in the future."[22] Comparing the assumption of risk doctrine with the informed consent process, both require a disclosure component[23] "which enables facility personnel to engage in a particular process with the participant or to lead the . . . participant in activity."[24] Contrasting the assumption of risk doctrine with the release/waiver process indicates, at least in theory, that an assumption of the risk "supplies evidence to establish a defense to a possible negligence action,"[25] whereas a release/waiver provided prospectively—in advance of contemplated activity—theoretically precludes successful suit because the participant has prospectively given up or relinquished his right to sue based on claims of negligence.[26]

If, however, research involving human subjects is carried out by facilities, the use of an institutional review board (IRB) may be a necessary prerequisite for the conduct of such research. Federal law requires that informed consent be obtained in reference to all such research. That requirement involves not only securing written consent from all participants, but requires the provision of information as to applicable risks associated with the research. The use of written assumption of risk documents may be permissible, but the use of waivers/releases in such settings would not be permissible.[27]

APPLICATION OF ASSUMPTION OF RISK IN AGREEMENTS TO PARTICIPATE

An agreement to participate is a type of an express assumption of risk document. Whether signed by adults or even minors, these documents may not amount to enforceable contracts or even operate like informed consents. However, they serve two major purposes. Such documents (a) help to establish the primary assumption of risk defense by providing documentary evidence that the plaintiff, whether an adult or a minor, knew, understood, and appreciated the inherent risks of activity and voluntarily assumed those risks; and (b) help to establish a type of secondary assumption of risk (contributory fault) by showing the plaintiff knew the rules, regulations, expected behaviors, and so on, of the activity and agreed to adhere to them.[28] Because such documents do not include exculpatory clauses as do waivers, they are often best used with minors and in states where waivers are against public policy or prohibited otherwise, such as by state statutory law as in New York.

STRENGTHENING THE ASSUMPTION OF RISK DEFENSE

As discussed earlier, the assumption of risk defense can be used as an effective strategy to help refute negligence claims and lawsuits in some situations. To strengthen this defense, health/fitness facilities should consider adopting the following procedures:

- To make effective use of this defense, assumption of risk documents should be secured in writing and signed by the participant and a staff member who participated in the process.
- Written assumption of risk documents should describe the inherent risks associated with the activity—minor and major injuries and even death, and supplement the delineation of risks with a catch-all phrase indicating there are also other nonspecific risks—and the process should be supplemented by an opportunity for questions to be answered by the administering staff member.
- When assumption of risk documents are secured, the advising staff member should provide sufficient information, especially to "new" participants, as to what they will be doing so they may realize, know, understand, and appreciate the inherent risks of the activity they will pursue. Facility records should be documented in this regard.
- Misuse of equipment, failures to follow instructions, to heed warnings, or to obey participation rules should be noted, and such behavior corrected by staff members and facility records noted accordingly.
- Periodic evaluation of staff service delivery should be observed, evaluated, and recorded by supervisors to help ensure that services are properly provided in accordance with the standard of care, and in so doing help avoid the creation of incidents that otherwise could be determined by a jury in the event of needless injury followed by an otherwise avoidable claim and suit.

Sample express assumption of risk documents are included in Appendix 4 as follows:

Form 4-1: Express Assumption of Risk for Participation in Specified Activity
Form 4-2: Express Assumption of Risk Combined with Prospective Waiver of Liability and Release Agreement

WHAT ARE WAIVERS/PROSPECTIVE RELEASES?

Prospectively executed releases or waivers of liability are contractual-type documents, which, like all contracts, must be supported by adequate consideration, something of value, by which one party—in advance of contemplated activity—agrees to release the other party for responsibility for mishaps—including those owing to ordinary negligence—which may occur during activity to be carried on thereafter. Although the law on this subject varies from state to state, and even though such documents are also referred to as "waivers," the requirements generally include execution by a competent adult party, possessed with the legal ability to contract (be of the age of majority and not under some disability) under circumstances where that party gives up and relinquishes claims related to defined, known, and/or reasonably contemplated acts or risks, so-called foreseeable events. It is different from an express assumption of risk because release/waiver documents also include the relinquishment of the right to assert a claim or institute successful suit as an additional contractual-type clause. Waiver and releases include an **exculpatory clause,** which basically means to relieve or clear one of blame.

As reviewed previously, most personal injury or wrongful death actions against health/fitness facilities are based on allegations of negligence. A legal cause of action for negligence requires certain elements, including proof of duty by one person toward another.

Waivers and releases, where effective, circumvent or nullify the duty element necessary to establish a cause of action for negligence. Once such documents are executed, the party so released is waived of his or her obligations imposed by the duty element otherwise required by law for negligence actions to be successfully prosecuted by an injured party. Waivers/releases are generally effective in most states for the release of ordinary negligence claims but not for gross negligence, willful, wanton, reckless, or criminal conduct. Assumption of risk concepts, in contrast, provide evidence of the acceptance of inherent risks associated with certain activity, or even the acceptance of the risk of the negligence of another, sometimes referred to as secondary assumption of risk.

The law surrounding the use of releases/waivers in the health/fitness setting has developed a substantial body of decisions that have accumulated over a significant number of years. Sometimes the question of whether or not such documents should be enforced depends on public policy considerations, which the courts are often asked to determine and balance against other considerations such as the right to freely contract. When public policy issues are raised, the balancing of interests—those of the consumer versus those of the provider—when viewed from an overall societal perspective are often examined by the courts to address whether prospectively executed waivers/releases of liability are in the public interest—in other words, whether such documents are contrary to or against **public policy.** Public policy is a difficult concept to define but amounts to a judicial determination of society's mores and views as to what is best for a civilized and enlightened community balanced against certain other constitutional interests and other basic concepts such as freedom of choice, freedom to contact, and other similar concepts.

Perhaps the seminal case used in determining whether or not prospectively issued waivers/releases should be enforced by the judicial system came from a 1963 California decision, *Tunkl v. Regents of the University of California*,[29] which concerned the validity of a "release from liability for future negligence imposed as a condition for admission to a charitable research hospital."[30] The California Supreme Court, which addressed this issue, concluded that these exculpatory contracts could only be valid if the public interest was not adversely impacted. To decide this question, the court developed a test to be used to make such determinations. In this regard, it decided that the following questions needed to be addressed in reviewing such contracts:

1. Is the business in question of a type generally thought suitable for public regulation?
2. Is the party seeking exculpation engaged in performing a service of great importance to the public, which is often a matter of practical necessity for some members of the public?
3. Does the party performing the service hold himself out as willing to perform this service for any member of the public who seeks it, or at least for any member coming within certain established standards?
4. As a result of the essential nature of the service and in the economic setting of the transaction, does the party invoking exculpation possess a decisive advantage of bargaining strength against any member of the public who seeks his services?
5. In exercising a superior bargaining power does the party seeking an adhesion contract of exculpation make no provision whereby a purchaser may pay additional reasonable fees and obtain protection against negligence?
6. As a result of the transaction, is the person or property of the purchaser placed under the control of the seller, thereby subject to the risk of carelessness by seller or his agents?[31]

Although the California Supreme Court determined that the contract in the *Tunkl* case could not withstand such an inquiry and it was against public policy, cases from that and other states that have been decided in the health/fitness industry have not usually reached such a conclusion. However, the *Tunkl* decision is often used to examine whether such contracts are violative of public policy considerations. For example, in the case of *Banfield v. Louis*,[32] a Florida court of appeals determined that a triathlon participant release used by the City of Fort Lauderdale was not against pubic policy because it was not "readily injurious to the public good" nor did it involve "an activity of great public interest" or "a necessary service" when analyzed through the *Trunkl* six-factor test. Therefore, the use of the release in that action was upheld. However, some states in this regard have determined that these documents will not be enforced in those states as they have been determined to be contrary to or against public policy. These states include Virginia, New Jersey, Louisiana, Montana, and Connecticut.

LANGUAGE CONSIDERATIONS IN WAIVERS

The language of release/waiver documents (see Appendix 4 for examples of waivers) generally includes a provision such as the following: "The undersigned does hereby waive, release, acquit, and discharge a named health/fitness facility from any responsibility or liability for any injury, damage, or loss of whatsoever description, which may arise or be sustained by one while engaged in any activities at the facility." Although actual release/waiver language is generally more comprehensive and detailed than this example and may vary from jurisdiction to jurisdiction, the general thrust of all releases is that they contain the same basic provisions.

Release/waiver documents generally are made binding on the party executing them and often others. Efforts are sometimes made to make waiver/release contracts binding on executors, administrators, heirs, and even spouses and other dependents. Sometimes, spouses of participants are also asked to execute such documents and thereby become parties to these contracts. Questions also arise as to whether such documents can be binding when signed by parents or guardians on behalf of their minor children. A somewhat substantial body of law on this subject is in the process of being developed and will be examined because a good many minors participate in activities carried on at most health/fitness facilities, particularly at YMCAs, YWCAs, and JCCs.

One of the earliest waiver/release cases to be reviewed in the health/fitness facility setting was reported in 1964. The *Owen v. Vic Tanny's Enterprises* case[33] involved a plaintiff who fell near the defendant's pool and subsequently brought suit claiming the defendant was negligent. A release containing an exculpatory provision—one purportedly releasing the defendant from liability—was executed by the plaintiff prior to his participation in activity. The court was faced with the question of whether or not the membership agreement containing the exculpatory clause—one releasing the defendant from liability for negligence—would be enforced so as to bar the plaintiff's lawsuit. The document in question provided as follows:

> *Member, in attending said gymnasiums and using the facilities and equipment therein, does so at his own risk. Tanny shall not be liable for any damages arising from personal injuries sustained by Member in, on or about the premises of any of the said gymnasiums. Member assumes full responsibility for any injuries or damages . . . which may occur to Member in, on or about the premises of said gymnasiums and he does hereby fully and forever release and discharge Tanny and all associated gymnasiums, their owners, employees and agents from any and all claims, demands, damages, rights of action, or causes of action, present or future, whether the same be known, anticipated or unanticipated, resulting from or arising out of the Member's use or intended use of the said gymnasium or the facilities and equipment thereof.*[34]

Even though the court ruled that such clauses should be "strictly construed against the party whom it favors" and that "other terms of the instrument may be considered in weighing the parties intent with regard to the clause," the court determined that the release should be enforced, and it overturned the trial court's determination that denied the defendant's request to grant judgment in its favor notwithstanding a jury's verdict of $2,000. In its response, the court viewed the contract, quoted from an earlier New York case[35] and stated,

> *The wording of the contract in the instant case expresses as clearly as language can the intention of the parties to completely insulate the defendant from liability for injuries sustained by plaintiff by reason of defendant's own negligence, and, in the face of the allegation of the complaint charging merely ordinary negligence, such agreement is valid.*[36]

The *Owen* court further stated,

> *We believe the foregoing pronouncements in Ciofalo v. Vic Tanney [sic]Gyms, Inc., apply here. The scarcity of facilities for gymnastic and reducing activities hardly creates such a disparity of bargaining power that plaintiff is forced to accept such terms without alternatives. If the public interest is involved, it is for the legislature to make such pronouncements. Absent appropriate legislative action, we must hold that the instant exculpatory clause barred plaintiff's suit, and the court erred in not directing a verdict for the defendant and in denying defendant's motion for a judgment notwithstanding the verdict.*[36]

In a case rendered some 20 years later, *Neumann v. Gloria Marshall Figure Salon,*[37] a court of appeals reviewed another similar case. In this case, the plaintiff joined the Gloria Marshall Figure Salon in 1982. Upon joining, she signed a contract agreeing to pay a specified sum for a specific number of visits. That membership contract also contained the following language:

> *Patron specifically assumes all risks of injury while using any equipment or facilities at the salon and waives any and all claims against Gloria Marshall Management Company and the owners and employees of the salon for any such injury.*[38]

Shortly after joining the facility, the plaintiff allegedly injured her back while using one of the defendant's exercise machines. She contended that one of the defendant's employees (after her selection of a machine) placed the leg portion of the machine in a downward position before turning it on and leaving the room. While the machine was activated, the plaintiff felt sharp, stabbing pains in her back but nevertheless continued with her exercises on the machine. She alleged that the defendant's employee did not determine whether or not she was lying properly on the table prior to leaving the room. After the initial session on the exercise machine, the plaintiff advised the spa employee that she had experienced the excruciating back pain while the machine was operating with the leg portion of the machine in a downward position. Allegedly the employee advised the plaintiff not to repeat the exercise with the machine in that position. However, the plaintiff completed the program that night, including the use of the same machine with the leg portion in the upward position, even though she continued to experience back pain. Thereafter the plaintiff obtained medical treatment that revealed a ruptured disk. A lumbar laminectomy was required in an effort to treat the plaintiff.

Suit was later filed alleging, among other things, negligence of the spa and its employees. Although the plaintiff attempted to raise several factual issues, the court determined that the exculpatory clause was enforceable because it clearly stated the range of activities to which it applied. In reviewing the Gloria Marshall exculpatory clause as contained within its membership application, the court noted, "The provision explicitly mentions 'injury while using any equipment' and waiving claims against defendant for 'any such injury.'"[39] Although finding the form was sufficient to bar the plaintiff's action, the court held that the use of the word "negligence" was not required. The court concluded,

> [I]n this case, plaintiff assumed the risk that due to an employee's negligence and whether or not the employee was an expert, she may be injured by using a machine. As a result, plaintiff could have reasonably altered her conduct, for example, by stopping the exercise immediately after experiencing the excruciating pain or by consulting an employee of defendant immediately regarding the possibility of improper usage.[39]

Inasmuch as the court found that the exculpatory clause in this case was not against public policy or otherwise invalid, the plaintiff's cause of action was dismissed. In yet another Illinois case, *Garrison v. Combined Fitness Center, Ltd.,*[40] the plaintiff signed a membership agreement that purported to release the club "of all liability for injury arising out of the use of its facilities and equipment." The document was couched in terms of an assumption of risk and indemnity agreement. It stated,

> It is further agreed that all exercise including the use of weights, number of repetitions, and use of any and all machinery, equipment and apparatus designed for exercising shall be at the Member's sole risk. Notwithstanding any consultation on exercise programs which may be provided by Center employees it is hereby understood that the selection of exercise programs, methods and types of equipment shall be Member's entire responsibility, and COMBINED FITNESS CENTER shall not be liable to Member for any claims, demands, injuries, damages, or actions arising due to injury to Member's person or property arising out of or in connection with the use by Member of the services and facilities of the Center or the premises where the same is located and Member hereby holds the Center, its employees and agents, harmless from all claims which may be brought against them by Member or on Member's behalf for any such injuries or claims aforesaid.[41]

The plaintiff club member was injured in early 1985 while doing bench presses with 295 pounds. In response to this suit, the health club moved for summary judgment, contending the plaintiff had previously released the club from all responsibility related to the use of this equipment by reason of the previously executed release. The trial court granted summary judgment in favor of the club, even though the plaintiff club member contended he did not contemplate releasing the club from liability stemming from defective equipment when he signed the release and that the document was in violation of public policy.

The appellate court disagreed with the plaintiff's argument and found the plaintiff's complaint to be without "substantive merit." The court found that according to Illinois law, "a party may contract to avoid liability for his own negligence and, absent fraud or willful or wanton negligence, the contract will be valid and enforceable."[41] Although the court did indicate that there were exceptions to this general rule, the contract in this case "could not have been more clear or explicit. It stated that each member bore the 'sole risk' of injury that might result form the use of weights, equipment or other apparatus provided and that the selection of the type of equipment to be used would be the 'entire responsibility' of the member."

In a number of other cases, analyzed and published in *The Exercise Standards and Malpractice Reporter* between 1987 and 2006, similar results have been reached. However, where gross negligence or intentional conduct is involved, such releases are not generally upheld. For example, in the case of *Universal Gym Equipment, Inc. v. Vic Tanny Intenational, Inc.,*[42] the court recognized that it would not enforce a release for grossly negligent conduct. In this case, the plaintiff, a member of a Vic Tanny health club, filed suit against Universal Gym Equipment, Inc. "after she was injured at a Vic Tanny health club while using an exercise machine manufactured by Universal." However, because she had signed a membership contract that contained a release, she did not name the club as a defendant. The plaintiff reached a settlement agreement with the equipment manufacturer for $225,000. Thereafter, the equipment manufacturer filed suit against the defendant club for failure to maintain safe premises and alleged it had an obligation to **indemnify** (or, in other words, to protect and hold another party harmless—to make them whole) the manufacturer or to contribute toward the settlement. The club moved for summary judgment in its favor on the basis that it could not be liable for indemnification or contribution where it possessed a valid defense to the member's action because of her execution of the release. The trial court granted the club's motion and the equipment manufacturer appealed.

On appeal, the club contended the release was unenforceable as against public policy and that the defense of the club based on the release was not a bar to its action. Although the manufacturer conceded on appeal that the release was enforceable in cases of ordinary negligence, it argued the release did not act so as to bar claims of gross negligence, which it contended existed in the case and to which argument the court agreed—if present—would be against public policy. The court also dealt with certain other procedural and substantive law issues but held that the club could only be liable for contribution if the club was grossly negligent because the release would not then be valid if such claims were proven.

These documents are also sometimes questioned on the basis that they do not indicate the real intentions of the parties with sufficient clarity so as to spell out unambiguously the matters to which the release applies. In some cases, release documents that propose to cover participation in exercise activity have been held not to apply to slips on a shower room floor so as to bar a lawsuit for injuries relating to such falls,[43] or to activities that were not spelled out in a release document.[44] Other similar decisions have also been reached in other cases where participant activities that caused injury were not delineated in release documents.[45]

Sometimes factual issues related to the question of whether or not releases cover an activity that results in injury are left for jury determination.[46] Failures to follow statutorily mandated language in release document can also result in rulings making such documents "unenforceable."[47] Agreements that are less than clear—ambiguous in their word choices and language—can also fail to protect health/fitness clubs from liability. In such a case from the state of Oregon, *Landgren v. Hood Rivers Sports Club, Inc.,*[48] a plaintiff club member was injured when a sauna bench, on which he was standing, collapsed and threw him to the floor causing injuries. He filed suit for negligence and the defense moved for summary judgment on the basis of a release he had signed. The release was part of "a membership contract that incorporated Defendants Policies and Procedures handout." At the top of the last page of this handout, a section was included, entitled *Use of Property*. The *Use of Property* section contained a paragraph entitled *Liability of the Club and the Members*. The language of this paragraph provided as follows:

> *Any member, guest, nominee member or other person who in any manner makes use of or accepts the use of any apparatus, appliance, facility, privileges or service whatsoever owned and operated by the club, or who engages in any contest, game, function, exercise, competition, or other activity operated or organized, arranged or sponsored by the club, either on or off the club's premises, shall do so at his or her own risk, waives any legal claims against the club, its agents or employees and shall [hold] the club, its owners, employees, representatives and agents harmless from any and all loss, cost, claim, injury, damages and all liability sustained or incurred by him or her resulting therefrom, and/or resulting from any act of any owner, employee, representative or agent of the club.[49]*

In response to the defendant's motion for summary judgment, the plaintiff responded. Although he acknowledged the existence of the language in the *Policies and Procedures* handout, he contended the release was unenforceable because he alleged it was inconspicuous and did not exonerate the defendant clearly and unambiguously for liability based on its own negligence. When it analyzed the language of the release, the court determined that the law of Oregon provided as follows:

> *A presumption exists against an intention to contract for immunity from the consequences of one's own negligence, and contracts will not be construed to provide immunity or indemnity unless the intention to do so is 'clearly and unequivocally expressed. . . . An ambiguous agreement is to be construed against the drafter. . . . Additionally, agreements to limit the ability of one party to a contract for its own tortuous conduct are enforceable only under three circumstances: (1) the limitation of the liability was bargained for; (2) the provision was called to the other party's attention; or (3) the provision is "conspicuous."[50]*

In applying this law to the facts of the case, the court determined that the language of the release was in the middle of a paragraph on the back page of the handout and the language of the release, except for the title section, was in the same typeface and size as all of the other information in the handout. Therefore, the court determined that the tort liability limitation section found in the handout was not conspicuous and should not be enforced. More importantly than the foregoing, however, the court examined the language of the release and compared it to what transpired when the plaintiff was injured and determined as follows:

> *The club is a place where the members go to work out and engage in physical activity, some of which involve a risk of injury. It is reasonable for a club of this type to limit its liability for members who exceed their physical limitations, misuse equipment or suffer usual sports-related injuries and most members would understand the language to cover these types of injuries. However, it is not reasonable for a club to limit its liability for injuries to its members that occur in the auxiliary areas [of such facilities], such as locker rooms, showers, saunas or restaurants, that result from the club's failure to appropriately maintain these areas.[51]*

Because the language of the release provision dealt with a member's physical use of equipment owned and operated by the club and participation in physical activities organized and sponsored by the club, the language of the release in the court's opinion, "does not clearly cover a member injured by a loose locker in the locker room or a broken chair in the reception area, or, as in the case at hand, a broken bench in a sauna." The court determined that the defendant failed to limit its liability for negligently maintaining the sauna, and as a consequence, its motion for summary judgment was denied. Therefore, the plaintiff was entitled to pursue his negligence claim against the defendant.

The preceding case is very similar to a previously determined California case that was not cited in the Oregon court's opinion but was based on very similar facts and resulted in essentially the same ruling, *Leon v. Family Fitness Center, Inc.*[52] In that case, a facility member was injured while he was lying on a sauna bench. The court determined that the release used in that case pertained to hazards "known to relate to the use of the health club facilities," which the court in that case defined as hazards related to equipment use or from slipping in the locker room shower. The *Leon* court determined, as did the Oregon court, that the release in question did not apply to injuries that resulted from "simply reclining on a sauna bench." As a consequence, the release used in the Leon case did not apply to bar his claims, just like the release in the Oregon case did not bar that plaintiff's claims. Facilities would be well advised to ensure that release language is not only conspicuous but clearly applies to those situations that might arise, including those that relate in some way to the use of ordinary furniture and other similar items that may be located in such facilities.

WAIVERS AND EXECUTION ISSUES

In other situations in which releases have been held unenforceable, courts have ruled that "contracts attempting to limit the liability of one of the parties will not be enforced unless the limitation [on liability] is fairly and honestly negotiated and understood by both parties."[53]

Releases have been used to bar actions related to injuries suffered on exercise machines,[54] facilities,[47] a hot tub,[55] falls from a treadmill,[56] injuries suffered in aerobics[2] or even water aerobics,[57] climbing gym walls,[58] and even as to allegedly defendant emergency response procedures[59] (although in this regard perhaps specific additional wording should be included in such releases to cover these circumstances; see Appendix 4). Sometimes certain expert testimony can assist in overcoming the defense provided by a release in a negligence claim such as where a questioned document examiner brings into issue the question of whether a release was *"easily readable"* by the party signing it.[60] The taking of medication that might also affect a signer's judgment can also call into question the validity of a release in particular circumstances.[61] Language added to release documents acknowledging that the participant is not under the influence of drugs, medication, or alcohol that impairs his or her ability to contract might be effective in avoiding such judgments. Even release documents that evidence indicates were signed but lost[62] and electronically "signed" release documents[63] might be valid and bar claims against health and fitness facilities in appropriate circumstances.

Some health/fitness facilities, as well as other business entities, provide for the execution of release/waiver documents by spouses, if any, of participants so as to bar their own causes of action for loss of consortium—interference with the marital relationship—in the event of injury to or death of their participant spouse. However, in other instances, no such execution by a spouse is required if such a cause of action depends on or, in other words, is "derivative" to the claim of the injured spouse. In those states where a **loss of consortium** claim—interference with a relationship, usually a marital one—depends on the injured spouse's right to sue—Alabama, Kansas, Maryland, New York, and others—separate execution of release documents by such a spouse is probably not necessary to bar a spouse's acts by loss of consortium. In other states, however, including Florida, Ohio, and Massachusetts, among others, one spouse's execution of a release document will probably not bar suit by the noninjured spouse for loss of consortium unless that spouse signs too, and then only under circumstances where the release is otherwise upheld since in those states the loss of consortium claim is an independent one.

To illustrate this concept, in the 1992 case of *Bowen v. Kil-Kare, Inc.*,[64] the Ohio Supreme Court determined that the wife's cause of action for loss of consortium due to the claimed negligence of another was not barred by her husband's execution of release documents for his participation in race car driving. The Ohio Supreme Court also indicated that the release might not bar any action by the couple's children for loss of parental consortium because of the injuries the husband/father suffered in the race accident. Even though the husband/father executed two separate express assumption of risk/indemnity/covenant not to sue agreements, the court noted that the wife's cause of action "is her separate and personal right arising from the damages she sustains as a result of the tortfeasor's conduct" and that "the right of the wife to maintain an action for loss of consortium occasioned by her husband's injury is a cause which belongs to her and which does not belong to her husband."[65] The court determined that her cause would continue even if her husband was ultimately barred from pursuing his claim due to his execution of the release documents. The court used this same reasoning as to the potential for a child's cause of action for loss of parental consortium and remanded the whole case to the trial court for full consideration of all of the issues.

Although this Ohio case was not definitive on the issue of a child's right to compensation for **loss of parental consortium**—interference with the parent-child relationship—it brings up some potentially troubling issues for health/fitness professionals. If a spouse/child's cause of action is not barred by a participant's/member's execution of release documents, much of the potential benefit of these documents to the facilities (e.g., avoidance of claim and suit, reduced insurance rates) may be lost, unless the spouse's signature on such release documents is secured or unless the member agrees to indemnify the facility from any action brought by the member's spouse or children/heirs.

As to minor children seeking to hold a facility or program liable for injuries to a parent or for death, the children's signatures on contract documents would be invalid because of their inability to contract as adults. However, facilities could include indemnification provisions within the documents, whereby the contracting party would agree to indemnify the facilities for any claim brought by any member's spouse, children, or heirs. So long as the member would be collectible in the event of suit by the spouse or child, such a provision may reduce the likelihood of suit and provide a source from which remuneration might be sought in the event of suit despite such a provision within a release document. Some such provisions, however, may be invalid as discussed later.

Despite the ruling in the Ohio case just cited, however, some states have ruled that a spouse's action for loss of consortium will be barred by an injured spouse's execution of a release. In the case of *Byrd v. Matthews*,[66] the Supreme Court of that state ruled:

> *This Court, until otherwise convinced, reaffirms long-established Mississippi case law by holding that a defense available against a plaintiff in his or her personal-injury action (in this case, assumption of risk) is available against the spouse's derivative consortium action. The circuit court, therefore, properly directed a verdict in favor of the defendants.*[67]

Given the differences in various laws, health/fitness programs should consider whether or not participant spouses need to execute such documents in addition to participants. Legal counsel has to be consulted in this regard.

The first edition of *ACSM's Health/Fitness Facility Standards and Guidelines* provided for the use of waiver/release documents for some clients where individuals who should have medical clearance prior to beginning an exercise or activity program refused to do so. The second and third editions of that publication included similar recommendations, as did the ACSM/AHA Scientific Statement from 1998. Although these latter two statements recognized that the legal system may limit a facility's ability to exclude a patron from participation when he or she refuses to obtain medical clearance or to sign a waiver/release/assumption of risk document, for the most part, only the federally enacted Americans with Disabilities Act (ADA) and any similar state local laws may affect such determinations. The ADA does, however, allow the use of safety requirements in eligibility criteria provided such requirements are not based on speculation, stereotypes, or generalizations about individuals with disabilities.[68]

In October 2000, the federal Electronic Signatures in Global and National Commerce Act (S. 761) became law. The new act allows for the enforceability of "internet contracts." Such contracts may well include those involving heath/fitness facility releases.

WAIVERS AND MINORS

Minors cannot lawfully contract owing to their legal incapacity because they are under the age of majority. As a consequence, they cannot sign binding and enforceable waivers of liability, and these documents are voidable by them at their election.[69] Questions also arise as to whether or not parents may execute binding releases on behalf of their children. Many facilities, including health and fitness clubs, use prospectively executed waivers of liability to limit their potential exposure to personal injury and wrongful death claims that may occur within their physical plants. Often, facilities have parents execute such documents on behalf of their children so as to provide a line of defense from claims related to injuries to or death of their children. Recent decisions from the states of Colorado and California indicate that in some jurisdictions, a parent may prospectively release a child's personal injury claims, whereas in other states they may not do so.

In the California cases, *Lashley v. East County Gymnastics*,[70] a minor (9-year-old) child was injured while participating in a gymnastics class in 1999. Prior to her participation in this instructional class, her mother executed a release and waiver of liability and indemnity agreement on her behalf. The injury occurred when, according to the plaintiff's complaint, the appellant fell from the upper bar of uneven parallel bars onto a portion of a floor not protected by a mat, resulting in a severe injury to her elbow with accompanying nerve damage. The complaint alleged that the defendants negligently failed to provide mats in the area where the appellant was working out and failed to adequately supervise and instruct the child or to provide a spotter. The complaint also alleged inadequate training of the defendant's employees. In response to these claims, the defendant facility asserted the release and moved for summary judgment on the basis of the release and on the alternative grounds of express and primary assumption of the risk. The trial court granted summary judgment, finding that the mother clearly signed the release with the intent to release the facility and to assume the risks of injury to her child. The court of appeals to which the injured child by and through her mother appealed held that "given the inherently dangerous nature of teaching gymnastics to young children, the requirement of this waiver as a condition of participation is reasonable," and therefore concluded that "the releases barred respondents' negligence liability for appellant's injuries."[71] The court reached this conclusion without any discussion of the ability of the parent to execute the waiver on behalf of the child.

In a second California case from March 15, 2002, *McGowan v. West End YMCA*,[72] another child, while participating in the defendant's summer day care camp, was injured when another child actually struck the plaintiff in the head with a baseball bat. Following the injury, the plaintiffs filed suit contending that the YMCA "negligently operated the daycare center and negligently supervised"[73] the child and other children enrolled in the program. The defendants moved for summary judgment on the ground that the plaintiff's lawsuit was barred by a release that the mother executed. The court determined "the uncontradicted extrinsic evidence established as a matter of law that the release was executed by Ms. McGowan on . . . [the child's] behalf and applied to him"[74] so as to bar the other claims that were asserted by the mother on behalf of her minor child. Again, the court did not include in its opinion any discussion of the ability of the mother to execute on behalf of her child a prospective waiver releasing the defendant from liability for negligence. This decision may be questioned because of later California court decisions.

In the Colorado case, *Cooper v. Aspen Skiing Company,* however,[75] the issue of a parent's ability to execute a prospective release or waiver of liability on behalf of a child was analyzed and discussed with some thoroughness. The Colorado Supreme Court based its decision on an analysis of not only Colorado law but the law from several other states, including Utah[76] and Washington,[77] both holding that parents lacked the ability to execute a release on a prospective basis barring their child's cause of action for personal injuries. The Colorado Supreme Court, in adopting the reasoning of these states, determined that the release the child's mother executed prior to his participation in training on a ski race course, where he lost control and suffered extreme injuries, including blindness, did not bar the 17-year-old's claim against the defendant because the court held that "Colorado's public policy disallows a parent or guardian to execute exculpatory provisions on behalf of his minor child for a prospective claim based on negligence."[78] The court further held "that a parent or guardian may not release a minor's prospective claim for negligence and may not indemnify a tortfeasor for negligence committed against his minor child."[79] Thus Colorado joined the states of Utah and Washington in prohibiting the execution on a prospective basis of such releases while rejecting decisions allowing such releases to be executed by parents including another decision like the California decisions, which was decision determined by the Ohio Supreme Court in *Zivich v. Mentor Soccer Club, Inc.*[80]

In another extremely significant decision from the state of California, a Court of Appeals determined that prospectively executed releases given in reference to child care are invalid and void as against public policy. In this case, *Gavin W. v. The YMCA of Metropolitan Los Angeles,*[81] a child and the child's parents sued the YMCA and certain of its employees for damages arising out of an incident of sexual touching between the child and another child in the YMCA's child care program. At the time that the child was enrolled in the child care program, on June 4, 1996, the child's parents signed a YMCA release and waiver of indemnity agreement that provided as follows:

1. THE UNDERSIGNED, HEREBY RELEASES, WAIVES, DISCHARGES AND COVENANTS NOT TO SUE the YMCA, its directors, officers, employees, and agents (hereinafter referred to as "releasees") from all liability to the undersigned, his personal representatives, assigns, heirs, and next of kin for any loss or damage, and any claim or demands therefore on account of injury to the person or property or resulting death of the undersigned, whether caused by the negligence of the releasees or otherwise while the undersigned or such children is in, upon, or about the premises or any facilities or equipment therein or participating in the program affiliated with the YMCA.
2. THE UNDERSIGNED HEREBY AGREES TO INDEMNIFY AND SAVE AND HOLD HARMLESS the releasees and each of them from any loss, liability, damage or cost they may incur due to the presence of the undersigned in, upon or about the YMCA premises or in any way observing or using any facilities or equipment of the YMCA or participating in any program affiliated with the YMCA whether caused by the negligence of the releasees or otherwise.
3. THE UNDERSIGNED HEREBY ASSUMES FULL RESPONSIBILITY FOR AND RISK OF BODILY INJURY, DEATH OR PROPERTY DAMAGE due to the negligence of releasee or otherwise while in, about or upon the premises of the YMCA and/or while using the premises or any facilities or equipment thereon or participating in any program affiliated with the YMCA.[82]

Despite the parents' execution of the agreement just cited, they instituted suit against the YMCA and some of its employees for breach of contract, negligence, fraud, and several other intentional torts following the incident as previously described. The complaint alleged that the YMCA had knowledge of the other child's propensities to inappropriate sexual conduct, and in light of that knowledge they contended the YMCA should have taken steps to protect their child from his assailant. The complaint was later amended to include certain other claims, including negligent supervision and failure to warn. In response to these claims, the YMCA set forth the executed release as a defense.

The trial court ruled that the release was enforceable and not void as against public policy. It therefore dismissed the cause of action based on breach of contract and the three negligence causes of action. Ultimately the trial court dismissed all claims but the one based on fraud, and a jury returned a unanimous verdict in favor of the YMCA on that issue. Judgment was entered in August 2001 and the appeal by the plaintiffs followed.

On appeal, the parents and child alleged that the release was void as against public policy. The court determined that "to permit a child care provider to contract away its duty to exercise ordinary care is, in any event, antithetical to the very nature of child care services."[83] In this regard the court also noted in its conclusion, "Because we believe child care should live up to its name, we hold that exculpatory agreements that purport to relieve child care providers of liability for their own negligence are void as against public policy."[83] As a consequence, the decision of the trial court was reversed, and the case was remanded to that court for further proceedings not inconsistent with the opinion.

Sports medicine clinics, health/fitness facilities, and a variety of other similar institutions often provide day care services while parents engage in rehabilitation or health and physical fitness activities within such facilities. The decision just described may clearly impact the use of releases in those settings and what services are provided in this regard. Perhaps language can be included within such releases to distinguish the impact of the case, but such a task requires very careful drafting and consideration.

Based on the holdings in these cases, facilities would be well advised to consult with their individual legal counsel to determine when and under what circumstances a parent may execute prospectively a waiver of liability or release agreement on behalf of a child. Even under circumstances in which such documents are not permissibly executed by a parent, there may be other defenses that can be asserted based on concepts such as express or primary assumption of the risk.

The law dealing with the legal nuances of prospectively executed waivers/releases varies from state to state and is subject to various judicial constructions of law principles and then application to particular facts. See Table 4-1 for a summary of the applicable state-by-state positions on the use of waivers/releases in this industry that demonstrates the various state positions in this regard.

Because of these requirements and other drafting principles applicable to the development of potentially enforceable prospective release documents, lawyers knowledgeable with the process should be involved in assisting programs considering the development and use of these documents. Where recognized, the use of these protective writings should be part of any risk management plan for health and fitness facilities. However, in those states where state statutory provisions or court decisions bar the use of waiver/release documents, other risk management techniques such as using written or express assumption of risk documents might be necessary. The following sections (Ten Tips for Writing a Waiver and Five Tips for Administering a Waiver) have been adapted with permission from an article published in *ACSM's Health & Fitness Journal.*[84]

TEN TIPS FOR WRITING A WAIVER

It is important that health/fitness facilities seek out a lawyer who is knowledgeable or willing to become knowledgeable to write a waiver. The "Sample Waivers" in the appendix to this chapter and the tips for writing and administering a waiver should assist all providers and their lawyers in this regard. However, no waiver should ever be used in any health/fitness facility without a legal analysis because it has to reflect the requirements of individual state law. Although waivers (and other protective documents) can be drafted by health/fitness professionals, they *must* at least be reviewed

TABLE 4-1	Review of the Enforceability of Prospectively Executed Waivers in Health and Fitness Facilities by State			
State	States Where Waivers Are Generally Permissible and Enforced	States Where Waivers May or May Not Be Readily Enforced But Subject to Close Judicial Examination	States Where Waivers Are Not Enforced or Are Prohibited	States Where the Enforceability of Waivers Is Unknown
AL	X			
AK		X		
AZ		X		
AR		X		
CA		X		
CO	X			
CT			X	
DE		X		
FL		X		
GA	X			
HA	X			
ID	X			
IL	X			
IN	X			
IA	X			
KS	X			
KY		X		
LA			X	
ME		X		
MD	X			
MA	X			
MI	X			
MN	X			
MS	X			
MO		X		
MT			X	
NE	X			
NV		X		
NH		X		
NJ		X		
NM				X
NY			X	
NC	X			
ND				X
OH	X			

(Continued)

TABLE 4-1	Review of the Enforceability of Prospectively Executed Waivers in Health and Fitness Facilities by State *(Continued)*			
State	States Where Waivers Are Generally Permissible and Enforced	States Where Waivers May or May Not Be Readily Enforced But Subject to Close Judicial Examination	States Where Waivers Are Not Enforced or Are Prohibited	States Where the Enforceability of Waivers Is Unknown
OK	X			
OR	X			
PA	X			
RI				X
SC	X			
SD	X			
TN	X			
TX		X		
UT		X		
VA			X	
VT		X		
WA	X			
WV	X			
WI		X		
WY	X			

and edited by a knowledgeable lawyer prior to their implementation. Many factors need to be considered when writing a waiver. The following 10 suggestions represent "major" factors to consider when writing a waiver:

1. Some experts recommend a stand-alone waiver or at least one that is conspicuous, which is titled in capitalized, bold, or large letters. This makes the waiver conspicuous.
2. Be sure the "consideration" requirement for a contract as discussed previously is adequately stated.
3. The exculpatory clause should be bold or otherwise conspicuous, and it may be best to include the note that is applies to "ordinary negligence" but not to gross negligence, willful/wanton, or intentional/criminal conduct.
4. The language should be broad. For example, phrases such as "any and all present and future claims" in the exculpatory clause as well as "using the facilities and equipment" and "activities or any activities incidental thereto" are broad to cover all types of situations. Some courts have not upheld certain waivers used by health/fitness facilities because they did not include broad enough language to clearly indicate "any and all" activities.
5. The duration of the waiver should be clear and apply to "present and future claims."
6. All parties (in addition to the signer) who are waiving any and all claims resulting from ordinary negligence should be clearly identified and stated. These include family, perhaps—spouses and children—the person's estate, executors, administrators, heirs, and assigns.

7. The document should include a clause covering inherent risks of activity as well as any specific tasks associated with participation.
8. An indemnification clause may be needed. Such a clause might be advisable, especially for cumulative clauses.
9. A "severability" clause should be included so that if a court finds any portion of the waiver to be invalid, the remainder of the waiver would still be in effect.
10. A clause in the waiver should indicate that the individual is of legal age (affirms "contractual capacity" discussed earlier) and that the individual has read and understands the form he or she is signing. It is best to place this statement right above the participant's signature. Courts generally assume that individuals take responsibility for documents they sign.

In addition to these tips for writing a waiver, there also needs to be some thought given to the administrative process surrounding the actual execution of the waiver.

FIVE TIPS FOR ADMINISTERING A WAIVER

Proper administration of the waiver is just as important as the content of the waiver. The following five tips should help health/fitness professionals establish practical and correct administrative procedures for the execution process of the actual signing of a waiver:

1. Explain verbally, in an honest and clear manner, the purpose of the waiver. Courts may not uphold waivers unless the signer is told the reason for his or her signature. If a different reason is given (e.g., this is just for insurance purposes), the waiver may be void because this may constitute "fraud" or "misrepresentation."
2. Allow adequate time for individuals to read the waiver because courts have invalidated waivers when individuals were asked to sign quickly. Health/fitness facilities should establish a set procedure for those administering waivers, asking each participant if they have read and understood the waiver. Documenting that this was done will help refute a claim of ignorance of what was signed. Also, take the time to obtain a copy of one piece of reliable identification verifying the age of the individual. This helps affirm that the individual is of legal age and free to enter into this contract.
3. Read the waiver to nonreaders. Even though courts generally rule that persons are responsible for what they sign, it may be best for health/fitness facility staff to establish a procedure to actually read the waiver to those who cannot read but understand English. Translation into other languages may also be necessary in some situations.
4. Develop a policy regarding the retention of waivers. Participants can file a lawsuit years after an injury occurs because many **statutes of limitations** allow for the filing of lawsuits within one, two, or more years of the time an untoward event occurs. The time allowed depends on the particular state's statutes of limitations. Therefore, the retention period depends on individual state law.
5. Preserve the waiver documents securely so they can be obtained quickly and easily. It will be difficult to demonstrate in a court of law that a waiver was administered if it is misplaced or destroyed. Also, be sure waivers are secure from access by unauthorized parties.

Sample Waiver/Release Documents and clauses are included in the appendix to this chapter as follows:

Form 4–7: User's Representations, Express Assumption of All Risks and Release of Liability Agreement
Form 4–8: Example of a Waiver Upheld Twice in a Rigorous State
Form 4–9: Illustrative Stand-Alone Waiver

SUMMARY

The application of the assumption of risk defense by health and fitness facilities can assist in the overall risk management process for such entities. Written documents evidencing such assumptions can help demonstrate knowledge and acquaintance of such an assumption by participants. The use of prospectively executed waivers/releases presents a very real risk management technique to be implemented to limit claim and suit from ever being asserted or filed, while also providing an effective bar to successful suits in many jurisdictions if those documents are properly drafted and executed. Such documents should be used where permissible and in those jurisdictions where these agreements have been upheld. The services of knowledgeable legal counsel familiar with the drafting and use of such documents are necessary to ensure that the agreements are properly prepared and executed.

RISK MANAGEMENT ASSIGNMENTS

1. Explain how assumption of risk defenses are used to negate personal injury/wrongful death lawsuits against facilities and personnel.

   _____

   _____

   _____

   _____

2. Describe those limitations that may be applicable to the assumption of risk defense in reference to health and fitness facilities.

   _____

   _____

   _____

   _____

3. Compare and contrast those benefits and drawbacks of the express assumption of risk doctrine when compared with the application of the doctrine without a written document.

   _____

   _____

   _____

   _____

4. Develop a list comparing and contrasting assumption of risk, informed consent, and waiver/release documents to be used by health/fitness facilities in their development of relationships with clients.

   _____

   _____

   _____

   _____

5. Delineate the risks that are applicable to one or more of the typical activities carried on in most health/fitness facilities that could be included within assumption of risk documents for these entities.

_____

_____

_____

_____

6. List those risks that should be described in facility waiver/release documents for a particular activity such as free weight lifting.

_____

_____

_____

_____

7. Determine if releases/waivers executed in advance of activity are valid in a particular state.

_____

_____

_____

_____

8. Decide if a parent may lawfully execute a prospective release/waiver of liability in a particular state on behalf of his or her children.

_____

_____

_____

_____

9. Determine how long an executed waiver/release should be retained by a facility based on a particular state's statute of limitation for personal injury and wrongful death actions.

_____

_____

_____

_____

10. List those states where releases/waivers may not be recognized when executed in advance of particular activities.

_____

_____

_____

_____

KEY TERMS

Exculpatory clause
Express/contractual assumption
of risk
Indemnify

Loss of consortium
Loss of parental consortium
Primary/no duty assumption
of risk

Public policy
Secondary assumption of risk/
implied assumption of risk
Statute of limitations

REFERENCES

1. *Hildreth v. Rogers,* 2006 WL 2795605 (Ohio App. Dist., 2006), 4.
2. *Santana v. Women's Workout and Weight Loss Centers, Inc.,* 2001 WL 1521959 (Cal. App. Dist., 2001).
3. *Santana v. Women's Workout and Weight Loss Centers, Inc.,* 2001 WL 1521959 (Cal. App. Dist., 2001), 1.
4. *Santana v. Women's Workout and Weight Loss Centers, Inc.,* 2001 WL 1521959 (Cal. App. Dist., 2001), 2.
5. *Santana v. Women's Workout and Weight Loss Centers, Inc.,* 2001 WL 1521959 (Cal. App. Dist., 2001), 8–9.
6. Herbert DL, Herbert WG. *Legal Aspects of Preventive, Rehabilitative and Recreational Programs.* 4th ed. Canton, Ohio: PRC; 2002:249, 250.
7. *Mathis v. New York health Club, Inc.,* 261 A.D.2d 345 (N.Y. App. Div., 1999).
8. *Mathis v. New York health Club, Inc.,* 261 A.D.2d 345 (N.Y. App. Div., 1999), 346.
9. *Corrigan v. Musclemakers, Inc.,* 258 A.D.2d 861 (N.Y. App. Div., 1999).
10. *Corrigan v. Musclemakers, Inc.,* 258 A.D.2d 861 (N.Y. App. Div., 1999), 862.
11. *Corrigan v. Musclemakers, Inc.,* 258 A.D.2d 861 (N.Y. App. Div., 1999), 862–863.
12. Herbert DL. New York statute may bar effectiveness of executed releases. *Exercise Standards and Malpractice Reporter.* 2002;16(4):60.
13. *Weithofer v. Unique Racquetball and Health Clubs, Inc.,* 621 N.Y.S.2d 384 (N.Y. App. Div., 1995).
14. *Weithofer v. Unique Racquetball and Health Clubs, Inc.,* 621 N.Y.S.2d 384 (N.Y. App. Div., 1995), 385.
15. *Rutnik v. Colonie Center Court Club, Inc.,* 672 N.Y.S.2d 451 (N.Y. App. Div. LEXIS 4845, 1998).
16. *Rutnik v. Colonie Center Court Club, Inc.,* 672 N.Y.S.2d 451 (N.Y. App. Div. LEXIS 4845, 1998), 452.
17. *Rostai v. Neste Enterprises,* 138 Cal. App.4th 326 (Cal. Ct. App., 2006).
18. *Rostai v. Neste Enterprises,* 138 Cal. App.4th 326 (Cal. Ct. App., 2006), 329.
19. *Rostai v. Neste Enterprises,* 138 Cal. App.4th 326 (Cal. Ct. App., 2006), 333.
20. *Rostai v. Neste Enterprises,* 138 Cal. App.4th 326 (Cal. Ct. App., 2006), 334.
21. *Smogor v. Enke,* 874 F.2d 295 (5th Fed. Cir., 1989).
22. The Practical Lawyer. 1986;32(6):58.
23. *Hildreth v. Rogers,* 2006 WL 2795605 (Ohio Ct. App., 2006).
24. Herbert DL. Express assumption of risk is a defense to negligence claims: A practical analysis. *Exercise Standards and Malpractice Reporter.* 1987;1(6):91–96.
25. Herbert DL. Express assumption of risk is a defense to negligence claims: A practical analysis. *Exercise Standards and Malpractice Reporter.* 1987;1(6):91–96, 92.
26. Herbert DL. The use of prospective releases containing exculpatory language in exercise and fitness programs. *Exercise Standards and Malpractice Reporter.* 1987;1(6):89–90.
27. Protection of Human Subjects, 21 C.F.R. § 50.20 General requirements for informed consent (1999).
28. Cotten DJ, Cotten MB. *Legal Aspects of Waivers in Sport, Recreation and Fitness Activities.* Canton, Ohio: PRC; 1997.
29. *Tunkl v. Regents of the University of California,* 60 Ca1.2d 92 (Cal., 1963).
30. *Tunkl v. Regents of the University of California,* 60 Ca1.2d 92 (Cal., 1963), 92.

31. *Tunkl v. Regents of the University of California*, 60 Ca1.2d 92 (Cal., 1963), 98–101.
32. *Banfield v. Louis*, 589 S0.2d 441 (Fla. Dist. Ct. App., 1991).
33. *Owen v. Vic Tanny's Enterprises*, 199 N.E.2d 280 (Ill. App. Ct., 1964).
34. *Owen v. Vic Tanny's Enterprises*, 199 N.E.2d 280 (Ill. App. Ct., 1964), 281.
35. *Ciofalo v. Vic Tanney Gyms, Inc.*, 10 N.Y.2d 294 (N.Y., 1961).
36. *Owen v. Vic Tanny's Enterprises*, 199 N.E.2d 280 (Ill. App. Ct., 1964), 286.
37. *Neumann v. Gloria Marshall Figure Salon*, 500 N.E.2d 1011 (Ill. App. Ct., 1986)
38. *Neumann v. Gloria Marshall Figure Salon*, 500 N.E.2d 1011 (Ill. App. Ct., 1986), 1012.
39. *Neumann v. Gloria Marshall Figure Salon*, 500 N.E.2d 1011 (Ill. App. Ct., 1986), 1014.
40. *Garrison v. Combined Fitness Centre Ltd.*, 201 Ill. App. 3d 581 (Ill. App. Ct., 1990).
41. *Garrison v. Combined Fitness Centre Ltd.*, 201 Ill. App. 3d 581 (Ill. App. Ct., 1990), 584.
42. *Universal Gym Equipment, Inc. v. Vic Tanny International, Inc.*, 207 Mich. App. 364 (Mich. Ct. App., 1994).
43. *Brown v. Racquetball Centers, Inc.*, 534 A.2d 842 (Pa. Super. Ct., 1987).
44. *Macek v. Schooner's, Inc.*, 586 N.E.2d 442 (Ill. App. Ct., 1991).
45. *Pastizzo v. Connecticut Valley Fitness Centers, Inc.*, WL 644870 (Conn. Super. Ct., 1997).
46. *Summers v. Slivinsky*, 141 Ohio App. 3d 82 (Ohio Ct. App., 2001).
47. *Dunlap v. Fortress Corporation*, 2000 WL 1599458 (Tenn. Ct. App., 2000).
48. *Landgren v. Hood River Sports Club, Inc.*, 2001 WL 34041883 (D. Or., 2001).
49. *Landgren v. Hood River Sports Club, Inc.*, 2001 WL 34041883 (D. Or., 2001), 1.
50. *Landgren v. Hood River Sports Club, Inc.*, 2001 WL 34041883 (D. Or., 2001), 2.
51. *Landgren v. Hood River Sports Club, Inc.*, 2001 WL 34041883 (D. Or., 2001), 3.
52. *Leon v. Family Fitness Center, Inc.*, 71 Cal.Rptr.2d 923 (Cal. Ct. App., 1998).
53. *Rigby v. Sugar's Fitness and Activity Center*, 803 S0.2d 497 (Miss. App., 2002).
54. *Martin v. Tan & Tone America*, 965 P.2d 995 (OK CIV. App. 148, 1998).
55. *White-Vondran v. Ruiz*, 2001 WL 1422347 (Cal. Ct. App., 2001).
56. *Smith v. Connecticut Racquetball Club*, 2002 WL 1446633 (Conn. Super. Ct., 2002).
57. *Intriligator v. PLC Santa Monica*, 2002 WL 31424522 (Cal. Ct. App., Unpub., 2002)
58. *Delk v. Go Vertical Inc.*, 303 F.Supp.2d 94 (D. Conn., 2004).
59. *Skotak v. Vic Tanny International, Inc.*, 203 Mich. App. 616 (Mich. Ct. App., 1994).
60. *Neumann v. Gloria Marshall Figure Salon*, 500 N.E.2d 1011 (Ill. App. Ct., 1986)
61. *Stalnaker v. McDermott*, 505 S0.3d 139 (La. Ct. App., 1987).
62. *Corso v. United States Surgical Corporation*, 2005 WL 1435905 (Conn. Super. Ct., 2005).
63. Gilbert RR, Wijesundera S. Are Internet recreational releases/waivers valid? *Exercise Standards and Malpractice Reporter.* 2000;14(5):70-71.
64. *Bowen v. Kil-Kare, Inc.*, 585 N.E.2d 384 (Ohio, 1992).
65. *Bowen v. Kil-Kare, Inc.*, 585 N.E.2d 384 (Ohio, 1992), 391.
66. *Byrd v. Matthews*, 571 So. 2d 258 (Miss., 1990).
67. *Byrd v. Matthews*, 571 So. 2d 258 (Miss., 1990), 261.
68. Nondiscrimination on the Basis of Disability by Public Accommodations and in Commercial Facilities, 28 C.F.R. § 36.301 Eligibility criteria (1991).
69. *Dilallo v. Riding Safely, Inc.*, 687 So. 2d 353 (Fla. Dist. Ct., 1997).
70. *Lashley v. East County Gymnastics*, 2001 Cal. App. Unpub. LEXIS 1729 (Cal. Ct. App., 2001).
71. *Lashley v. East County Gymnastics*, 2001 Cal. App. Unpub. LEXIS 1729 (Cal. Ct. App., 2001), 19.
72. *McGowan v. West End YMCA*, 2002 WL 414341 (Cal. Ct. App., 2002).
73. *McGowan v. West End YMCA*, 2002 WL 414341 (Cal. Ct. App., 2002), 1.
74. *McGowan v. West End YMCA*, 2002 WL 414341 (Cal. Ct. App., 2002), 3.
75. *Cooper v. Aspen Skiing Company*, 2002 Colo. LEXIS 528 (Colo., 2002).
76. *Hawkins v. Peart*, 37 P.3d 1062 (Utah, 2001).
77. *Scott v. Pacific West Mountain Resort*, 119 Wash. 2d 484 (Wash., 1992).
78. *Cooper v. Aspen Skiing Company*, 2002 Colo. LEXIS 528 (Colo., 2002), 28.
79. *Cooper v. Aspen Skiing Company*, 2002 Colo. LEXIS 528 (Colo., 2002), 28–29.

80. *Zivich v. Mentor Soccer Club, Inc.,* 82 Ohio St. 3d 367 (Ohio, 1998).
81. *Gavin W. v. The YMCA of Metropolitan Los Angeles,* 106 Cal. App. 4th 662 (Cal. Ct. App. 2003)
82. *Gavin W. v. The YMCA of Metropolitan Los Angeles,* 106 Cal. App. 4th 662 (Cal. Ct. App. 2003), 668.
83. *Gavin W. v. The YMCA of Metropolitan Los Angeles,* 106 Cal. App. 4th 662 (Cal. Ct. App. 2003), 676.
84. Eickhoff-Shemek J, Forbes F. Waivers are usually worth the effort. *ACSM's Health Fitness J* 1999;3(4):24-30.

A P P E N D I X   4

EDITORIAL NOTE: CAUTION!

No form should be adopted by any program until it has first been reviewed by legal counsel in the state where the form is to be used, as well as by the medical director/adviser/risk manager for the program. To be acceptable, each form must be written in accordance with prevailing state laws by knowledgeable legal counsel and should state to the participant the reasons for the procedure, the risks and benefits, etc., in a manner specific to the program activities for which consent or other form of contractual document is being obtained. The forms here reproduced are protected by copyright and may not be reproduced in any form, by any means. They are reproduced here with permission of the copyright holder (PRC Publishing, Inc., 3976 Fulton Drive NW, Canton, OH 44718, 1-800-336-0083, www.prcpublishingcorp.com) from those publications identified later herein.

FORM 4-1
Express Assumption of Risk for Participation In Specified Activity

I, the undersigned, hereby expressly and affirmatively state that I wish to participate in _____. I realize that my participation in this activity involves risks of injury, including but not to limited to *(list)* _____ and even the possibility of death. I also recognize that there are many other risks of injury, including serious disabling injuries, which may arise due to my participation in this activity and that it is not possible to specifically list each and every individual injury risk. However, knowing the material risks and appreciating, knowing, and reasonably anticipating that other injuries and even death are a possibility, I hereby expressly assume all of the delineated risks of injury, all other possible risk of injury, and even death which could occur by reason of my participation.

I have had an opportunity to ask questions. Any questions which I have asked have been answered to my complete satisfaction. I subjectively understand the risks of my participation in this activity and knowing and appreciating these risks I voluntarily choose to participate, assuming all risks of injury or even death due to my participation.

_____   _____   Dated:_____
Witness   Participant

NOTES OF QUESTIONS AND ANSWERS

_____

_____

This is, as stated, a true and accurate record of what was asked and answered.

_____
Participant

TO BE CHECKED BY PROGRAM STAFF

	CHECKED	INITIALS
I. RISKS WERE ORALLY DISCUSSED	_____	_____
II. QUESTIONS WERE ASKED AND THE PARTICIPANT INDICATED COMPLETE UNDERSTANDING OF THE RISKS	_____	_____
III. QUESTIONS WERE NOT ASKED, BUT AN OPPORTUNITY TO QUESTION WAS PROVIDED AND THE PARTICIPANT INDICATED COMPLETE UNDERSTANDING OF THE RISKS	_____	_____

_____   _____
Staff Member   Date

FORM 4-2
Express Assumption of Risk/Prospective Waiver of Liability and Release Agreement

I, the undersigned, hereby expressly and affirmatively state that I wish to participate in fitness assessments, activities and programs and in the use of exercise equipment at various sites, including home, club or worksite, that may be provided or recommended by (_____ _____) (hereinafter "Facility"). I realize that my participation in these activities or in the use of equipment involves various risks of injury including but not limited to *(list)* _____ and even the possibility of death. I also recognize that there are many other risks of injury, including serious disabling injuries, that may arise due to my participation in these activities or in the use of equipment and that such risks, including remote ones, have been reviewed with me. I also understand, that under some circumstances I may choose to engage in activity in a non-supervised setting under circumstances where there is no one to respond to any emergency that may arise as a result of my participation or use of equipment on an individual basis, in an unsupervised setting. Despite the fact that I have been duly cautioned as to such unsupervised and unattended activity or equipment use, and despite the fact that I have been advised against such activity and equipment use in an unsupervised and unattended setting, I, knowing the material risks and appreciating, knowing, and reasonably anticipating that other injuries and even death are a possibility as a result of my participation in fitness assessments, activities, or programs or in the use of equipment in supervised/attended and unsupervised/unattended settings (within which settings I acknowledge that the risks of injury or death may be greater than in other settings), I hereby expressly assume all of the delineated risks of injury, all other possible risks of injury and even the risk of death which could occur by reason of my participation in any of the assessments, activities or programs or in the use of equipment in any or all settings.

IF YOU UNDERSTAND AND AGREE, PLEASE INITIAL _____.

I have had an opportunity to ask questions regarding my participation in various activities and in the use of exercise equipment. Any questions I have asked have been answered to my complete satisfaction. I subjectively understand the risks of my participation in various activities or in the use of equipment and knowing and appreciating these risks, I voluntarily choose to participate, assuming all risks of injury and death which may arise due to my participation.

IF YOU UNDERSTAND AND AGREE, PLEASE INITIAL _____.

I further acknowledge that my participation in the activities and use of equipment is completely voluntary and that it is my choice to participate and/or use equipment or not to participate as I see fit.

IF YOU UNDERSTAND AND AGREE, PLEASE INITIAL _____.

In consideration of being allowed to participate in the activities and programs provided through (Facility) and/or in the use of its facilities, equipment and machinery, I do hereby waive, release and forever discharge (Facility), and all of its directors, officers, agents, employees, representatives, successors and assigns, and all others from any and all responsibility or liability for injuries or damages resulting from my participation in any activities at Facility or elsewhere. I do also hereby release all of those mentioned and any others acting upon their behalf from any responsibility or liability for any injury or damage to myself, including those caused by the negligent act or omission of any of those mentioned or others acting on their behalf or in any way arising out of or connected with my participation in any of the contemplated activities or in the use of equipment and machinery through the Facility or otherwise. I understand that this release is given in advance of any injury or damage to me and that it includes injury or damage to me caused by the ordinary negligence of those released hereby but not from gross negligence, willful/wanton/intentional or criminal conduct. **IF YOU UNDERSTAND AND AGREE, PLEASE INITIAL _____.**

I understand and am aware that strength, flexibility and aerobic exercise including the use of equipment is a potentially hazardous activity. I also understand that fitness activities involve a risk of injury and even death and that I am voluntarily participating in these activities and using equipment with knowledge of the dangers involved. **IF YOU UNDERSTAND AND AGREE, PLEASE INITIAL _____.**

I do further declare myself to be physically sound and suffering from no condition, impairment, disease, infirmity or other illness that would prevent my participation in any of the activities and programs provided through Facility or in the use of equipment and machinery except as hereinafter stated: _____ _____. I do hereby acknowledge that I have been informed of the need or desirability for a physician's approval for my participation in exercise/fitness activity or in the use of exercise equipment. I also acknowledge that it has been recommended that I have a yearly or more frequent physical examination and consultation with my physician as to physical activities, exercise and as to the use of exercise equipment so that I might have recommendations concerning these physical activities and equipment use. I acknowledge that I have either had a physical examination and have been given my physician's permission to participate or that I have decided to participate in activity and/or use of equipment without the approval of my physician and do hereby assume all responsibility for my participation and activities or in the utilization of equipment without that approval. **IF UNDERSTAND AND YOU AGREE, PLEASE INITIAL _____.**

I, the undersigned spouse of the participant, do hereby further acknowledge that my spouse/participant wishes to engage in certain activities and programs provided by Facility including the use of various facilities and equipment. In consideration of my spouse's/participant's voluntary decision to engage in such activities, and in consideration of the provision of such activities and equipment to spouse by Facility, I the undersigned do hereby waive, release and forever discharge Facility and its directors, officers, agents, employees, representatives, successors and assigns and all others from any and all responsibility or liability for any injuries or damages resulting from my spouse's participation in any activities or in my spouse's use of equipment as a result of participation in any such activities or otherwise arising out of that participation. I do further release all of those above mentioned and any others acting upon their behalf from any responsibility or liability for any injury to or even death of my spouse including those caused by the negligent act or omission of any of those mentioned or others acting upon their behalf or in any way arising out of or connected with my spouse's participation in any of the activities provided by Facility or in the use of any equipment at any location. I specifically acknowledge that my execution of this prospective Waiver and Release relinquishes any cause of action that I may have either directly, through my spouse or independently by way of a loss of consortium or other type of action of any kind or nature whatsoever and I do hereby further agree to my spouse's participation in the activities as above mentioned and in the use of any equipment at any location. **IF SPOUSE UNDERSTANDS AND AGREES, SPOUSE TO INITIAL HERE _____.**

IN WITNESS WHEREOF, the participant and the participant's spouse, if any, have executed this Express Assumption of Risk/Prospective Waiver of Liability and Release Agreement this _____ day of _____, 20___, which shall be binding upon each of them and their respective heirs, executors, administrators and assigns. Each does hereby further agree to indemnify and hold Facility and all those identified or named herein absolutely harmless in the event that anyone claiming any cause of action as a result of any injury and/or death to participant or spouse attempts at any time to institute any claim or suit against the Facility arising out of any of the activities or programs herein or in the use of any equipment.

Signed in the presence of:

_____

_____   _____
                                                   Participant

_____   _____
                                                   Participant's Spouse
_____

*Reproduced and adapted with permission from Herbert & Herbert, LEGAL ASPECTS OF PREVENTIVE, REHABILITATIVE AND RECREATIONAL EXERCISE PROGRAMS, FOURTH EDITION (PRC Publishing, Inc., Canton, Ohio 2002). All other rights reserved.

FORM 4-3
Example of an Agreement to Participate†
Agreement to Participate
(Acknowledgement of Risks)

I am aware that the activities I am participating in, under the arrangements of Brown's Fort family recreation center; its agents, employees, and associates, involves certain inherent risks. I recognize that white water rafting . . . and other activities, scheduled or unscheduled have an element of risk which combined with the forces of nature, acts of commission, or omission, by participants or others, can lead to injury or death.

I also state and acknowledge that the hazards include, but are not limited to the loss of control, collisions with rocks, trees and other man made or natural objects, whether they are obvious or not obvious, flips, immersions in water, hypothermia, and falls from vessels, vehicles, animals, or on land.

I understand that any route or activity, chosen as a part of our outdoor adventure may not be the safest, but has been chosen for its interest and challenge . . . I . . . understand and agree that any bodily injury, death or loss of personal property, and expenses thereof, as a result of my . . . participation in any scheduled or unscheduled activities, are my responsibility. I hereby acknowledge that I and my family . . . have voluntarily applied to participate in these activities. I do hereby agree that I and my family . . . are in good health with no physical defects that might be injurious to me and that I and my family are able to handle the hazards of traffic, weather conditions, exposure to animals, walking, riding, and all and any similar conditions associated with the activities we have contracted for . . .

I and my family . . . agree to follow the instructions and commands of the guides, wranglers, and others in charge at Brown's Fort recreation center with conducting activities in which I and my family are engaged.

Further, and in consideration of, and as part payment for the right to participate in such trips or other activities . . . I have and do hereby assume all the above risks and will hold Brown's Fort . . . its agents, employees, and associates harmless from any and all liability, action, causes of action, debts, claims, and demands of any kind or nature whatsoever which I now have or which may arise out of, or in connection with, my trip or participation in any other activities.

The terms of this contract shall serve as a release and assumption of risk for my heirs, executors and administers and for all members of my family, including any minors accompanying me . . .

I have carefully read this contract and fully understand its contents. I am aware that I am releasing certain legal rights that I otherwise may have and I enter into this contract in behalf of myself and my family of my own free will.

†Based on the case report of *Formen v. Brown* 1996 Colo.App.LEXIS 343.

FORM 4-4
Illustrative Agreement to Participate
(for Use with Adults)
Agreement to Participate in Racquetball
(Substitute Information Appropriate to Other Activities for Italicized Sections)

Participation in all sports and physical activities involves certain inherent risks and, regardless of the care taken, it is impossible to ensure the safety of the participant. *Racquetball* is an activity requiring *considerable coordination, agility,* and a *high level of cardiovascular fitness.* It involves *vigorous activity for as long as an hour or more, many quick bursts of speed, and being alert to fast moving objects in a confined space.* While it is a reasonably safe sport as long as safety guidelines are followed, some elements of risk cannot be eliminated from the activity.

A variety of injuries may occur to a *racquetball* participant. Some examples of those injuries are: *1. Minor injuries such as scrapes, bruises, strains, and sprains; 2. More serious injuries such as broken bones, cuts, concussions, and loss of vision; 3. Catastrophic injuries such as heart attacks, paralysis, and death.*

These, and other injuries, sometime occur in *racquetball* as a result of hazards or accidents such as *slips, being struck by a ball, being struck by a racquet, colliding with another player, colliding with the wall, falling to the floor, or stress placed on the cardiovascular system.*

To help reduce the likelihood of injury to yourself and to other participants, participants are expected to follow the following rules:

1. *All participants are expected to wear proper footwear.*

2. *All participants are expected to keep the racquet strap around the wrist during play.*

3. *All participants are expected to wear protective eyewear during play.*

4. *All participants are expected to avoid swinging when it might endanger another player.*

5. *All participants are expected to follow all posted safety rules plus the rules of racquetball.*

I agree to follow the preceding safety rules, all posted safety rules, and all rules common to the sport of *racquetball.* Further, I agree to report any unsafe practices, conditions, or equipment to the management.

I certify that 1) I possess a sufficient degree of physical fitness to safely participate in *racquetball*; 2) I understand that I am to discontinue activity at any time I feel undue discomfort or stress; and 3) I will indicate below any health related conditions that might affect my ability to play *racquetball* and I will verbally inform activity management immediately.

Circle: Diabetes   Heart Problems   Seizures   Asthma   Other _____

I have read the preceding information and it has been explained to me. I know, understand, and appreciate the risks associated with participation in *racquetball* and I am voluntarily participating in the activity. In doing so, I am assuming all of the inherent risks of the sport. I further understand that in the event of a medical emergency, *management will call EMS to render assistance and that I will be financially responsible for any expenses involved.*

_____   _____
Signature of Participant   Date

WAIVER OF LIABILITY: In consideration of being permitted to play *racquetball,* on behalf of myself, my family, my heirs, my assigns, my executors, and administrators, **I hereby release the service provider from liability for injury, loss, or death to myself,** while *using the facility, equipment, or in any way associated with participating in the activity of racquetball now or in the future,* **resulting from the ordinary negligence of the service provider, its agents, or employees.**

_____   _____
Signature of Participant   Date

*Reproduced and adapted with permission from Cotten and Cotten, LEGAL ASPECTS OF WAIVERS IN SPORT, RECREATION AND FITNESS ACTIVITIES (PRC Publishing, Inc., Canton, Ohio 1997). All other rights reserved.

FORM 4-5
Illustrative Agreement to Participate
(for Use with Minors)
Agreement to Participate in Racquetball
(Substitute Information Appropriate to other Activities for Italicized Sections)

Participation in all sports and physical activities involves certain inherent risks and, regardless of the care taken, it is impossible to ensure the safety of the participant. *Racquetball* is an activity requiring *considerable coordination, agility, and a high level of cardiovascular fitness.* It involves *vigorous activity for as long as on hour or more, many quick bursts of speed, and being alert to fast moving objects in a confined space.* While it is a reasonably safe sport as long as safety guidelines are followed, some elements of risk cannot be eliminated from the activity.

A variety of injuries may occur to a *racquetball* participant. Some examples of those injuries are: *1. Minor injuries such as scrapes, bruises, strains, and sprains; 2. More serious injuries such as broken bones, cuts, concussions, and loss of vision; 3. Catastrophic injuries such as heart attacks, paralysis, and death.*

These, and other injuries, sometime occur in *racquetball* as a result of hazards or accidents such *as slips, being struck by a ball, being struck by a racquet, colliding with another player, colliding with the wall, falling to the floor, or stress placed on the cardiovascular system.*

To help reduce the likelihood of injury to yourself and to other participants, participants are expected to follow the following rules:

1. *All participants are expected to wear proper footwear.*

2. *All participants are expected to keep the racquet strap around the wrist during play.*

3. *All participants are expected to wear protective eye wear during play.*

4. *All participants are expected to avoid swinging when it might endanger another player.*

5. *All participants are expected to follow all posted safety rules plus the rules of racquetball.*

I agree to follow the preceding safety rules, all posted safety rules, and all rules common to the sport of *racquetball.* Further, I agree to report any unsafe practices, conditions, or equipment to the management.

I certify that 1) I possess a sufficient degree of physical fitness to safely participate in *racquetball,* 2) I understand that I am to discontinue activity at any time I feel undue discomfort or stress, and 3) will indicate below any health related conditions that might affect my ability to play *racquetball* and I will verbally inform activity management immediately.

Circle: Diabetes   Heart Problems   Seizures   Asthma   Other _____

I have read the preceding information and it has been explained to me. I know, understand, and appreciate the risks associated with participation in *racquetball* and I am voluntarily participating in the activity. In doing so, I am assuming all of the inherent risks of the sport. I further understand that in the event of a medical emergency, *management will call EMS to render assistance and that I will be financially responsible for any expenses involved.*

_____   _____

Signature of Participant   Date

_____   _____

Signature of Parent   Date

FORM 4-6
**Informed Consent for Participation
in an Exercise Program for
Apparently Healthy Adults**
(without known or suspected heart disease)

1. Purpose and Explanation of Procedure

I hereby consent to voluntarily engage in a program of exercise conditioning. I also give consent to be placed in program activities which are recommended to me for improvement of my general health and well-being. These may include dietary counseling, stress reduction, and health education activities. The levels of exercise which I will perform will be based upon my cardiorespiratory (heart and lungs) fitness as determined through my recent laboratory graded exercise evaluation. I will be given exact instructions regarding the amount and kind of exercise I should do. I agree to participate three times per week in the formal program sessions. Professionally trained personnel will provide leadership to direct my activities, monitor my performance, and otherwise evaluate my effort. Depending upon my health status, I may or may not be required to have my blood pressure and heart rate evaluated during these sessions to regulate my exercise within desired limits. I understand that I am expected to attend every session and to follow staff instructions with regard to exercise, diet, stress management, and smoking cessation. If I am taking prescribed medications, I have already so informed the program staff and further agree to so inform them promptly of any changes which my doctor or I have made with regard to use of these. I will be given the opportunity for periodic assessment with laboratory evaluations at 6 months after the start of my program. Should I remain in the program thereafter, additional evaluations will generally be given at 12 month intervals. The program may change the foregoing schedule of evaluations if this is considered desirable for health reasons.

I have been informed that during my participation in exercise, I will be asked to complete the physical activities unless symptoms such as fatigue, shortness of breath, chest discomfort or similar occurrences appear. At that point, I have been advised it is my complete right to decrease or stop exercise and that it is my obligation to inform the program personnel of my symptoms. I hereby state that I have been so advised and agree to inform the program personnel of my symptoms, should any develop.

I understand that during the performance of exercise, a trained observer will periodically monitor my performance and, perhaps measure my pulse, blood pressure or assess my feelings of effort for the purposes of monitoring my progress. I also understand that the observer may reduce or stop my exercise program, when any of these findings so indicate that this should be done for my safety and benefit.

2. Risks

It is my understanding, and I have been informed, that there exists the remote possibility during exercise of adverse changes including abnormal blood pressure, fainting, disorders of heart rhythm, and very rare instances of heart attack, stroke or even death. Often injuries to bones, muscles, tendons, ligaments and other parts of my body may also occur. Every effort, I have been told, will be made to minimize these occurrences by proper staff assessment of my condition before each exercise session, through staff supervision during exercise and by my own careful control of exercise efforts. I have also been informed that emergency equipment and personnel are readily available to deal with unusual situations should these occur. I understand that there is a risk of injury, heart attack or even death as a result of my exercise, but knowing those risks, it is my desire to participate as herein indicated.

3. **Benefits to be Expected and Alternatives Available To Exercise**

I understand that this program may or may not benefit my physical fitness or general health. I recognize that involvement in the exercise sessions will allow me to learn proper ways to perform conditioning exercises, use fitness equipment and regulate physical effort. These experiences should benefit me by indicating how my physical limitations may affect my ability to perform various physical activities. I further understand that if I closely follow the program instructions, that I will likely improve my exercise capacity after a period of three (3) to six (6) months.

4. **Confidentiality and Use of Information**

I have been informed that the information which is obtained in this exercise program will be treated as privileged and confidential and will consequently not be released or revealed to any person without my express written consent or as required bylaw. I do however agree to the use of any information which is not personally identifiable with me for research and statistical purposes so long as same does not identify my person or provide facts which could lead to my identification. Any other information obtained however, will be used only by the program staff in the course of prescribing exercise for me and evaluating my progress in the program.

5. **Inquiries and Freedom of Consent**

I have been given an opportunity to ask certain questions as to the procedures of this program. Generally these requests which have been noted by the interviewing staff member and his/her responses are as follows:

_____

_____

   I further understand that there are also other remote risks that may be associated with this program. Despite the fact that a complete accounting of all these remote risks is not entirely possible, I am satisfied with the review of these risks which was provided to me and it is still my desire to participate.

   I acknowledge that I have read this document in its entirety or that it has been read to me if I have been unable to read same.

   I consent to the rendition of all services and procedures as explained herein by all program personnel.

Date _____   _____
                                                 Participant's Signature

_____
Witness' Signature

_____
Test Supervisor's Signature

FORM 4-7
[Club Name]
[address]
[address]

User's Representations, Express Assumption of All Risks, and Release of Liability Agreement

PURPOSE OF THIS BINDING AGREEMENT:

By reading and signing this document, "You", the undersigned, sometimes also referred to as "User" or "I", will agree to release and hold __[Club Name]__ ("Club" or "We") harmless from, and assume all responsibility for all claims, demands, injuries, damages, actions or causes of action to persons or property, arising out of, or connected with your use of the Club's facilities, premises or services. The agreement and release is for the benefit of the Club, its employees, agents, independent contractors, other users of the Club and all persons on the Club's premises. This agreement includes your release of these persons from responsibility for injury, damage or death to yourself because of those acts or omissions claimed to be related to the ordinary negligence of these persons. This agreement also includes your representations as to important matters which the Club will rely upon.

A. REPRESENTATIONS

The undersigned, You, represent: (a) that you understand that use of the Club premises, facilities, equipment, services and programs includes an inherent risk of injury to persons and property, (b) that you are in good physical condition and have no disabilities, illnesses, or other conditions that could prevent you from exercising and using the Club's equipment/facilities without injuring yourself or impairing your health, and (c) that you have consulted a physician concerning an exercise program that will not risk injury to yourself or impairment of your health. Such risk of injury includes, but is not limited to, injuries arising from or relating to use by you or others of exercise equipment and machines, locker rooms, spa and other wet areas, and other Club facilities; injuries arising from or relating to participation by you or others in supervised or unsupervised activities or programs through the Club; injuries and medical disorders arising from or relating to use of the Club's facilities such as heart attacks, sudden cardiac arrest, strokes, heat stress, sprains, strains, broken bones, and torn muscles, tendons, and ligaments, among others, and accidental injuries occurring anywhere in the Club including lobbies, hallways, exercise areas, locker rooms, steam rooms, pool areas, Jacuzzis, saunas, and dressing rooms. Accidental injuries include those caused by you, those caused by other persons, and those of a "slip-and-fall" nature. If you have any special exercise requirements or limitations, you agree to disclose them to the Club before using the Club's facilities and when seeking help in establishing an exercise program, you hereby agree that all exercise and use of the Club's facilities, services, programs, and premises are undertaken by you at your sole risk. As used herein, the terms "include," "including," and words of similar import are descriptive only, and are not limiting in any manner.

You also acknowledge and represent that you realize and appreciate that access to and use of the Club's facilities during non-supervised times increases and enhances certain risks to you. You realize that if you use the Club during non-supervised hours, any emergency response to you in the event of need for same may be impossible or delayed. While we encourage you to use the Club's facility with a partner during non-supervised times, you may choose to do so without a partner, therefore enhancing and increasing the risks to you as to the provision of first aid and emergency response. You realize that a delay in the provision of first aid and/or emergency response may result in greater injury and disability to you and cause or contribute to your death. Use of the Club with no one else present to supervise or watch your activities is not recommended and would not be allowed unless you agree to assume all risks of injury, whether known or unknown to you.

You do hereby further declare yourself to be physically sound and suffering from no condition, impairment, disease, infirmity or other illness that would prevent your participation or use of equipment or machinery except as hereinafter stated. You do hereby acknowledge that you have been informed of the need for a physician's approval for your participation in an exercise/fitness activity or in the use of exercise equipment and machinery. You also acknowledge that it has been recommended that you have a yearly or more frequent physical examination and consultation with your physician as to physical activity, exercise and use of exercise and training equipment so that you might have his recommendations concerning these fitness activities and equipment use. You acknowledge that you have either had a physical examination and have been given your physician's permission to participate, or that you have decided to participate in activity and use of equipment and machinery without the approval of your physician and do hereby assume all responsibility for your participation and activities, and utilization of equipment and machinery in your activities.

YOU HAVE READ THE FOREGOING, ACKNOWLEDGE THAT YOU UNDERSTAND THE TERMS AND CONDITIONS SET FORTH IN THE PRECEDING PARAGRAPHS AND AGREE TO SAME.
Initials:_____

B. EXPRESS ASSUMPTION OF ALL RISKS

You have represented to us and acknowledged that you understand and appreciate all of the risks associated with your participation in various activities at the Club and in the use of equipment/facilities at the Club, including the risks of injury, disability, and death. You have also acknowledged that there are greater, enhanced, and even other risks to you if you decide to use the Club's facility during non-supervised times. Knowing and appreciating all of these risks and enhanced risks, you have knowingly and intelligently determined to expressly assume all risks associated with all of your activities and use of equipment/facilities at the Club.

You understand and are aware that strength, flexibility and aerobic exercise, including the use of equipment is a potentially hazardous activity. You also understand that fitness activities involve the risk of injury and even death, and that you are voluntarily participating in these activities and using equipment and machinery with knowledge of the dangers involved. We have also reviewed the risks with you on the date when you signed this Agreement and answered any questions that you may have had. You hereby agree to expressly assume and accept any and all risks of injury or death including those related to your use of or presence at this facility, your use of equipment, and your participation in activity, including those risks related to the ordinary negligence of those released by this Agreement, and including all claims related to ordinary negligence in the selection, purchase, set up, maintenance, instruction as to use, use and/or supervision of use, if any, associated with all equipment and facilities.

YOU HAVE READ THE FOREGOING, ACKNOWLEDGE THAT YOU UNDERSTAND THE TERMS AND CONDITIONS SET FORTH IN THE PRECEDING PARAGRAPHS AND AGREE TO SAME.
Initials:_____

C. AGREEMENT AND RELEASE OF LIABILITY

In consideration of being allowed to participate in the activities and programs of the Club and to use its equipment/facilities, machinery in addition to the payment of any fee or charge, you do hereby waive, release and forever discharge the Club and its directors, officers, agents, employees, representatives, successors and assigns, administrators, executors, and all others from any and all responsibilities or liability from injuries or damages resulting from your participation in any activities or your use of equipment/facilities or machinery in the above-mentioned activities. You do also hereby release all of those mentioned and any others acting upon their behalf from any responsibility or liability for any injury or damage to yourself, including those caused by the negligent act or omission of any of those mentioned or others acting on their behalf or in any way arising out of or connected with your participation in any activities of the Club. This provision shall apply to ordinary acts of negligence but shall not apply to gross acts/omissions of negligence, willful or wanton acts/omissions or those of an intentional/criminal nature.

YOU HAVE READ THE FOREGOING, ACKNOWLEDGE THAT YOU UNDERSTAND THE TERMS AND CONDITIONS SET FORTH IN THE PRECEDING PARAGRAPHS AND AGREE TO SAME.
Initials:_____

D. LOSS OR THEFT OF PROPERTY

The Club is not responsible for lost or stolen articles. You should keep any valuables with you at all times while using the facilities. Storage space or lockers do not always protect valuables. Consequently, by executing this Agreement and any accompanying documents, you do hereby agree to assume all responsibility for your own property and that of any dependent(s) and to insure that property against risk of loss as you see fit. By the execution hereof, you expressly, on behalf of yourself, and any dependents, do hereby knowingly agree to forego, waive, release and prospectively give up any right to institute any claim or action against the Club relating to lost or stolen property, including property lost or stolen due to the negligent act or omission of the Club. You agree to indemnify and save the Club and all of its personnel harmless from any action, claim, suit or subrogated claim or suit instituted at any time hereafter against the Club related to the theft or loss of your or your dependents' property at the Club. The Club shall be indemnified by you for all costs, expenses, fees, including attorney fees, incurred by the Club or its personnel by reason of any such action.

YOU HAVE READ THE FOREGOING, ACKNOWLEDGE THAT YOU UNDERSTAND THE TERMS AND CONDITIONS SET FORTH IN THE PRECEDING PARAGRAPHS AND AGREE TO SAME.
Initials:_____

User shall receive a copy of the foregoing Agreement at the time of its initialing and signing and hereby acknowledges User's receipt of same.

YOU HAVE READ THE FOREGOING, ACKNOWLEDGE THAT YOU UNDERSTAND THE TERMS AND CONDITIONS SET FORTH IN THE PRECEDING PARAGRAPHS AND AGREE TO SAME.
Initials: :_____

This Agreement shall be interpreted according to the laws of the State of_____. If any part of this Agreement should ever be determined by a court of final jurisdiction to be invalid, the remaining portions hereof shall be deemed to be valid and enforceable.

YOU HAVE READ THE FOREGOING, ACKNOWLEDGE THAT YOU UNDERSTAND THE TERMS AND CONDITIONS SET FORTH IN THE PRECEDING PARAGRAPHS AND AGREE TO SAME.
Initials:_____

ACKNOWLEDGMENT

I have read and received a completed copy of this Agreement and all of its Exhibits, as well as any Rules and Regulations of the Club which are incorporated herein by reference. I agree to be bound by the terms and conditions of the Agreement and the Rules and Regulations of the Club, as same exist or as same may be amended from time to time hereafter. This Agreement shall be binding upon me and my spouse, my heirs, my estate, my executors, my administrators and my successors and/or assigns. I realize that this Agreement is designed to prevent me and/or them from filing any personal injury or other lawsuit based upon ordinary negligence, including negligent battery, or even negligent wrongful death, loss of consortium or any other similar lawsuit arising out of any injury to me which I or they may possess hereafter.

The undersigned, on behalf of myself and my heirs, executors, administrators, successors and assigns hereby agree to indemnify the Club and all those hereby released and to hold them absolutely harmless if anyone, including the undersigned, should hereafter file suit against the Club or those released hereby for any matter intended to be released by this Agreement including claims based upon ordinary negligence such as but not limited to personal injury, wrongful death, loss of consortium or other similar actions.

Signature_____ Date:_____

Print Name:_____

Address: _____

Phone Number: (_____) _____

FORM 4-8
Example of a Waiver Upheld Twice in a Rigorous State*

"YMCA OF METROPOLITAN LOS ANGELES"
RELEASE AND WAIVER OF LIABILITY AND
INDEMNITY AGREEMENT

IN CONSIDERATION of being permitted to enter the YMCA for any purpose, including, but not limited to observation, use of facilities or equipment or participation in any way, the undersigned; hereby acknowledges, agrees and represents that he or she has or immediately upon entering will, inspect such premises and facilities. It is further warranted that such entry in the YMCA for observation, participation or use of any facilities or equipment constitutes an acknowledgment that such premises and all facilities and equipment thereon have been inspected and that the undersigned finds and accepts same as being safe and reasonably suited for the purposes of such observation or use.

IN FURTHER CONSIDERATION OF BEING PERMITTED TO ENTER THE YMCA FOR ANY PURPOSE INCLUDING, BUT NOT LIMITED TO OBSERVATION, USE OF FACILITIES OR EQUIPMENT, OR PARTICIPATION IN ANY WAY, THE UNDERSIGNED HEREBY AGREES TO THE FOLLOWING:

THE UNDERSIGNED HEREBY RELEASES, WAIVES, DISCHARGES AND COVENANTS NOT TO SUE the YMCA; (hereinafter referred to as releasees") from all liability to the undersigned: for any loss or damage, and any claim or demands therefor on account of injury to the person or property or resulting in death of the undersigned, whether caused by the negligence of the releasees or otherwise, while the undersigned is in, upon, or about the premises or any facilities or equipment therein.

THE UNDERSIGNED HEREBY AGREES TO INDEMNIFY AND SAVE AND HOLD HARM-LESS the releasees and each of them from any loss, liability, damage or cost they may incur due to the presence of the undersigned in, upon or about the YMCA premises or in any way observing or using any facilities or equipment of the YMCA whether caused by the negligence of the releasees or otherwise.

THE UNDERSIGNED HEREBY ASSUMES FULL RESPONSIBILITY FOR AND RISK OF BODILY INJURY, DEATH OR PROPERTY DAMAGE due to the negligence of releasees or otherwise while in, about or upon the premises of the YMCA and/or while using the premises or any facilities or equipment hereon.

THE UNDERSIGNED further expressly agrees that the foregoing RELEASE, WAIVER AND INDEMNITY AGREEMENT is intended to be as broad and inclusive as is permitted by the law of the State of California and that if any portion thereof is held invalid, it is agreed that the balance shall, notwithstanding, continue in full legal force and effect.

THE UNDERSIGNED HAS READ AND VOLUNTARILY SIGNS THE RELEASE AND WAIVER OF LIABILITY AND INDEMNITY AGREEMENT, and further agrees that no oral representations, statements, or inducement apart from the foregoing written agreement have been made.

I HAVE READ THIS RELEASE

Date:_____

_____

Signature of Applicant

*This waiver has been upheld in two separate cases in California (a state classified as Rigorous): *Randas v. YMCA of Metropolitan Los Angeles, Cal.,* 1993; and *Los Angeles v. The Superior Court of Los Angeles County,* Cal., 1997.

Reproduced with permission from Cotten & Cotten, LEGAL ASPECTS OF WAIVERS IN SPORT, RECREATION AND FITNESS ACTIVITIES (PRC Publishing, Inc., Canton, Ohio 1997). All other rights reserved.

FORM 4-9
Illustrative Stand-Alone Waiver
WAIVER AND RELEASE OF LIABILITY

Disclaimer: Winner's Health and Fitness Club (WHFC) is not responsible for any injury (or loss of property) suffered while participating in club activities, using equipment, or on club premises, for any reason whatsoever, including ordinary negligence on the part of WHFC, its agents, or employees.

In consideration of my membership and being able to use Winner's Health and Fitness Club (WHFC) facilities and equipment, **I hereby release and covenant not to sue** WHFC, its owners, its employees, instructors, or agents **from any and all present and future claims resulting from ordinary negligence on the part of WHFC or others listed** for loss, damage, or theft of personal property, personal injury or death, arising as a result of using the facilities and equipment of WHFC and engaging in any WHFC activities or any activities incidental thereto, wherever, whenever, or however the same may occur. **I hereby voluntarily waive any and all claims resulting from ordinary negligence,** both present and future that may be made by me, my family, estate, heirs, or assigns.

Further, I am aware that health and fitness club activities may range from vigorous cardiovascular activity (*i.e.,* aerobics, bicycles, steppers, or racquetball) to the strenuous exertion of strength training (*i.e.,* free weights, weight machines). I understand that these and other physical activities at WHFC involve certain risks, including but not limited to, death, serious neck and spinal injuries resulting in complete or partial paralysis, heart attacks, and injury to bones, joints, or muscles. I am voluntarily participating in club activities with knowledge of dangers involved and hereby agree to accept any and all inherent risks of property damage, personal injury, or death.

I further agree to indemnify and hold harmless WHFC and others listed for any and all claims arising as a result of my engaging in club activities or any activities incidental thereto, wherever, whenever, or however the same occur.

I understand that this waiver is intended to be as broad and inclusive as permitted by the laws of this state (specify) and agree that if any portion is held invalid, the remainder of the waiver will continue in full legal force and effect. I further affirm that the venue for any legal proceedings shall be in this state (specify).

I affirm that I am of legal age and am freely signing this agreement. I have read this form and fully understand that by signing this form. I am giving up legal rights and/or remedies which may be available to me for the ordinary negligence of WHFC or any of the parties listed above.

_____   Date:_____
Signature of Participant

_____   Date:_____
Signature of Parent or Minor

PART II

ASSESSMENT OF MAJOR LIABILITY EXPOSURES AND DEVELOPMENT OF RISK MANAGEMENT STRATEGIES

CHAPTER 5

Employment Issues

LEARNING OBJECTIVES After reading this chapter, health/fitness students and professionals will be able to:

1. Understand certain existing federal, state, and local laws and regulations applicable to employment issues.

2. Appreciate the importance of complying with employment laws and regulations.

3. Understand why it is essential to hire qualified and competent personnel to carry out health/fitness programs and services.

4. Understand the difference between employees and independent contractors, both of which categories of personnel work in and/or staff most health/fitness facilities.

5. Understand liability issues that can arise from employer–employee and other relationships and understand the legal doctrines of vicarious liability and ostensible agency.

6. Learn the types of allegations that are frequently put forth in claims and litigation against health/fitness personnel and facilities that deal with negligent hiring/training.

7. Distinguish between general and professional liability insurance and understand the importance of having both.

8. Describe credentialing issues related to accreditation, certification, statutory certification, national board examinations, and licensure.

A variety of people work or provide service within health/fitness facilities. Laws and regulations at the federal, state, and even local level impact the relationship between employers and employees in this setting. These laws include Title VII of the Civil Rights Act of 1964, the Equal Pay Act of 1963, the Age Discrimination Employment Act of 1967, and countless other laws that deal with employment, rates of pay, benefits, tax and other withholdings issues, and a number of other matters. Some of these laws and regulations are clearly beyond the scope of this text but can be reviewed in a number of other publications, including Fried and Miller, *Employment Law: A Guide for Sport, Recreation, and Fitness Industries* (Durham: Carolina Academic Press, 1998).

Personnel who work and/or provide service within health/fitness facilities include the following:

- **Employees:** Those who work in and are on the payroll of such facilities, subject to the direction and control of employers, for whom the employer provides space, facilities, and equipment, and for whom employers withhold payroll taxes and other deductions for such employees as required by law. Such employees are usually paid by the hour or on a salary basis.
- **Independent contractors:** Those who provide services for participants of a facility but under circumstances where they are not under the direction of facility personnel as would be the case with an employer–employee relationship, and who are generally paid on a nonhourly/nonsalary basis but on a set compensation basis, which in some circumstances may be established by reference to an hourly or daily rate. Service is generally provided to participants by such independent contractors where such services are delivered by the contractor using his or her own equipment even though such services may be delivered at the employer's premises. Sometimes such independent contractors in health/fitness facility settings pay facilities for the right to train the contractor's participants in facility buildings.

Substantial legal questions and concerns can often be raised in litigation or administrative settings, whereby the status of service providers as either employees or independent contractors is called into question. Such inquiries can include claims by governmental entities that payroll taxes and other withholdings should have been withheld from such individuals as employees, and as a consequence that monies are due from such employers, as well as claims that facilities are "legally responsible" or liable for the actions and services of such individuals to those for whom services are provided. This chapter discusses these legal questions and concerns and presents risk management strategies that will help minimize liability associated with these types of personnel issues. Moreover, this chapter also addresses the qualifications and training of health/fitness facility staff, issues that are frequently raised in litigation against these facilities. Staff qualifications, training, board examination, certification, and even licensing or the lack thereof are often called into question in these lawsuits, all of which also need to be examined.

STEP 1 ASSESSMENT OF LEGAL LIABILITY EXPOSURES

The legal concerns just described need to be explored and assessed to evaluate the risk exposures presented by these matters. Thereafter, risk management suggestions can be offered to ideally avoid or reduce—at least where possible—these concerns.

DISTINGUISHING EMPLOYEES AND INDEPENDENT CONTRACTORS

From the perspective of a business entity's compliance with laws, rules, and regulations of governmental entities such as the Department of Treasury and Internal Revenue Service (IRS), employers and prospective service providers can consult Form SS-8 to answer a series of questions to lead to a determination if a proposed service provider is an employee or an independent contractor. This Form SS-8 (see Appendix 5; also available from https://www.irs.gov/pub/ins-pdf/p1779.pdf) is used to request a delineation of the status of a worker for purposes of federal employment taxes and income tax withholding. In response to the submission of a Form SS-8, the IRS issues an information letter as an advisory that, although not binding on the IRS, may be helpful in determining the employment or independent contractor status of an individual, but only for federal tax purposes. The IRS also publishes an informational brochure, Publication 1779, entitled *Independent Contractor or Employee . . .* which is also available from the same website. This publication states, "The courts have considered many facts in deciding whether a worker is an **independent contractor** or an **employee.** These relevant facts fall into three main categories: *behavioral control; financial control;* and *relationship* *of the parties.* In each case, it is very important to consider all the facts—no single fact provides the answer. [emphasis and italics in the original]"; see Appendix 5.

Case Law

Aside from these employment status questions addressed from a federal income tax and federal withholding perspective, similar issues also arise as to other federal laws or even as related matters at the state and local level. For example, in the case of *Donovan v. Unique Racquetball and Health Clubs, Inc.,*[1] the U.S. Secretary of Labor instituted suit against the defendant health and fitness facility and others for alleged violations of the Fair Labor Standards Act (FLSA). Although a default judgment was taken against the defendants in this case because of their failure to answer the complaint in a timely fashion, the defendants appealed and the case was remanded or, in other words, sent back to the trial court. At the trial court level on remand, the court looked to determine if "locker room attendants" and "front desk receptionists" were employees for the purposes of the FLSA or independent contractors as the defendants contended. If classified as employees, such individuals would be entitled to be compensated at a rate of 1.5 times their regular rate of pay for certain overtime work. Although certain other issues were also involved as to some allegations involving minor workers, the court examined the facts and determined, among other things, that the locker room attendants were employees of the defendants rather than independent contractors. As the court noted, the determination of the employment relationship does not depend on "isolated factors, but rather upon the circumstances of the whole activity." In this regard the court concluded that the defendant owner of the corporation was, "in active control and management of defendant corporation, regulated the employment of all persons employed . . . and thus an employer of said employees"[2] within the meaning of the FLSA. This conclusion was based on the fact that the locker room attendants' primary responsibility was "to keep the locker rooms clean, open up lockers, and hand out towels and toiletries to customers in the locker rooms. They would wash the sinks, showers, and toilets. In addition, it was an important part of their job to keep other parts of the club clean. They frequently did such things as vacuum the carpets in the lounge and aisle areas, sweep the courts, clean the whirlpool, take out the garbage, and police the trash from the parking lots."[2]

As to the front desk receptionists, the court found that they "attended a desk at each club where they would greet customers coming to play racquetball, take their money in payment, take telephone reservations, show prospective members the club facilities, and give instructions to the locker room attendants. They received payroll checks from the Unique Racquetball bank account. They were rarely paid overtime wages for hours worked over forty despite the fact that they were regularly working such hours."[3] As a result of these and other findings and conclusions of law, the defendants were ordered to pay almost $135,000 in compensation due.

An analogous case brought against another similar facility by a tennis professional contended that the defendant club failed to pay him overtime compensation in violation of the FLSA and Maryland law (*Paukstis v. Kenwood Golf & Country Club, Inc., et al.*[4]). That case and others like it often depend on factual determinations that must be assessed by juries or judges.

ADDITIONAL LEGAL PRINCIPLES RELATED TO EMPLOYER–EMPLOYEE RELATIONSHIPS

The creation of principal–agent relationships can also create liability concerns. These relationships can be created by fact or by the imposition of certain legal principles and concepts.

Liability for Employees/Agents

Putting aside those issues dealing with tax withholdings and labor matters, employers are liable for the activities carried out by their employees which are within the scope of the employees' duties and job descriptions. Employers can also be responsible for the activities of those who can appear to be their employees or agents under some special circumstances. These circumstances include situations where "apparent agents" or **ostensible agents**—because of particular circumstances—are deemed to be agents of a third party who is held liable or responsible for their actions just like in the situation of an employer–employee relationship. These circumstances arise where it appears that the person providing services is an employee or is otherwise so closely connected with the facility that the entity should be liable for his or her actions.

Notwithstanding the preceding, however, employers are not liable for the actions of employees that are not within the scope of their job duties and requirements, such as, for example, where an employee for his or her own benefit determines to stop at a dry cleaners on his or her daily route to pick up clothes. Should such an individual commit a negligent act or omission that harms another person while on such a "side" trip, the employer would generally not be liable for that person's actions.

Likewise, facilities that contract with third parties for someone else to deliver service to customers/clients are generally not liable for the actions or omissions of those independent contractors. There are exceptions to this general rule, such as where it appears the contractor is really an employee or agent of the facility under circumstances mentioned earlier, and where another party claims to be injured or damaged by the act or omission of that party. This situation can occur, for example, where contractors provide service at a facility but do not divulge their status to clients/customers, wear facility clothing, provide service using facility equipment in facility buildings, and so on.

Liability for the actions/omissions of employees, or sometimes for those who are agents, is based on a legal concept referred to in law as *respondeat superior*, which means masters are liable for the acts of their servants. Under this doctrine, programs are vicariously liable for the negligent acts/omissions of their employees, agents, and even ostensible/apparent agents, whose clients may consider them to be agents of a facility, particularly where such a facility allows the impression to be made that such persons are agents of the facility.

Claims are frequently put forth against employees and employers and even contractors and agents whereby it is alleged that both are liable for negligent service delivery/hiring/supervision/direction/care. These allegations can include claims, according to the court in *Seigneur v. National Fitness Institute, Inc.*, that the service providers "lacked sufficient training, experience, certification and/or other qualifications and knowledge to properly, reasonably and safely instruct, direct or guide [consumers] in lifting weights and in the use of weight equipment . . . [as well as negligence in failing to provide instruction] with sufficient training and knowledge to properly, reasonably and safely instruct, direct and guide."[5] See Chapter 8 for more information on liability issues associated with instruction and supervision.

Case Law   Claims based on *respondeat superior* principles can also be put forth in other situations against health/fitness facilities. In one such case, *Chai v. Sports & Fitness Clubs of America, Inc.*, it was alleged, among other things, that the defendant:

- Negligently failed to have personnel adequately trained to recognize cardiac arrest and to subsequently start CPR.
- Negligently failed to have employees adequately trained in the administration of CPR, available to assist . . . [the member] when he collapsed while exercising.
- Negligently failed to have employees adequately trained in the use and operation of an automated external defibrillator, available to assist . . . [the member] when he collapsed while exercising.
- Negligently failed to have automated external defibrillators on the premises and available for use at all times.
- Negligently failed to promptly perform CPR, on . . . [the member] when he collapsed while exercising.

- Negligently failed to promptly use an automated external defibrillator, on . . . [the member] when he collapsed while exercising.
- Negligently failed to properly monitor . . . [the member] while he was exercising in the cardiovascular room.
- Negligently failed to promptly call for emergency medical assistance for . . . [the member] when he collapsed while exercising.
- Negligently failed to require prescreening of members, including . . . [the member], to assess his fitness and health, prior to his use of the Defendant's exercise facilities.
- Negligently failed to require sufficient certification or training of staff members designated to train and monitor . . . [the member] when he was using the cardiovascular exercise equipment.[6]

When claims are made that fitness personnel are really employees of a health/fitness facility, for which that facility should be liable, courts must review applicable facts to determine the existence or lack of the relationship before a facility can be potentially responsible for the acts or omissions of the individual in question. For example, in the case of *Aydelotte v. BQE Racquetball Club, Inc.,*[7] the plaintiff claimed that she suffered certain back injuries while working out with a personal trainer at the defendant club. Despite the claim that the trainer was employed by the club, the court determined,

> *Contrary to the plaintiff's contentions, the record is devoid of any evidence that [the trainer] was employed by . . . [the club]. [The trainer] . . . was merely a member . . . [himself] . . . and there is no proof that any other relationship existed . . . Furthermore, no evidence was submitted to establish that . . . [the club] had control over the manner or method in which . . . [the trainer] performed his work.*[8]

Very serious allegations in health/fitness cases can be and have been raised against employees and employers alike, based claims of employer liability based on a *respondeat superior* basis. For example, in *Capati v. Crunch Fitness International, et al.,*[9] a $320 million lawsuit filed in the state of New York against Crunch Fitness, a personal trainer, his employer, and others, a 37-year-old mother and fashion designer died while working out under the guidance of a personal trainer employed by the defendant facility.[10] Allegedly the decedent was taking a variety of nutritional supplements, some of which contained ephedrine, which the suit alleged the personal trainer recommended to her. Although the facility contended that its trainers were not permitted to recommend supplements and the trainer denied doing so, the trainer did admit during his deposition that he never advised the decedent that there might be adverse health consequences to her taking these dietary supplements while working out or discontinuing her blood pressure medication. The decedent allegedly died from a cerebral vascular incident after working out with the trainer in 2004. The case settled for a multimillion dollar amount.[11]

Although damage claims like the preceding related to negligence or untoward death complaints are typically filed against facilities, employers, and agents, such claims can also even be asserted against other third parties, including standards setting organizations[12] and even volunteers.[13] Claims and lawsuits related to personnel can also be directed at the facilities themselves as well as other personnel. These claims and suits can deal with alleged violations of federal and state law such as those brought under federal and state civil rights acts, Equal Employment Opportunity Commission (EEOC)–type claims, sexual harassment claims, Americans with Disabilities Act (ADA)–type claims and suits, and potentially a myriad of other assertions. A claim by a former employee that he was discriminated against in employment at a health/fitness facility in violation of EEOC laws and regulations and the ADA will be tried to a jury when a court concludes that a reasonable jury could find in favor of the employee on his claims related to demotion and termination (see *Stewart v. Bally Total Fitness*[14]).

Employee/Agent Qualification Issues

The lack of clear, uniform, industrywide standards, discussed previously in this text, may have contributed to industry efforts to improve the education, training, and qualifications of fitness professionals and even to some state governmental efforts to license fitness professionals. This may be especially true when some industry events and/or practices have been the subject of media scrutiny as to a variety of concerns and issues that may in some situations be clearly substandard.[15]

One way that some of these concerns have been addressed is through educational programs at institutions of higher learning or to otherwise "professionalize" those in the fitness industry. Many colleges and universities in the United States and Canada offer programs leading to bachelors, masters, and doctoral degrees in exercise/clinical physiology, kinesiology, and sports medicine/administration, as well as various fitness professional designations and other degrees. Typically these programs prepare students in related scientific disciplines associated with the profession, but rarely include comprehensive course work in personal fitness training, risk management, legal/business issues, and related topics.

As a consequence, a number of fitness educational entities have stepped forward to provide training for professionals in the fitness industry. These include ACSM, AFAA, NSCA, American Council on Exercise (ACE), the Cooper Institute, and many others. All of these groups, profit and nonprofit alike, provide certifications for various categories of fitness professionals, such as personal fitness trainers, aerobics instructors, group exercise leaders, and so on. Perhaps because of the diversity of the groups involved in this process, there appears to be no uniform standards against which compliance is judged for any particular professional designation. In 2004 the National Board of Fitness Examiners (NBFE) was organized to provide such a nationally based and uniform test, as discussed later.

Based on perhaps all of the preceding, the industry in the early 2000s began an effort to attempt to raise the bar as to the qualifications and capabilities of some exercise professionals—mainly personal fitness trainers. In 2002 IHRSA gathered together the fitness industry's top professional fitness certification agencies—among them ACSM, ACE, NSCA, AFAA, and the Cooper Institute, among others[16]—to look for ways to improve the qualifications of such fitness professionals. Ultimately, some in this group opted to focus on the process by which personal fitness trainers were certified as contemplated by IHRSA. As a result, IHRSA's board of directors adopted a corporate resolution in 2005 that recommended to all of its member clubs that they hire only personal trainers who were certified by a group that had obtained (or had begun) third-party accreditation of its certification, such as the National Commission for Certifying Agencies (NCCA).[17]

Not everyone in the profession agreed with this recommendation.[18] At about the same time, efforts were being made by a newly formed organization, the NBFE (**www.nbfe.org**), to develop a uniform national test to determine the competencies of personal fitness trainers. The testing program became viable in 2006 and is to be followed by a practical testing component for all testing candidates who pass the written examination. Ultimately, NBFE's efforts will result in the creation of a national register of personal fitness trainers who successfully pass the examination.[19] At least one state legislative proposal (Georgia, 2006) to license such personnel has suggested that the NBFE examination process be used in reference to proposed fitness professional licensing in that state, but that proposal itself was later changed in 2007. For more on licensure issues for exercise/fitness professionals, see a three-part article published in *ACSM's Health & Fitness Journal*.[20-22]

Many of the published standards of practice (listed in Chapter 3 and described in more detail in subsequent chapters) indicate certain credentials that health/fitness professionals should possess. In addition to credentials, health/fitness professional must be aware of their potential legal duties and know how to carry them out. Negligence claims and lawsuits against facilities and personnel typically include the following allegations in reference to service delivery:

- Failed to properly disclose certain risks during the informed consent process preceding graded exercise stress testing or exercise activity.
- Failed to properly monitor an exercise test.
- Failed to properly stop a graded exercise stress test in the exercise of competent professional judgment.
- Failed to adequately and competently instruct/supervise participants as to the safe performance of the recommended conditioning activities or in the proper use of exercise equipment.
- Failed to properly and competently evaluate participants' capacities or physical impairments as these would limit or contraindicate certain types of exercise.
- Failed to prescribe a proper exercise intensity in terms of metabolic and cardiovascular demand.
- Failed to properly supervise the participants' exercise during program sessions or advise individuals regarding any restrictions or modifications that should be followed in modifying physical activities during unsupervised periods.
- Failed to assign participants to an exercise setting with a proper level of physiological monitoring, supervision and emergency medical support.
- Failed to provide or secure employee response in the event of an untoward occurrence.
- Failed to properly train staff.
- Failed to provide emergency aid or response, including first aid, CPR, and perhaps even AEDs.
- Failed to perform or rendered performance in a negligent manner in a variety of other situations.[23]

Negligent Hiring

To illustrate a negligent hiring claim, consider the case of *Seigneur v. National Fitness Institute*.[24] In this case, the plaintiff decided to join the defendant exercise and fitness facility to begin a weight loss and fitness program. She joined the defendant facility in part based on the recommendation of her chiropractor, and because of her allegation that the facility promoted itself as a fitness facility that "employed degreed, certified fitness, clinical exercise and health specialists."[25] While she was undergoing an initial evaluation by a facility staff member, she was allegedly injured on a weight machine and later filed suit. The contention, among other things, was that the defendant facility breached its duty to her "by negligently hiring . . . [a defendant employee who performed the initial evaluation] who [she contended] lacked sufficient training, experience, certification and/or other qualifications and knowledge to properly, reasonably and safely instruct, direct and guide [her] in lifting weights and in the use of the weight equipment."[26] Despite these and similar claims made against the facility, the court granted the defendant's motion to dismiss the action owing to an exculpatory release that the plaintiff signed when she joined the facility, purportedly releasing the facility from claim and suit (see Chapter 4 for more on releases/waivers).

In cases where negligent hiring claims make their way through a trial court for judge or jury determination, the proper evaluation standard is based on "an employer's duty to use reasonable care in the employment, training and supervision of its employees" (*Mathis v. New York Health Club, Inc.*[27]). In this case, the plaintiff's claims included negligent hiring allegations because there were questions as to whether the plaintiff, "who was not a novice to weight training, did assume those risks ordinarily entailed by properly supervised weight training."[28] In this regard, the court noted,

> [H]e [the plaintiff] cannot be said to have assumed risks in excess of those usually encountered in the activity, particularly unreasonably increased risks attributable to lapses in judgment by a trainer whose qualifications, plaintiff

alleges, were not all they had been represented to be by defendant health club at the time plaintiff purchased the club's specialized training package. According to plaintiff, defendant trainer increased the weight on the training machine plaintiff had been using to 270 pounds and, despite plaintiff's repeatedly expressed doubts as to whether he could handle so much weight, urged plaintiff to continue with his repetitions. Given this scenario, factual issues are raised as to whether plaintiff's injury, which allegedly occurred in the course of the repetitions urged upon him by defendant trainer, was not the consequence of risks which, although inherent in weight training, were unreasonably augmented by culpable misjudgment as to plaintiff's capacity to bear so much weight.[28]

Criminal Background Checks   Health/fitness facilities, particularly those that serve vulnerable populations, such as children, older adults, and people with disabilities, should perform background checks on all employees who will be working with these populations. Employees who work closely with clients, such as personal trainers, massage therapists, and so on, may need to be closely evaluated in this regard because of the nature of their work. Claims related to negligence in hiring and supervising such employees can arise if such employees are not adequately screened on hiring and/or are negligently supervised. For example, in the case of *Geiger v. McClurg Court Associates,*[29] a suit was filed dealing with negligent hiring and supervision of a massage therapist who allegedly sexually molested the plaintiff. Similar kinds of claims have been asserted in other cases that should serve as a reminder to all facilities to check out staff members prior to their employment.[30] In an effort to assist their facilities in preventing these kinds of potential claims, the YMCA Medical Advisory Committee has issued guidelines dealing with child abuse prevention, children in adult locker rooms, massage therapy, and personal training.[31]

Employers are generally not liable for the criminal actions of an employee toward their patrons[32] even where, for example in the health/fitness setting, it is alleged that the employer should be held liable for a sexual assault by a massage therapist who the plaintiff claimed—but did not prove—was negligently hired, as in *Geiger.* However, procedures such as conducting criminal background checks should be conducted prior to hiring of certain employees to help minimize potential civil claims associated with negligent hiring.

LIABILITY INSURANCE

Although there are many types of insurance that health/fitness professionals and facilities should consider, this discussion focuses on "general" and "professional" liability insurance and the protection each provides from financial losses owing to negligence. As described in Chapter 2, if a health/fitness professional and/or facility is found negligent, the judge or jury can award the plaintiff (a) economic damages (e.g., medical expenses, portion of loss wages), (b) noneconomic damages (e.g., pain of suffering, loss of consortium), and perhaps (c) punitive damages for gross negligence (also referred to as willful/wanton or reckless conduct). Both economic and noneconomic damages are paid by the insurance company (protecting the financial assets of the health/fitness professional and/or facility) up to the limits established in the policies. Generally, neither general nor professional liability insurance policies pay for punitive damages.

Liability insurance is an important risk management strategy that is an example of a **contractual transfer of risks** (or liability). Like a waiver, the liability is "transferred" to someone other than the health/fitness professional and/or facility. The insurance provider agrees to pay damages awarded to a plaintiff. An individual who signs a waiver agrees to assume any liability for negligence on part of the professional and/or facility.

General liability insurance is obtained through a commercial general liability (CGL) policy and protects health/fitness professionals and facilities from conduct that would be classified as "ordinary" negligence. Professional liability insurance (also termed errors and omissions insurance) protects health/fitness professionals and facilities from conduct classified as "professional" negligence. Professional liability insurance is similar to malpractice insurance for physicians. The following article about the case of *Jacob v. Grant Life Choices Center,* reprinted with permission from *The Exercise Standards and Malpractice Reporter,*[33] is an excellent illustration of why health/fitness professionals and facilities need both general and professional liability insurance.

Jacob v. Grant Life Choices

In this case, *Jacob v. Grant Life Choices Center,* Case No. 93 CVC-06–4353 (Franklin County, Ohio Court of Common Pleas, Complaint filed June 21, 1993 against the named defendant, as well as Club Management, Inc. (CMI) and employee Robert Getz, amended complaint filed October 6, 1993, adding a new party, Grant Medical Center), the plaintiff club member allegedly suffered a heart attack after exercising at the defendant facility. The facility was managed by CMI and located within the defendant Medical Center hospital. On the day of his heart attack, the plaintiff, who was not in any medically based program, engaged in his regular routine of running 5 to 6 miles and using weight machines thereafter for 15 to 20 minutes. He also sat in a sauna for a while after his exercise routine but began to feel ill. He experienced nausea and light-headedness and believed he suffered a lapse of consciousness after he lay down on a bench in the men's locker room. According to his deposition testimony he described discomfort across his upper body to the defendant employee of the facility. Allegedly the employee asked some cardiac history–related questions, took the plaintiff's blood pressure, drew some blood via a finger prick and analyzed it for blood sugar, and gave the plaintiff some orange juice and a banana. According to certain court papers, the employee defendant determined that the plaintiff was not experiencing any chest pains but was disoriented, lightheaded, and nauseous. In addition, the defendant employee determined that the plaintiff's breathing was normal but his blood pressure and blood sugar (from the blood test results) were low. The employee defendant determined that the plaintiff's condition was related to a decrease in blood sugar because of a vigorous workout. The employee defendant asked the plaintiff to drink lots of orange juice, to eat a banana, and to go home and rest. The plaintiff followed these instructions, got dressed, and drove himself home. However, once there, he began to have difficulty breathing, and he drove himself to a local hospital. He was eventually determined to have suffered an acute myocardial infarction (MI).

After his diagnosis, the plaintiff filed suit against the facility, CMI, and the employee (later adding the defendant hospital where the facility was located), alleging that the defendants were negligent in not summoning and providing appropriate emergency medical aid for him in light of his symptoms and complaints. The plaintiff complained that in accordance with the appropriate standard of care and because of the defendant's position within a hospital-based exercise facility, that the defendant had a duty to properly train personnel to respond to emergencies and that as a consequence of the defendant's negligence, the plaintiff suffered more severe heart damage than would have been the case if he had received timely and appropriate care. The plaintiff, who was 47 years of age at the time, further alleged that he will require a heart transplant in the future because of the defendant's alleged breach of care.

While these allegations were pending, the insurance carrier for CMI, Meridian Mutual Insurance Company, moved to intervene in the case. The carrier sought a declaration from the trial court that the carrier did not have a duty to defend or indemnify the facility, CMI, or the employee if they were found liable because the policy of insurance that it supplied excluded coverage for "professional services." The carrier contended that such services had been rendered by the employee in his care and assessment of the plaintiff following his postexercise untoward event and in his failure to summon medical assistance.

After the insurance carrier's motion to intervene was granted by the trial court, CMI and the employee filed counterclaims against it, seeking a declaration that they were entitled to a defense and indemnification. Cross motions for summary judgment were then filed. The trial court granted the motion of CMI and the employee, finding that the essence of the plaintiff's complaint was one for negligence for failing to implement an emergency response plan and not one for acts or omissions related to the provision or nonprovision of professional services. In this regard, the trial court noted,

> *Common experience also demonstrates that rendering first aid and or even simply making a decision to call a rescue squad generally is not 'professional in nature.' Presumably, these acts and decisions are made by any person coming upon another in distress. Although a person in need of assistance would hope the actor rendering the aid or involved in the decision making process was the most knowledgeable, this most likely does not occur in the course of human events. While rendering first aid requires some skill and decision making, it does not require an educational degree or lengthy training of specialized instruction.*

Therefore, the trial court determined that CMI and the employee were entitled to a legal defense and indemnification, if necessary, from the carrier.

The insurance carrier then appealed this decision to an Ohio Court of Appeals (Tenth Appellate District, Case No. 94APE10-1436) in late 1994. The Court of Appeals upheld the trial court decision and determined that what the employee did amounted to first aid services that

> *did not rise to the level of professional service within the purview of the professional service exclusion [in the insurance policy]. The mere exercise of judgment as was involved in the decision to call or not to call for medical help does not convert the inaction to a professional service [or omission]. At most, the term [as used in the insurance policy and due to the fact that the term, as the trial court found, has received only 'sparse attention' by Ohio courts] is ambiguous in regard to what is professional in this respect and it must be construed to the benefit of the insured.*

As a consequence, the trial court's ruling on the insurance carrier's complaint was upheld.

While the insurance coverage question was being considered on appeal, the underlying personal injury case of the plaintiff was placed on inactive status. However, once the insurance carrier's appeal of the trial court's ruling was determined, the plaintiff's case became active once again. At that point the defendants moved for summary judgment.

In response to the plaintiff's allegations, the defendants contended in their motion for summary judgment that a waiver of liability clause contained in the plaintiff's membership application as signed by the plaintiff barred his suit. The waiver of liability claims paragraph as contained within the membership contract provided as follows:

> **Waiver of claims.** *It is expressly agreed that all use of the Center facilities and any transportation provided by the Center should be undertaken by a member or guest at his/her sole risk, and the Center shall not be liable for any injuries or any damage to any member or guest, or the property of any member or guest, or be subject to any claim, demand, injury or damages whatsoever, including, without any limitation, those damages resulting from acts of active or passive negligence on the part of the Center, its officers or agents. The member, for himself-herself and on behalf of his/her executors, administrators, heirs, assigns and successors, does hereby expressly forever release and discharge the Center, its owners, officers, employees, agents, assigns and successors from all such claims, demands, injuries, damages, actions or causes of action. The Center shall not be responsible or liable to members or their guests for articles damaged, lost or stolen in or about the Center, or in lockers, or for loss of damages to any property including but not limited to automobiles and the contents thereof.*

and prevailed in a subsequent court ruling because the insurance coverage in question stated that it did not apply to bodily injury arising out of the "failure to render any service, treatment, advice or instruction relating to the physical fitness . . . or physical training programs." Because of decisions like this one, facilities and professionals need to make sure they have the proper and appropriate insurance coverages in place to protect them from potential untoward events and lawsuits that may arise from these events.[35-37]

Purchasing Considerations for General and Professional Liability Insurance

As demonstrated in the *Jacob* case, CMI purchased a Commercial General Liability (CGL) policy but had not obtained a professional liability insurance policy to cover the programs and services offered. This case illustrates that programs/services provided by health/fitness professionals and facilities are largely legally undefined. This means there is not adequate case law to determine if the services provided by health/fitness staff members would be covered under a CGL policy, or whether a Professional Liability (PL) insurance policy is needed to provide the necessary added protection for so-called professional negligence. In *York*, the insurance policy specified that it excluded advice and instructional services related to physical fitness. Although this describes what many health/fitness professionals do, this facility should have addressed this exclusion by perhaps purchasing PL insurance. Therefore, it may be prudent for health/fitness professionals and facilities to obtain PL insurance. Because CGL policies generally do not cover "professional" services, PL insurance needs to be purchased separately or through an endorsement that is added to the CGL policy. In all cases, health/fitness professionals and facilities should review their liability insurance needs with insurance and legal experts who are familiar with the types of health/fitness services provided. If at any time, the types of health/fitness services change or a new program is being planned (e.g., an event like a triathlon), it will be important to determine if any changes/additions with the current policies need to be made.

When they are hired, health/fitness professionals should ask their employer the types of liability insurance provided. Generally, health/fitness facilities have CGL policies in place, but they may or may not have a PL insurance policy to cover their employees. If the employer does not provide PL insurance, it may be wise for the health/fitness professional to obtain it on their own or ask their employer to provide it. Also, CGL policies do not cover independent contractors; they only cover employees and perhaps others such as volunteers. Therefore, health/fitness facilities should require independent contractors to have both general and professional liability insurance.

Health/fitness students and professionals who are members of a professional organization can often obtain PL insurance at a low cost through a group plan. For example, the ACSM has an arrangement with an insurance provider, Forrest T. Jones & Company (FTJ), for their group plan that provides coverage up to $2 million in liability protection for each incident and up to $4 million annual aggregate. In addition, ACSM "certified" members can receive a lower premium in some cases. Application forms for students and employed/self-employed health/fitness professionals are available on the FTJ website, www.ftj.com/acsm. This website also contains helpful information about professional liability insurance: See Commonly Asked Questions About Professional Liability Insurance.

Students in academic exercise science (or related areas) programs can also obtain a blanket professional liability insurance policy through Marsh Affinity Group Services (1–800–621–3008) that covers "all" students in the program at a very low cost, e.g., $15 per student). This is especially helpful for students because many internship sites require proof that students have professional liability insurance. Once the blanket policy is purchased, copies of the declarations page can be given to students, who can in turn make a copy for their internship site as proof of coverage.

STEP **2** DEVELOPMENT OF RISK MANAGEMENT STRATEGIES

The preceding section presented relevant laws related to a variety of employment issues. Several case laws examples were described that addressed issues such as employee versus independent contractor status, employer–employee relationship principles such as ostensible agency and *respondeat superior,* employee/agent qualifications, and negligent hiring. The following management risk strategies can be developed that can lead to a reduction in the occurrence of untoward events as well as claims and suits related to these types of employment issues. The following sample documents are included in Appendix 5 and referred to in some of the risk management strategies that follow:

Form 5-1: IRS Form SS-8
Form 5-2: IRS Publication 1779, *Independent Contractor or Employee . . .*
Form 5-3: Sample Employment Agreement
Form 5-4: Sample Independent Contractor Agreement

Risk Management Strategy 1: Comply with existing employment laws and regulations.

Although many employment laws exist to which health/fitness facilities must comply, issues surrounding who is or is not an employee for tax withholding, overtime compensation, and related purposes should be established and followed by each organization using personnel. The use of available resources, including IRS publications (e.g., see Forms 5-1 and 5-2) and informal rulings will assist in the delineation process for such personnel. Such information should be used to address questions about whether service providers are likely to be determined to be employees or independent contractors. When in doubt, legal counsel should be consulted and his or her advice followed.

Risk Management Strategy 2: Hire qualified and competent personnel who provide health/fitness programs and services.

Health/fitness facilities should only hire those professionals who have achieved the necessary requirements, education, training, certifications, and/or licensure (if required). The credentials of all prospective employees should be checked and verified prior to hiring and all credentials including certifications kept up to date. Copies of these documents should be maintained in employer files for all employees. Consider the use of employment contracts for some employees, particularly professionals. See Form 5-3 for an example of such an agreement.

Regardless of whether services are provided by employees, agents, or independent contractors, only those who are competent should provide services within health/fitness facilities. Competence may be based on education, experience, training, certifications, successful completion of a national examination, and/or perhaps even licensure if that comes to pass in the future. Factors such as these, used to demonstrate competence, cannot usually be achieved through short duration training programs, some of which may be superficial at best. In addition, these factors alone do not determine competence. Competence is also based on whether or not a health/fitness professional carried out his or her duties properly. For example, the question may be—did the health/fitness professional know how to properly *apply* principles of safe and effective exercise when providing services to participants?

Risk Management Strategy 3: Ensure that employees have employer-provided liability insurance coverage.

To provide important risk management protection, facilities should make sure that employees are covered by the facilities' liability insurance coverage. If there are exclusions in the provided insurance coverage that may result in a denial of coverage, or if certain employees are excluded, questions should be submitted to the carrier for determination in writing in advance of any event resulting in a claim or suit. If there is no coverage in such general liability insurance policies for certain employees, other liability insurance such as professional liability insurance may need to be secured.

Risk Management Strategy 4: Identify independent contractors as nonemployees.

To avert claims and suits against facilities based on claims that those who were really independent contractors were justifiably and reasonably believed to be employees for which facilities can potentially be held liable, certain steps should be taken. These include the provision or written communications to facility members/users identifying those who serve in independent contractor capacities. The use of different wearing apparel, identification badges, signage, and similar visual aids to notify others of the status of such individuals should be required.

Risk Management Strategy 5: Use written contracts with independent contractors.

The use of signed written contracts that provide and specify the independent contractor relationship between the parties should be secured in advance of service delivery. If such individuals are really independent contractors, the agreement should provide that the facility cannot control or direct the manner and/or method of service delivery. Clients of independent contractors may also need to sign similar contract documents with service providers to protect both the facility and the contractor as to the relationship between the client and the facility and between the client and the independent contractor, all of which should be specified in these contract documents. From a facility perspective, its contracts with independent contractors should require that independent contractors indemnify and hold facilities harmless from suit by those to whom service is provided by the contractors or otherwise and backed up with written proof of liability insurance along with those requirements previously specified. See Form 5-4 for an example of such a contract.

Risk Management Strategy 6: Ensure that independent contractors secure and prove their own liability insurance coverage.

Those who provide service within health and fitness facilities as independent contractors must secure their own liability insurance coverage and provide proof of such coverage to the facilities where service is provided. Insurance binders referred to as ACORD forms can be issued by authorized insurance agents to provide evidence of such coverage in writing and even name others as additional insureds. Insurance coverage contract requirements must also provide 30 or 60 days of advance written notice to facilities of any lapse in or cancellation of coverage.

Risk Management Strategy 7: Perform criminal background checks prior to hiring certain personnel.

Although health/fitness facilities generally are not held liable for criminal acts (e.g., sexual assault) of their employees while performing job tasks, facilities could be held liable for civil claims associated with negligent hiring and supervision. Therefore, health/fitness facilities, particularly those that serve vulnerable populations such as children, older adults, and people with disabilities, should perform background checks on all employees who will be working with these populations. Employees who work closely with clients, such as personal trainers, massage therapists, and so on, may need to be closely evaluated in this regard owing to the nature of their work. Therefore, proper supervision of these employees is also important. Guidelines and training programs such as those published by the YMCA[31] can be helpful in this regard.

✓ PUT INTO PRACTICE CHECKLIST 5-1

Rate your phase of development for each of following risk management strategies related to employment issues:

	Developed	Partially Developed	Not Developed
1. Complying with existing employment laws and regulations.			
2. Hiring qualified and competent personnel who provide health/ fitness programs and services.			
3. Ensuring that employees have employer-sponsored liability insurance coverage.			
4. Identifying independent contractors as nonemployees.			
5. Using written contracts with independent contractors.			
6. Ensuring that independent contractors secure and prove their own liability insurance.			
7. Performing criminal background checks prior to hiring certain personnel.			

SUMMARY

Health/fitness facilities employ and/or contract with a number of professionals to provide programs and services within these settings. The employing entities are responsible for the activities of their employees which are carried out within the scope and course of their employment. Facilities that contract with professionals to provide services within these facilities may not be liable for such professionals' activities if those providing service are truly independent contractors rather than employees. In either case, facilities need to select individuals to render services to their clients who are properly trained and prepared to provide such services. Although evidence of competence in this regard can take several forms, only those who are truly qualified should render these services. Other employment issues were also addressed in this chapter, such as hiring procedures (e.g., performing criminal background checks and using written contracts) and securing appropriate liability insurance for personnel.

RISK MANAGEMENT ASSIGNMENTS

1. Conduct a comprehensive search of available health/fitness certifications. What are the most valid/best certifications? Why?

   _____

   _____

   _____

   _____

2. Continuing education for health/fitness professionals is important. Identify the opportunities that exist in your area.

   _____

   _____

   _____

   _____

3. Develop an in-house staff training program on a specific topic.

_____

_____

_____

_____

4. If independent contractors are providing services at your facility and you do not have them sign a written independent contract, obtain a competent lawyer who specializes in contract law to develop one for your facility that your independent contractors would sign before providing any services.

_____

_____

_____

_____

5. If you do have independent contractors sign an independent contract agreement, have a knowledgeable lawyer who specializes in contract law critique each "section" and make any necessary changes.

_____

_____

_____

_____

6. It appears that licensure may be required for health/fitness professionals in the future. This is a controversial issue in the field. Develop a list of the pros and cons of licensure, and then draw a conclusion which you think is best using a sound rationale.

_____

_____

_____

_____

7. Develop a job description for a personal fitness trainer who is an employee in your health/fitness facility.

_____

_____

_____

_____

8. Develop a contract for a personal fitness trainer who will provide services to health/fitness facility members.

_____

_____

_____

_____

9. Prepare a list of factors that compare and contrast an employee and an independent contractor.

_____

_____

_____

_____

10. Delineate the kind of allegations that might be put forth by an injured party against an employer and an employed personal fitness trainer who allegedly rendered negligent fitness services to that client.

_____

_____

_____

_____

11. Draft a risk management plan for a fitness facility to use to minimize those risks arising from the provision of services by an independently retained personal fitness trainer.

_____

_____

_____

_____

12. Describe what is meant by ostensible agents and _respondeat superior_ and how these legal principles can apply in the health/fitness field.

_____

_____

_____

_____

KEY TERMS

Contractual transfer of risks   Independent contractor   _Respondeat superior_

Employee   Ostensible agents

REFERENCES

1. _Donovan v. Unique Racquetball and Health Clubs, Inc.,_ 674 F.Supp.77 (D. Ct., E.D. N.Y., 1987).
2. _Donovan v. Unique Racquetball and Health Clubs, Inc.,_ 674 F.Supp.77 (D. Ct., E.D. N.Y., 1987), 79.
3. _Donovan v. Unique Racquetball and Health Clubs, Inc.,_ 674 F.Supp.77 (D. Ct., E.D. N.Y., 1987), 80.
4. _Paukstis v. Kenwood Golf & Country Club, Inc., et al.,_ 241 F.Supp.2d 551 (D. Ct., Md., 2003).
5. _Seigneur v. National Fitness Institute, Inc.,_ 132 Md. App. 271 (Md. Ct. Spec. App., 2000). Analyzed in: Herbert DL. Release bars yet another suit. _Exercise Standards and Malpractice Reporter_ 2000;14(6):93–94.
6. _Chai v. Sports & Fitness Clubs of America, Inc.,_ Case No. 98–16053 CA (Broward County Circuit Court, Florida, 17th Judicial District, 2005). Analyzed in: Failure to defibrillate results in new litigation. _Exercise Standards and Malpractice Reporter_ 1999;13:55–56.

7. *Aydelotte v. BQE Racquetball Club, Inc.,* 283 A.D.2d 600 (N.Y. App. Div., 2001).
8. *Aydelotte v. BQE Racquetball Club, Inc.,* 283 A.D.2d 600 (N.Y. App. Div., 2001), 601.
9. *Capati v. Crunch Fitness International, et al.,* Supreme Court of New York, County of New York, 1999. See also *Capati v. Crunch Fitness International, Inc.,* 743 N.Y.S.2d 474 (N.Y. App. Div., 2002).
10. Herbert DL. $300 million lawsuit filed against health club. *Exercise Standards and Malpractice Reporter* 1999;13(3):33, 36.
11. Herbert DL. Wrongful death case of Anne Marie Capati settled for in excess of $4 million. *Exercise Standards and Malpractice Reporter* 2006;20(3):36.
12. Standards setting organizations may be liable to consumer. *Exercise Standards and Malpractice Reporter* 1991;5(1):13.
13. *Parks v. Gilligan,* Docket Number OCN-L-1945–96, Supreme Court of New Jersey, Law Division, Ocean County, February 6, 1998. Analyzed in: Volunteer spotter may be liable for weight lifter's injury. *Exercise Standards and Malpractice Reporter* 1998;12(2):24. (Note: Both volunteer and health club joined in suit—both settled).
14. *Stewart v. Bally Total Fitness,* 2000 WL 1006936 (D. Ct., E.D. Pa., 2000).
15. International Health, Racquet & Sportsclub Association (IHRSA). Who's training your trainers? Available at: https://cms.ihrsa.org/index.cfm?fuseaction=Page.viewPage&pageId=15559&nodeID=15 Accessed December 12, 2007.
16. News release . . . IHRSA establishes position on third-party accreditation for personal training certification programs. *Exercise Standards and Malpractice Reporter* 2004;18(1):10–11.
17. International Health, Racquet & Sportsclub Association (IHRSA). IHRSA provides update on its resolution on third party accreditation of personal training certification programs. Available at: https://cms.ihrsa.org/index.cfm?fuseaction=Page.viewPage&pageID=1806&nodeID=15. Accessed December 12, 2007.
18. President's message regarding personal trainer certification. Available at: http://www.afaa.org. Accessed November 2, 2007.
19. National Board of Fitness Examiners (NBFE). Important Information about the NBFE Registry of Personal Fitness Trainers. n.d. Available at: http://www.nbfe.org/registry/registry_terms.cfm. Accessed November 2, 2007.
20. Eickhoff-Shemek J, Herbert D. Is licensure in your future? Issues to consider—Part 1. *ACSM's Health Fitness J* 2007;11(5):35–37.
21. Eickhoff-Shemek J, Herbert D. Is licensure in your future? Issues to consider—Part 2. *ACSM's Health Fitness J* 2008;12(1):36–38.
22. Eickhoff-Shemek J, Herbert D. Is licensure in your future? Issues to consider—Part 3. *ACSM's Health Fitness J* 2008;12(3):36–38.
23. Herbert DL, Herbert WH. *Legal Aspects of Preventive, Rehabilitative and Recreational Exercise Programs.* 4th ed. Canton, Ohio: PRC; 2002:80–81.
24. *Seigneur v. National Fitness Institute,* 132 Md. App. 271 (Md. Ct. Spec. App., 2000).
25. *Seigneur v. National Fitness Institute,* 132 Md. App. 271 (Md. Ct. Spec. App., 2000), 271, 276.
26. *Seigneur v. National Fitness Institute,* 132 Md. App. 271 (Md. Ct. Spec. App., 2000), 271, 277.
27. *Mathis v. New York Health Club, Inc.,* 288 A.D.2d 56 (N.Y. App. Div., 2001).
28. *Mathis v. New York Health Club, Inc.,* 288 A.D.2d 56 (N.Y. App. Div., 2001), 346.
29. *Geiger v. McClurg Court Associates,* 1988 WL 26853 (D. Ct., N.D. Ill., 1998).
30. Herbert DL. Potential claims of sexual impropriety against health/fitness personnel and facilities. *Exercise Standards and Malpractice Reporter* 1995;9(3): 40–43.
31. *Medical Advisory Committee Recommendations: A Resource Guide for YMCAs.* Chicago: YMCA of the USA; February 2007.
32. Moorman A, Eickhoff-Shemek, J. Risk management strategies for avoiding and responding to sexual assault complaints. *ACSM's Health Fitness J* 2007;11(3):35–37.
33. Herbert DL. Liability insurance for health and fitness facilities: Making sure you're covered—while knowing what's at stake. *Exercise Standards and Malpractice Reporter* 1996;10(3):33, 36–38. (Reprinted with permission, all other rights reserved, PRC Publishing, Inc. Canton, Ohio.)
34. *York Insurance Company v. Houston Wellness Center, Inc.,* 261 Ga. App. 854 (Ga. Ct. App., 2003).
35. Herbert DL. When your insurance company won't pay. *Fitness Management* 2007;23(2):52.
36. Herbert DL. Picking the right liability insurance. *Fitness Management* 1996;12(9):48.
37. Herbert DL. Appeals court determines liability insurance coverage is not available to health club. *Exercise Standards and Malpractice Reporter* 2006;20(6):81, 84.

APPENDIX 5

Form **SS-8**
(Rev. November 2006)
Department of the Treasury
Internal Revenue Service

**Determination of Worker Status
for Purposes of Federal Employment Taxes
and Income Tax Withholding**

OMB No. 1545-0004

Name of firm (or person) for whom the worker performed services

Worker's name

Firm's address (include street address, apt. or suite no., city, state, and ZIP code)

Worker's address (include street address, apt. or suite no., city, state, and ZIP code)

Trade name

Daytime telephone number
(   )

Worker's social security number

Telephone number (include area code)
(   )

Firm's employer identification number

Worker's employer identification number (if any)

Note. If the worker is paid by a firm other than the one listed on this form for these services, enter the name, address, and employer identification number of the payer. ►

Disclosure of Information

The information provided on Form SS-8 may be disclosed to the firm, worker, or payer named above to assist the IRS in the determination process. For example, if you are a worker, we may disclose the information you provide on Form SS-8 to the firm or payer named above. The information can only be disclosed to assist with the determination process. If you provide incomplete information, we may not be able to process your request. See *Privacy Act and Paperwork Reduction Act Notice* on page 5 for more information. **If you do not want this information disclosed to other parties, do not file Form SS-8.**

Parts I–V. All filers of Form SS-8 must complete all questions in Parts I–IV. Part V must be completed if the worker provides a service directly to customers or is a salesperson. If you cannot answer a question, enter "Unknown" or "Does not apply." If you need more space for a question, attach another sheet with the part and question number clearly identified.

Part I   **General Information**

1   This form is being completed by: ☐ Firm ☐ Worker; for services performed _____ (beginning date) to _____ (ending date).

2   Explain your reason(s) for filing this form (for example, you received a bill from the IRS, you believe you erroneously received a Form 1099 or Form W-2, you are unable to get worker's compensation benefits, or you were audited or are being audited by the IRS).

3   Total number of workers who performed or are performing the same or similar services _____.

4   How did the worker obtain the job? ☐ Application ☐ Bid ☐ Employment Agency ☐ Other (specify) _____

5   Attach copies of all supporting documentation (contracts, invoices, memos, Forms W-2 or Forms 1099-MISC issued or received, IRS closing agreements, IRS rulings, etc.). In addition, please inform us of any current or past litigation concerning the worker's status. If no income reporting forms (Form 1099-MISC or W-2) were furnished to the worker, enter the amount of income earned for the year(s) at issue $ _____.

If both Form W-2 and Form 1099-MISC were issued or received, explain why.

6   Describe the firm's business.

7   Describe the work done by the worker and provide the worker's job title.

8   Explain why you believe the worker is an employee or an independent contractor.

9   Did the worker perform services for the firm in any capacity before providing the services that are the subject of this determination request?
☐ Yes ☐ No ☐ N/A
If "Yes," what were the dates of the prior service?
If "Yes," explain the differences, if any, between the current and prior service.

10   If the work is done under a written agreement between the firm and the worker, attach a copy (preferably signed by both parties). Describe the terms and conditions of the work arrangement.

For Privacy Act and Paperwork Reduction Act Notice, see page 5.   Cat. No. 16106T   Form **SS-8** (Rev. 11-2006)

Form SS-8 (Rev. 11-2006) Page **2**

Part II Behavioral Control

1 What specific training and/or instruction is the worker given by the firm? ....

2 How does the worker receive work assignments? ....

3 Who determines the methods by which the assignments are performed? ....

4 Who is the worker required to contact if problems or complaints arise and who is responsible for their resolution? ....

5 What types of reports are required from the worker? Attach examples. ....

6 Describe the worker's daily routine such as, schedule, hours, etc. ....

7 At what location(s) does the worker perform services (e.g., firm's premises, own shop or office, home, customer's location, etc.)? Indicate the appropriate percentage of time the worker spends in each location, if more than one. ....

8 Describe any meetings the worker is required to attend and any penalties for not attending (e.g., sales meetings, monthly meetings, staff meetings, etc.). ....

9 Is the worker required to provide the services personally? . . . . ☐ Yes ☐ No

10 If substitutes or helpers are needed, who hires them? ....

11 If the worker hires the substitutes or helpers, is approval required? . . . . ☐ Yes ☐ No
If "Yes," by whom? ....

12 Who pays the substitutes or helpers? ....

13 Is the worker reimbursed if the worker pays the substitutes or helpers? . . . . ☐ Yes ☐ No
If "Yes," by whom? ....

Part III Financial Control

1 List the supplies, equipment, materials, and property provided by each party:
The firm ....
The worker ....
Other party ....

2 Does the worker lease equipment? . . . . ☐ Yes ☐ No
If "Yes," what are the terms of the lease? (Attach a copy or explanatory statement.) ....

3 What expenses are incurred by the worker in the performance of services for the firm? ....

4 Specify which, if any, expenses are reimbursed by:
The firm ....
Other party ....

5 Type of pay the worker receives: ☐ Salary ☐ Commission ☐ Hourly Wage ☐ Piece Work
☐ Lump Sum ☐ Other (specify) ....
If type of pay is commission, and the firm guarantees a minimum amount of pay, specify amount $ _____ .

6 Is the worker allowed a drawing account for advances? . . . . ☐ Yes ☐ No
If "Yes," how often? ....
Specify any restrictions. ....

7 Whom does the customer pay? . . . . ☐ Firm ☐ Worker
If worker, does the worker pay the total amount to the firm? ☐ Yes ☐ No If "No," explain. ....

8 Does the firm carry worker's compensation insurance on the worker? . . . . ☐ Yes ☐ No

9 What economic loss or financial risk, if any, can the worker incur beyond the normal loss of salary (e.g., loss or damage of equipment, material, etc.)? ....

Form **SS-8** (Rev. 11-2006)

Form SS-8 (Rev. 11-2006)   Page **3**

Part IV Relationship of the Worker and Firm

1   List the benefits available to the worker (e.g., paid vacations, sick pay, pensions, bonuses, paid holidays, personal days, insurance benefits). ....

2   Can the relationship be terminated by either party without incurring liability or penalty? . . . . □ Yes □ No
    If "No," explain your answer. ....

3   Did the worker perform similar services for others during the same time period? . . . . □ Yes □ No
    If "Yes," is the worker required to get approval from the firm? . . . . □ Yes □ No

4   Describe any agreements prohibiting competition between the worker and the firm while the worker is performing services or during any later period. Attach any available documentation. ....

5   Is the worker a member of a union? . . . . □ Yes □ No

6   What type of advertising, if any, does the worker do (e.g., a business listing in a directory, business cards, etc.)? Provide copies, if applicable.
    ....

7   If the worker assembles or processes a product at home, who provides the materials and instructions or pattern? ....

8   What does the worker do with the finished product (e.g., return it to the firm, provide it to another party, or sell it)? ....

9   How does the firm represent the worker to its customers (e.g., employee, partner, representative, or contractor)? ....

10 If the worker no longer performs services for the firm, how did the relationship end (e.g., worker quit or was fired, job completed, contract ended, firm or worker went out of business)? ....

Part V For Service Providers or Salespersons. Complete this part if the worker provided a service directly to customers or is a salesperson.

1   What are the worker's responsibilities in soliciting new customers? ....

2   Who provides the worker with leads to prospective customers? ....

3   Describe any reporting requirements pertaining to the leads. ....

4   What terms and conditions of sale, if any, are required by the firm? ....

5   Are orders submitted to and subject to approval by the firm? . . . . □ Yes □ No

6   Who determines the worker's territory? ....

7   Did the worker pay for the privilege of serving customers on the route or in the territory? . . . . □ Yes □ No
    If "Yes," whom did the worker pay? ....
    If "Yes," how much did the worker pay? . . . . $ _____

8   Where does the worker sell the product (e.g., in a home, retail establishment, etc.)? ....

9   List the product and/or services distributed by the worker (e.g., meat, vegetables, fruit, bakery products, beverages, or laundry or dry cleaning services). If more than one type of product and/or service is distributed, specify the principal one. ....

10 Does the worker sell life insurance full time? . . . . □ Yes □ No

11 Does the worker sell other types of insurance for the firm? . . . . □ Yes □ No
    If "Yes," enter the percentage of the worker's total working time spent in selling other types of insurance . . . . _____%

12 If the worker solicits orders from wholesalers, retailers, contractors, or operators of hotels, restaurants, or other similar establishments, enter the percentage of the worker's time spent in the solicitation . . . . _____%

13 Is the merchandise purchased by the customers for resale or use in their business operations? . . . . □ Yes □ No
    Describe the merchandise and state whether it is equipment installed on the customers' premises. ....

Sign Here ▶   Under penalties of perjury, I declare that I have examined this request, including accompanying documents, and to the best of my knowledge and belief, the facts presented are true, correct, and complete.

_____   Title ▶ _____   Date ▶ _____
Type or print name below signature.

Form **SS-8** (Rev. 11-2006)

General Instructions

Section references are to the Internal Revenue Code unless otherwise noted.

Purpose

Firms and workers file Form SS-8 to request a determination of the status of a worker for purposes of federal employment taxes and income tax withholding.

A Form SS-8 determination may be requested only in order to resolve federal tax matters. If Form SS-8 is submitted for a tax year for which the statute of limitations on the tax return has expired, a determination letter will not be issued. The statute of limitations expires 3 years from the due date of the tax return or the date filed, whichever is later.

The IRS does not issue a determination letter for proposed transactions or on hypothetical situations. We may, however, issue an information letter when it is considered appropriate.

Definition

Firm. For the purposes of this form, the term "firm" means any individual, business enterprise, organization, state, or other entity for which a worker has performed services. The firm may or may not have paid the worker directly for these services.

 If the firm was not responsible for payment for services, be sure to enter the name, address, and employer identification number of the payer on the first page of Form SS-8, below the identifying information for the firm and the worker.

The SS-8 Determination Process

The IRS will acknowledge the receipt of your Form SS-8. Because there are usually two (or more) parties who could be affected by a determination of employment status, the IRS attempts to get information from all parties involved by sending those parties blank Forms SS-8 for completion. Some or all of the information provided on this Form SS-8 may be shared with the other parties listed on page 1. The case will be assigned to a technician who will review the facts, apply the law, and render a decision. The technician may ask for additional information from the requestor, from other involved parties, or from third parties that could help clarify the work relationship before rendering a decision. The IRS will generally issue a formal determination to the firm or payer (if that is a different entity), and will send a copy to the worker. A determination letter applies only to a worker (or a class of workers) requesting it, and the decision is binding on the IRS. In certain cases, a formal determination will not be issued. Instead, an information letter may be issued. Although an information letter is advisory only and is not binding on the IRS, it may be used to assist the worker to fulfill his or her federal tax obligations.

Neither the SS-8 determination process nor the review of any records in connection with the determination constitutes an examination (audit) of any federal tax return. If the periods under consideration have previously been examined, the SS-8 determination process will not constitute a reexamination under IRS reopening procedures. Because this is not an examination of any federal tax return, the appeal rights available in connection with an examination do not apply to an SS-8 determination. However, if you disagree with a determination and you have additional information concerning the work relationship that you believe was not previously considered, you may request that the determining office reconsider the determination.

Completing Form SS-8

Answer all questions as completely as possible. Attach additional sheets if you need more space. Provide information for all years the worker provided services for the firm. Determinations are based on the entire relationship between the firm and the worker. Also indicate if there were any significant changes in the work relationship over the service term.

Additional copies of this form may be obtained by calling 1-800-829-4933 or from the IRS website at *www.irs.gov*.

Fee

There is no fee for requesting an SS-8 determination letter.

Signature

Form SS-8 must be signed and dated by the taxpayer. A stamped signature will not be accepted.

The person who signs for a corporation must be an officer of the corporation who has personal knowledge of the facts. If the corporation is a member of an affiliated group filing a consolidated return, it must be signed by an officer of the common parent of the group.

The person signing for a trust, partnership, or limited liability company must be, respectively, a trustee, general partner, or member-manager who has personal knowledge of the facts.

Where To File

Send the completed Form SS-8 to the address listed below for the firm's location. However, only for cases involving federal agencies, send Form SS-8 to the Internal Revenue Service, Attn: CC:CORP:T:C, Ben Franklin Station, P.O. Box 7604, Washington, DC 20044.

Firm's location:	Send to:
Alaska, Arizona, Arkansas, California, Colorado, Hawaii, Idaho, Illinois, Iowa, Kansas, Minnesota, Missouri, Montana, Nebraska, Nevada, New Mexico, North Dakota, Oklahoma, Oregon, South Dakota, Texas, Utah, Washington, Wisconsin, Wyoming, American Samoa, Guam, Puerto Rico, U.S. Virgin Islands	Internal Revenue Service SS-8 Determinations P.O. Box 630 Stop 631 Holtsville, NY 11742-0630
Alabama, Connecticut, Delaware, District of Columbia, Florida, Georgia, Indiana, Kentucky, Louisiana, Maine, Maryland, Massachusetts, Michigan, Mississippi, New Hampshire, New Jersey, New York, North Carolina, Ohio, Pennsylvania, Rhode Island, South Carolina, Tennessee, Vermont, Virginia, West Virginia, all other locations not listed	Internal Revenue Service SS-8 Determinations 40 Lakemont Road Newport, VT 05855-1555

Instructions for Workers

If you are requesting a determination for more than one firm, complete a separate Form SS-8 for each firm.

 Form SS-8 is not a claim for refund of social security and Medicare taxes or federal income tax withholding.

If the IRS determines that you are an employee, you are responsible for filing an amended return for any corrections related to this decision. A determination that a worker is an employee does not necessarily reduce any current or prior tax liability. For more information, call 1-800-829-1040.

Time for filing a claim for refund. Generally, you must file your claim for a credit or refund within 3 years from the date your original return was filed or within 2 years from the date the tax was paid, whichever is later.

Filing Form SS-8 does not prevent the expiration of the time in which a claim for a refund must be filed. If you are concerned about a refund, and the statute of limitations for filing a claim for refund for the year(s) at issue has not yet expired, you should file Form 1040X, Amended U.S. Individual Income Tax Return, to protect your statute of limitations. File a separate Form 1040X for each year.

On the Form 1040X you file, do not complete lines 1 through 24 on the form. Write "Protective Claim" at the top of the form, sign and date it. In addition, you should enter the following statement in Part II, Explanation of Changes: "Filed Form SS-8 with the Internal Revenue Service Office in (Holtsville, NY; Newport, VT; or Washington, DC; as appropriate). By filing this protective claim, I reserve the right to file a claim for any refund that may be due after a determination of my employment tax status has been completed."

Filing Form SS-8 does not alter the requirement to timely file an income tax return. Do not delay filing your tax return in anticipation of an answer to your SS-8 request. In addition, if applicable, do not delay in responding to a request for payment while waiting for a determination of your worker status.

Instructions for Firms

If a **worker** has requested a determination of his or her status while working for you, you will receive a request from the IRS to complete a Form SS-8. In cases of this type, the IRS usually gives each party an opportunity to present a statement of the facts because any decision will affect the employment tax status of the parties. Failure to respond to this request will not prevent the IRS from issuing a determination letter based on the information he or she has made available so that the worker may fulfill his or her federal tax obligations. However, the information that you provide is extremely valuable in determining the status of the worker.

If you are requesting a determination for a particular class of worker, complete the form for one individual who is representative of the class of workers whose status is in question. If you want a written determination for more than one class of workers, complete a separate Form SS-8 for one worker from each class whose status is typical of that class. A written determination for any worker will apply to other workers of the same class if the facts are not materially different for these workers. Please provide a list of names and addresses of all workers potentially affected by this determination.

If you have a reasonable basis for not treating a worker as an employee, you may be relieved from having to pay employment taxes for that worker under section 530 of the 1978 Revenue Act. However, this relief provision cannot be considered in conjunction with a Form SS-8 determination because the determination does not constitute an examination of any tax return. For more information regarding section 530 of the 1978 Revenue Act and to determine if you qualify for relief under this section, you may visit the IRS website at *www.irs.gov.*

Privacy Act and Paperwork Reduction Act Notice. We ask for the information on this form to carry out the Internal Revenue laws of the United States. This information will be used to determine the employment status of the worker(s) described on the form. Subtitle C, Employment Taxes, of the Internal Revenue Code imposes employment taxes on wages. Sections 3121(d), 3306(a), and 3401(c) and (d) and the related regulations define employee and employer for purposes of employment taxes imposed under Subtitle C. Section 6001 authorizes the IRS to request information needed to determine if a worker(s) or firm is subject to these taxes. Section 6109 requires you to provide your taxpayer identification number. Neither workers nor firms are required to request a status determination, but if you choose to do so, you must provide the information requested on this form. Failure to provide the requested information may prevent us from making a status determination. If any worker or the firm has requested a status determination and you are being asked to provide information for use in that determination, you are not required to provide the requested information. However, failure to provide such information will prevent the IRS from considering it in making the status determination. Providing false or fraudulent information may subject you to penalties. Routine uses of this information include providing it to the Department of Justice for use in civil and criminal litigation, to the Social Security Administration for the administration of social security programs, and to cities, states, and the District of Columbia for the administration of their tax laws. We may also disclose this information to other countries under a tax treaty, to federal and state agencies to enforce federal nontax criminal laws, or to federal law enforcement and intelligence agencies to combat terrorism. We may provide this information to the affected worker(s), the firm, or payer as part of the status determination process.

You are not required to provide the information requested on a form that is subject to the Paperwork Reduction Act unless the form displays a valid OMB control number. Books or records relating to a form or its instructions must be retained as long as their contents may become material in the administration of any Internal Revenue law. Generally, tax returns and return information are confidential, as required by section 6103.

The time needed to complete and file this form will vary depending on individual circumstances. The estimated average time is: Recordkeeping, 22 hrs.; Learning about the law or the form, 47 min.; and Preparing and sending the form to the IRS, 1 hr., 11 min. If you have comments concerning the accuracy of these time estimates or suggestions for making this form simpler, we would be happy to hear from you. You can write to the Internal Revenue Service, Tax Products Coordinating Committee, SE:W:CAR:MP:T:T:SP, 1111 Constitution Ave. NW, IR-6406, Washington, DC 20224. Do not send the tax form to this address. Instead, see *Where To File* on page 4.

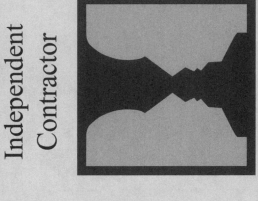

Independent Contractor
or Employee . . . .

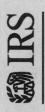

**Department of the Treasury
Internal Revenue Service**

www.irs.gov

Publication 1779 (Rev. 1-2005)
Catalog Number 16134L

IRS Tax Publications

If you are not sure whether you are an employee or an independent contractor, get Form SS-8, *Determination of Worker Status for Purposes of Federal Employment Taxes and Income Tax Withholding.* Publication 15-A, *Employer's Supplemental Tax Guide,* provides additional information on independent contractor status.

IRS Electronic Services

You may download and print IRS publications, forms, and other tax information materials on the Internet at www.irs.gov and you may call the IRS at 1-800-829-3676 (1-800-TAX-FORM) to order free tax publications and forms.

From a fax machine, dial (703) 368-9694 and you will immediately get a list of IRS tax forms faxed back to you. Follow the voice prompts to get specific forms faxed to you.

Publication 1796, *Federal Tax Products on CD-ROM,* of current and prior year tax publications and forms, can be purchased from the National Technical Information Service (NTIS). You may order Publication 1796 toll-free through the IRS at 1-877-233-6767 or via the Internet at www.irs.gov/cdorders.

Call 1-800-829-4933, the Business and Specialty Tax Line, if you have questions related to employment tax issues.

INDEPENDENT CONTRACTOR OR EMPLOYEE

Which are you?

For federal tax purposes, this is an important distinction. Worker classification affects how you pay your federal income tax, social security and Medicare taxes, and how you file your tax return. Classification affects your eligibility for employer and social security and Medicare benefits and your tax responsibilities. If you aren't sure of your work status, you should find out now. This brochure can help you.

The courts have considered many facts in deciding whether a worker is an **independent contractor** or an **employee**. These relevant facts fall into three main categories: *behavioral control; financial control;* and *relationship of the parties.* In each case, it is very important to consider all the facts – no single fact provides the answer. Carefully review the following definitions.

BEHAVIORAL CONTROL

These facts show whether there is a right to direct or control how the worker does the work. A worker is an employee when the business has the right to direct and control the worker. The business does not have to actually direct or control the way the work is done – as long as the employer has the right to direct and control the work.

- **Instructions** – if you receive extensive instructions on how work is to be done, this suggests that you are an employee. Instructions can cover a wide range of topics, for example:
  - how, when, or where to do the work
  - what tools or equipment to use

- what assistants to hire to help with the work
- where to purchase supplies and services

If you receive less extensive instructions about what should be done, but not how it should be done, you may be an **independent contractor.** For instance, instructions about time and place may be less important than directions on how the work is performed

- **Training** – if the business provides you with training about required procedures and methods, this indicates that the business wants the work done in a certain way, and this suggests that you may be an **employee.**

FINANCIAL CONTROL

These facts show whether there is a right to direct or control the business part of the work. For example:

- **Significant Investment** – if you have a significant investment in your work, you may be an **independent contractor.** While there is no precise dollar test, the investment must have substance. However, a significant investment is not necessary to be an **independent contractor.**

- **Expenses** – if you are not reimbursed for some or all business expenses, then you may be an **independent contractor,** especially if your unreimbursed business expenses are high.

- **Opportunity for Profit or Loss** – if you can realize a profit or incur a loss, this suggests that you are in business for yourself and that you may be an **independent contractor.**

RELATIONSHIP OF THE PARTIES

These are facts that illustrate how the business and the worker perceive their relationship. For example:

- **Employee Benefits** – if you receive benefits, such as insurance, pension, or paid

leave, this is an indication that you may be an **employee.** If you do not receive benefits, however, you could be either an **employee** or an **independent contractor.**

- **Written Contracts** – a written contract may show what both you and the business intend. This may be very significant if it is difficult, if not impossible, to determine status based on other facts.

When You Are an *Employee*

- Your employer must withhold income tax and your portion of social security and Medicare taxes. Also, your employer is responsible for paying social security, Medicare, and unemployment (FUTA) taxes on your wages. Your employer must give you a Form W-2, *Wage and Tax Statement,* showing the amount of taxes withheld from your pay.

- You may deduct unreimbursed employee business expenses on Schedule A of your income tax return, but only if you itemize deductions and they total more than two percent of your adjusted gross income.

When You Are an *Independent Contractor*

- The business may be required to give you Form 1099-MISC, *Miscellaneous Income,* to report what it has paid to you.

- You are responsible for paying your own income tax and self-employment tax (Self-Employment Contributions Act – SECA). The business does not withhold taxes from your pay. You may need to make estimated tax payments during the year to cover your tax liabilities.

- You may deduct business expenses on Schedule C of your income tax return.

FORM 5-3
Personal Fitness Trainer's Sample
EMPLOYMENT AGREEMENT†

This Agreement ("Agreement") is made this _____ day of _____, 20____ between _____ ("Employer") and _____ ("Employee").

RECITALS

The purpose of this Agreement is to state the terms and conditions under which the Employer/Employee relationship is created herein and to protect Employer's time and energy expended over the past years in developing its personal fitness training/consulting business, programs and clientele.

The fitness programs, business forms, subscribing client list, and any other related documents are considered trade secrets developed by Employer.

Employer is in the business of providing personal fitness training services, exercise and nutritional counseling, and sales of fitness equipment, products, and services.

Employer desires to have the above services performed by an Employee.

Employee agrees to perform those services for Employer under the terms and conditions set forth in this agreement.

Employer agrees to provide Employee with valuable training, experience, and knowledge in order to perform Employee's services hereunder.

THEREFORE, in consideration of the mutual promises and covenants set forth herein, Employer and Employee agree as follows:

1. NATURE OF WORK

Employee shall be employed as a PERSONAL FITNESS TRAINER. Employee shall perform services including, but not limited to, the following:
   a. Instructing Employer's clients in safe, effective and proper exercise programs;
   b. Training Employer's staff in safe, effective and proper exercise programs;
   c. Promoting Employer's products and services at all times while in the employment of the Employer; and
   d. Furthering and promoting Employer's business, fitness philosophy and policies and procedures.

2. COMPENSATION

Employer shall pay as compensation to Employee for services rendered hereunder, $_____ per client consultation session. In addition, Employer shall pay to Employee _____ percent (__%) of the fee for any of Employer's products sold or additional services provided.

3. OTHER BENEFITS

Employer shall provide Employee with other benefits as outlined in Exhibit "A" attached hereto and incorporated herein by reference.

4. EXPENSES

Employer will further reimburse Employee for all reasonable expenses documented sufficiently for purposes of allowing Employer to deduct said expenses pursuant to the Internal Revenue Code as may be amended from time to time, and properly incurred by Employee after the date hereof and in the performance of Employee's duties hereunder.

5. WITHHOLDING

Employer shall be entitled to withhold amounts from any compensation, or other form of remuneration or benefit payable by Employer to Employee which Employer reasonably believes it is required to withhold under any federal, state, local or foreign tax law to which Employer may be subject.

6. TIME AND EFFORTS

Employee shall devote his/her productive time, energies and abilities to the proper and efficient performance of his/her duties. Without the prior express written authorization of Employer, Employee shall not, directly or indirectly, during the term of this Agreement:
   a. Render services to any other person or firm, whether for compensation or otherwise, or;
   b. Engage in any activity competitive with or adverse to Employer's business, whether alone, as a partner, or as an officer, director or employee of any other corporation.

7. SOLICITING CLIENTS AFTER TERMINATION OF EMPLOYMENT

Upon termination of this Agreement, Employee shall immediately cease training and consulting with any and all of Employer's clients. Employee shall not for a period of two (2) years immediately following the termination of employment with Employer, either directly or indirectly:
   a. make known to any person, firm, or corporation the names and addresses of any of the clients of Employer or any other information pertaining to them; and/or
   b. call on, solicit or take away, or attempt to call on, solicit, or take away any client of the Employer, past, present or future whom Employee knows of or has become acquainted with during Employee's employment with Employer, either for Employee or for any other person or corporation; and/or
   c. call on, solicit or take away, or attempt to call on, solicit, or take away potential clients of the Employer.

8. COMPETING WITH EMPLOYER

Employee shall not for a period of two (2) years immediately following the termination of employment with Employer attempt in any manner either directly or indirectly to compete, or attempt to compete with Employer in personal fitness training activities in Employer's territories in the state of _____.

9. RETURN OF EMPLOYER'S PROPERTY

On the termination of Employee's employment or whenever requested by Employer, Employee shall immediately deliver to Employer all property in Employee's possession or control belonging to Employer.

10. OWNERSHIP OF RECORDS, FORMS AND DOCUMENTS

Any and all records, books, forms, accounts, programs and other documents relating in any manner whatsoever to the clients (past, present, future or potential) and/or business of Employer, whether purchased, prepared or developed by Employee or otherwise coming into Employee's possession, shall be the sole and exclusive property of Employer regardless of who actually prepared, developed or purchased the records, books, forms, accounts, programs or other documents. All such documents shall be immediately returned to Employer by Employee on any termination of Employee's employment or whenever requested by Employer.

11. REFERRALS

Employee understands that any referrals from clients of Employer are the sole property and business of the Employer. Employee shall not solicit for himself or herself, or on the behalf of any other person, corporation, partnership or business, referrals from Employer's clients during employment with Employer, and for a period of two (2) years immediately following termination of employment with the Employer.

12. RECRUITING EMPLOYEES AFTER TERMINATION OF EMPLOYMENT

Employee shall not for a period of two (2) years immediately following the termination of employment with Employer attempt in any manner either directly or indirectly to recruit, or attempt to recruit, any of the officers or employees, present or future, of Employer.

13. DURATION

This Agreement shall commence upon the date first written above and terminate upon the happening of any of the following events:
  a. Upon the death or permanent disability of Employee.
  b. Whenever Employer and Employee shall mutually agree to termination.
  c. Upon thirty (30) days prior written notice by either Employer or Employee to the other, with or without cause.
  d. Immediately upon written notice by Employer to Employee.

14. REMEDIES

Employee agrees that in the event of breach of any provisions of this Agreement, Employee shall be liable to Employer for any and all expenses, costs and reasonable attorneys' fees incurred to enforce Employer's rights under this Agreement plus the amount of loss, both direct and consequential, to Employer arising from or related to such breach.

15. SEVERABILITY

In the event that any one or more of the provisions contained in this Agreement shall for any reason be held to be invalid, illegal or unenforceable in any respect, such invalidity, illegality or unenforceability shall not affect any other provision thereof and this Agreement shall be construed as if such invalid, illegal, or unenforceable provision had never been contained herein.

16. GOVERNING LAW

This Agreement shall be construed in accordance with and governed by the laws of the State of _____.

17. AMENDMENTS

This Agreement may not be modified or amended or any term or provision thereof waived or discharged except in writing and signed by both Employer and Employee.

18. **ENTIRE AGREEMENT**

This Agreement embodies the entire agreement between Employer and Employee and supersedes all prior written and/or oral agreements and understandings between Employer and Employee.

19. **ADDITIONAL PROVISIONS**

Employee shall maintain the following:
a. Current membership in, and certification by:

_____

b. Current CPR certification.

IN WITNESS WHEREOF, the parties hereto have executed this Agreement as of the date above first written.

_____
Name of Company

by: _____
its Authorized Representative
"EMPLOYER"

_____
"EMPLOYEE"

FORM 5-4
Personal Fitness Trainer's Sample
INDEPENDENT CONTRACTOR AGREEMENT

This Agreement ("Agreement") is made this _____ day of _____, 20____ between _____ ("Employer") and _____ ("Independent Contractor").

RECITALS

The purpose of this Agreement is to state the terms and conditions under which the Employer/Independent Contractor relationship is created herein and to protect Employer's time and energy expended over the past years in developing its personal fitness training/consulting business, programs and clientele.

The fitness programs, business forms, subscribing client list, and any other related documents are considered trade secrets developed by Employer.

Employer is in the business of providing personal fitness training services, exercise and nutritional counseling, and sales of fitness equipment, products, and services.

Employer desires to have the above services performed by an Independent Contractor.

Independent Contractor agrees to perform those services for Employer under the terms and conditions set forth in this agreement.

Employer agrees to provide Employee with valuable raining, experience, and knowledge in order to perform Employee's services hereunder.

THEREFORE, in consideration of the mutual promises and covenants set forth herein, Employer and Employee agree as follows:

1. NATURE OF WORK

Independent Contractor shall be employed as a PERSONAL FITNESS TRAINER. Contractor shall perform services including, but not limited to, the following:
   a. Instructing Employer's clients in safe, effective and proper exercise programs;
   b. Providing safe, effective and proper nutritional counseling to Employer's clients;
   c. Promoting Employer's products and services at all times while in the employment of the Employer; and,
   d. Furthering and promoting Employer's business, fitness philosophy and policies and procedures.

2. COMPENSATION

As a PERSONAL FITNESS TRAINER, Employer shall pay as compensation to Independent Contractor for services rendered hereunder, $_____ per client consultation session. In addition, Employer shall pay to Independent Contractor, _____ percent (___%) of the fee for any of Employer's products sold or additional services provided.

3. STATUS OF INDEPENDENT CONTRACTOR

The parties intend that an Employer/Independent Contractor relationship be created by this Agreement. Employer is only interested in the results to be achieved, and the conduct and control of the work will lie solely with the Independent Contractor. Independent Contractor is not to be considered an agent or employee of Employer for any purpose. It is understood that Employer does not agree to use Independent Contractor exclusively. It is further understood that Independent Contractor is free to engage in the performance of his own personal client consultation pursuant to the terms and conditions of this Agreement. Independent Contractor agrees and covenants that in the performance of training, counseling, or advising personal clients, Independent Contractor shall not:

   a. Train any personal client simultaneously with any of Employer's clients;
   b. Wear Employer's uniform while training a personal client;
   c. Use any of Employer's forms, charts, business cards, stationary, or any other related documents pertaining to Employer's business;
   d. Represent to a personal client or act in any manner that tends to represent to the personal client that the client is being trained under the guidelines, principles, or formulas of Employer;
   e. Engage in the unauthorized sale of any services, goods, or products on behalf of Employer. Independent Contractor agrees not to sell, offer to sell, or distribute, with or without compensation, any services, goods, or products of Employer except with the express approval of Employer.

4. SOLICITING CLIENTS AFTER TERMINATION OF EMPLOYMENT

Upon termination of this Agreement, Independent Contractor shall immediately cease training any and all of Employer's clients. Independent Contractor shall not for a period of one (1) year immediately following the termination of employment with Employer, either directly or indirectly:

   a. make known to any person, firm, or corporation the names and addresses of any of the clients of the Employer or any other information pertaining to them; and/or
   b. call on, solicit or take away, or attempt to call on, solicit, or take away any client of the Employer, past, present or future whom the Independent Contractor knows of or has become acquainted with during the Independent Contractor's employment with the Employer, either for the Independent Contractor or for any other person or corporation; and/or
   c. call on, solicit or take away, or attempt to call on, solicit, or take away potential clients of the Employer.

5. COMPETING WITH EMPLOYER

Independent Contractor shall not both during Employment with Employer and for a period of one (1) year immediately following the termination of employment with Employer, attempt to compete with Employer in the personal fitness/consultation business in Employer's territories.

6. RETURN OF EMPLOYER'S PROPERTY

On the termination of Independent Contractor's employment or whenever requested by Employer, Independent Contractor shall immediately deliver to Employer all property in Independent Contractor's possession or control belonging to Employer.

7. OWNERSHIP OF RECORDS, FORMS AND DOCUMENTS

Any and all records, books, forms, accounts, programs and other documents relating in any manner whatsoever to the clients (past, present, future or potential) and/or business of Employer, whether purchased, prepared or developed by Independent Contractor or otherwise coming into Independent Contractor's possession, shall be the sole and exclusive property of Employer regardless of who actually prepared, developed or purchased the records, books, forms, accounts, programs or other documents. All such documents shall be immediately returned to Employer by Independent Contractor on any termination of Independent Contractor's employment or whenever requested by Employer. If Independent Contractor purchases any such original books or documents, he/she shall immediately notify Employer, who then shall immediately reimburse him/her.

8. REFERRALS

Independent Contractor understands that any referrals from clients of Employer are the sole property and business of the Employer. Independent Contractor shall not solicit for himself or herself, or on the behalf of any other person, corporation, partnership or business, referrals from Employer's clients during employment with Employer, and for a period of one (1) year immediately following termination of employment with Employer.

9. RECRUITING EMPLOYEE'S AFTER TERMINATION OF EMPLOYMENT

Independent Contractor shall not for a period of one (1) year immediately following the termination of employment with Employer attempt in any manner either directly or indirectly to recruit, or attempt to recruit, any of the officers or employees, present or future, of Employer.

10. LIABILITY AND INDEMNIFICATION

The work to be performed under this Agreement will be performed entirely at Independent Contractor's risk and independent Contractor agrees to provide his own professional liability insurance. Independent Contractor agrees to indemnify Employer for any and all liability or loss arising in any way out of the performance of the services of Independent Contractor under this Agreement.

11. LIABILITY FOR TAXES

Independent Contractor agrees that all state and federal withholding taxes, social security taxes, unemployment insurance contributions and assessments, worker's compensation insurance, general excise and sales taxes, self-employment taxes, and any and all other taxes, fees, assessments or contributions covering Independent Contractor, if any, shall be the sole responsibility of Independent Contractor.

12. DURATION

Either party may cancel this Agreement upon fifteen (15) days notice to the other.

13. MINIMUM COMMITMENT

Independent Contractor agrees to make himself or herself available to Employer to train a minimum of five (5) clients per week. Employer is not obligated to provide Independent Contractor with the minimum commitment stated above, but will make a good faith attempt to provide Independent Contractor with as many clients as Independent Contractor desires.

14. REMEDIES

Independent Contractor agrees that in the event of breach of any provision of this Agreement, Independent Contractor shall be liable to Employer for any and all expenses, costs and reasonable attorneys' fees incurred to enforce Employer's rights under this Agreement plus the amount of loss, both direct and consequential, to Employer arising from or related to such breach.

15. SEVERABILITY

In the event that any one or more of the provisions contained in this Agreement shall for any reason be held to be invalid, illegal, or unenforceable in any respect, such invalidity, illegality, or unenforceability shall not affect any other provision thereof and this Agreement shall be construed as if such invalid, illegal, or unenforceable provision had never been contained herein.

16. ADDITIONAL PROVISIONS

Independent Contractor shall maintain the following:
a. Current membership in, and certification by:
b. Current CPR certification;
c. His/her own professional liability insurance and health insurance;

IN WITNESS WHEREOF, the parties hereto have executed this Agreement as of the date above first written.

_____

By: _____
Its Authorized Representative
"EMPLOYER"

_____

"INDEPENDENT CONTRACTOR"

CHAPTER 6

The Pre-Activity Health Screening Process

LEARNING OBJECTIVES After reading this chapter, health/fitness students and professionals will be able to:

1. Identify applicable laws related to the pre-activity health screening process and use them in the development of risk management strategies.

2. Describe the various published standards of practice that address the pre-activity health screening process and apply them in the development of risk management strategies.

3. Understand the three major steps in the pre-activity screening process and develop risk management strategies that address each step.

This chapter describes statutory, administrative, and case law, as well as various standards of practice published by professional organizations relevant to the pre-activity health screening process. In addition, specific risk management strategies are presented to guide health/fitness professionals and their risk management advisory committees in the development of their own risk management strategies related to the pre-activity health screening process.

STEP 1 ASSESSMENT OF LEGAL LIABILITY EXPOSURES

This section presents laws and published standards of practice related to the pre-activity health screening process, but first it is important to understand the reasons for conducting pre-activity health screening. In Chapter 1, we discussed both health risks and injury risks as two categories of risks associated with physical fitness activities. The major purpose of pre-activity health screening is to identify those individuals who may have any health risks—medical conditions and/or risk factors that could lead to life-threatening situations such as cardiac arrest and stroke.

According to the American Heart Association (AHA), one in three American adults has one or more forms of cardiovascular disease (CVD), for example, high blood pressure, coronary heart disease, congestive heart failure, stroke, and so on.[1] In the United States, CVD accounts for more deaths each year than any other single cause or group of causes of death.[1] As most health/fitness professionals know, regular physical activity can decrease the incidence of CVD. However, vigorous exercise can increase the risk of sudden cardiac death (SCD) and acute myocardial infarction (AMI) in individuals with preexisting CVD.[2] Pre-activity health screening identifies those individuals who have known CVD, but it also attempts to identify those who may be at risk for CVD but are not aware of it by assessing signs/symptoms and risk factors associated with CVD. For more information about exercise and cardiovascular risks, health/fitness professionals should refer to a recent ACSM/AHA joint position paper.[3] According to ACSM, the purposes of pre-activity health screening are as follows:

- Identification and exclusion of individuals with medical contraindications to exercise.
- Identification of individuals at increased risk for disease because of age, symptoms, and/or risk factors who should undergo a medical evaluation and exercise testing before starting an exercise program.
- Identification of persons with clinically significant disease who should participate in a medically supervised exercise program.
- Identification of individuals with other specific needs.[4]

For most health/fitness facilities, the **pre-activity health screening process** involves three steps: (1) obtaining health information from a participant using some type of a screening device, (2) determining from the health information obtained whether or not the participant should obtain physician clearance, and (3) informing participants of the inherent risks associated with physical activity prior to participation. Certain federal and state laws should be reviewed and discussed by health/fitness professionals and their risk management advisory committees to determine if such screening processes are applicable to their health/fitness facilities.

The Law

Health/fitness professionals need to be aware of federal and state statutory and administrative laws that apply to the pre-activity health screening process. These include the Health Insurance Portability and Accountability Act (HIPAA), Americans with Disabilities Act (ADA), and state privacy laws. In addition, health/fitness professionals should understand that failure to conduct pre-activity health screening has been a claim made by plaintiffs in various legal cases and may be contrary to published standards of practice.

Administrative and Statutory Law

The Health Insurance Portability and Accountability Act (HIPAA) of 1996 contained provisions that mandated the protection of private individual health information. These provisions were included in the legislation because of the many advances in electronic technology and the risks this technology could impose on an individual's privacy. Therefore, what has become known as HIPAA's Privacy Rule[5] was published by Health and Human Services (HHS) and became effective on April 14, 2001. It required covered entities that provide health care services and who bill electronically (i.e., health plans, health care clearinghouses, and health care providers) to be compliant by April 14, 2003. Generally, most health/fitness facilities may not be considered covered entities according to HIPAA's definition, but some health promotion and disease prevention programs may be subject to the act's provisions.[6]

HIPAA's Privacy Rule protects all individually identifiable health information known as *protected health information* (PHI) and includes demographic data related to:

- "the individual's past, present or future physical or mental health, or condition,
- the provision of health care to the individual, or
- the past, present, or future payment for the provision of health care to the individual."[7]

Therefore, any type of data that can identify an individual or could reasonably be expected to identify an individual, such as name, telephone number, Social Security number, address, and birthdate, must be protected. Health/fitness professionals should be familiar with the following HIPAA-related definitions and should discuss with their risk management advisory committees how they could ensure these three basic elements are implemented when handling an individual's PHI electronically, by paper, or orally.

> **Privacy:** Privacy is the right of an individual to enjoy freedom from intrusion or observation; the right to maintain control over certain personal information; and the right to expect health care providers to respect the individual's rights.
> **Confidentiality:** Confidentiality is the practice of permitting only certain authorized individuals to access information, with the understanding that they will disclose it only to other authorized individuals.
> **Security:** Security refers to the physical, technical, and administrative safeguards used to control access and protect information from accidental or intentional disclosure to unauthorized person(s), and from alteration or destruction to maintain the integrity of the information.[8]

Sanctions for not complying with HIPAA's Privacy Rule can result in severe criminal penalties, including incarceration, large fines, or both. An individual can file a complaint with the Department of Health and Human Services Office of Civil Rights, HIPAA's enforcement agency. In addition to criminal penalties, the failure to keep PHI private, confidential, and secure can result in a civil claim/lawsuit under state law (e.g., an invasion-of-privacy tort).[6] For more information on HIPAA, visit http://dhhs.gov/ocr/hipaa. The site includes a summary of the HIPAA Privacy Rule published by the Office of Civil Rights (OCR).

State privacy statutes should also be reviewed by legal counsel with regard to their applicability to health information obtained during pre-activity health screening. Generally these statutes apply to health care providers and their patients and therefore may not apply to health/fitness professionals. However, whether or not state privacy laws (or HIPAA) apply to health/fitness facilities, it is best to take steps to keep health information obtained in pre-activity health screening (or by other means through fitness testing, educational programs, accident report forms, etc.) private, confidential, and secure to prevent any unintended uses. For example, unintended uses can include the sale to others (e.g., businesses seeking member profile information) or disclosure to individuals who do not have a need or requirement to know.[9] Failure to keep health information private, confidential, and secure can result in civil claims such as "breach of contract, intentional or negligent infliction of emotional distress, invasion of privacy, libel, slander, or even disparagement."[10]

In 1990 the ADA was enacted, prohibiting discrimination against persons with disabilities.[11] The ADA defines a person with a disability as someone who (a) has a physical or mental impairment that substantially limits one or more of the major life activities (*an actual disability*), (b) has a record of such an impairment (*a history of a physical or mental disability*), or (c) is regarded as having such an impairment (*a perceived disability*).[12] See Table 6-1 for definitions provided in the ADA that further describe these three categories of persons with disabilities.

The ADA is made up of five titles, two of which are applicable to health/fitness facilities: Title I—Employment and Title III—Public Accommodations and Services Operated by Private Entities.[13] Title III applies to the pre-activity health screening process. In addition to addressing architectural barriers such as steps/curbs (versus ramps), conventional doors (versus automatic doors), and stairs (versus elevators), Title III also prohibits discrimination with regard to programs and services offered by places of public accommodation. Title III lists 12 categories of places of public accommodation. One of these includes "a gymnasium, health spa, bowling alley, golf course, or other place of exercise or recreation."[14] Therefore, health/fitness facilities are considered

TABLE 6-1	ADA Definitions

(1) The phrase physical or mental impairment means—

(i) Any physiological disorder or condition, cosmetic disfigurement, or anatomical loss affecting one or more of the following body systems: neurological; musculoskeletal; special sense organs; respiratory, including speech organs; cardiovascular; reproductive; digestive; genitourinary; hemic and lymphatic; skin; and endocrine;

(ii) Any mental or psychological disorder such as mental retardation, organic brain syndrome, emotional or mental illness, and specific learning disabilities;

(iii) The phrase physical or mental impairment includes, but is not limited to, such contagious and noncontagious diseases and conditions as orthopedic, visual, speech, and hearing impairments, cerebral palsy, epilepsy, muscular dystrophy, multiple sclerosis, cancer, heart disease, diabetes, mental retardation, emotional illness, specific learning disabilities, HIV disease (whether symptomatic or asymptomatic), tuberculosis, drug addiction, and alcoholism;

(iv) The phrase physical or mental impairment does not include homosexuality or bisexuality.

(2) The phrase major life activities means functions such as caring for one's self, performing manual tasks, walking, seeing, hearing, speaking, breathing, learning, and working.

(3) The phrase has a record of such an impairment means has a history of, or has been misclassified as having, a mental or physical impairment that substantially limits one or more major life activities.

(4) The phrase is regarded as having an impairment means—

(i) Has a physical or mental impairment that does not substantially limit major life activities but that is treated by a private entity as constituting such a limitation;

(ii) Has a physical or mental impairment that substantially limits major life activities only as a result of the attitudes of others toward such impairment; or

(iii) Has none of the impairments defined in paragraph (1) of this definition but is treated by a private entity as having such an impairment.

ADA Title III, Part 36—Nondiscrimination on the Basis of Disability by Public Accommodation and in Commercial Facilities. Part 36.104 Definitions, pp. 5–6. Available at: http://www.ada.gov/reg3a.html. Accessed June 26, 2006.

places of public accommodation under the ADA, which requires them to make "reasonable accommodations" with regard to their programs and services. With reference to pre-activity health screening, it means that persons with disabilities are treated the same way as other participants (e.g., the procedures and the criteria used to determine if physician clearance is needed must be the same for all individuals). For example, in *Larsen v. Carnival Corp., Inc.*, the court ruled that the defendant's screening actions were not discriminatory under the ADA.[15] In Herbert's analysis of *Larsen*, he stated that "applying the same reasoning to the situation where a health and fitness facility excludes an individual from participation absent a medical clearance, it appears such action may be justifiable, and non-discriminatory under the ADA so long as such actions are actually based upon neutral, non-discriminatory and appropriate criteria."[16]

Failure to comply with the ADA can result in serious consequences for property owners such as **injunctions,** a court order that requires the property owner to do something (e.g., installing a ramp) or to refrain from doing something, and civil penalties in the form of monetary damages that the ADA establishes (e.g., up to $50,000 for the first violation and up to $100,000 for subsequent violations).[17] In addition to the ADA, health/fitness professionals and their risk management advisory committees should also review other federal laws (e.g., the Rehabilitation Act of 1973) as well as similar state and local laws to determine applicability to their facility and programs.

Case Law

Several cases exist in which plaintiffs have claimed that the defendant health/fitness facility failed to conduct pre-activity health screening. To date, it appears from a review of published cases regarding litigation over the participant screening issue that it has infrequently been raised. No health/fitness facilities have been found liable for negligence, via omission or commission, related *solely* to pre-activity health screening. However, the fact that this issue has been raised in legal cases and because of the many published standards of practice that address pre-activity health screening (discussed later), it is essential that health/fitness professionals develop and implement pre-activity health screening procedures into their overall risk management plan.

In *Contino v. Lucille Roberts Health Spa*,[18] Linda Contino was advised by her chiropractor (who treated her for back problems) to take an aerobic dance class to relieve her tension headaches. During an aerobics dance class, she fell and injured her back. She claimed the class was overcrowded, improperly supervised, negligently conducted by the defendants' personnel, and that the defendants' failed to use due care in screening her to determine if she was physically capable of taking such classes or if any physical conditions disqualified her. She also claimed the defendants (Lucille Roberts Health Spa and Spa Shop Management Inc.) failed to warn her of the dangers of aerobics for people with back problems.

The defendants then brought a third-party action against the appellant (the chiropractor) for indemnification and/or contribution alleging that his improper advice to Contino to take an aerobics class contributed to the plaintiff's injury. The chiropractor moved to dismiss this third-party complaint, arguing that the primary defendants' alleged torts were successive and independent and therefore they could not obtain contribution (for negligence) from him. The court disagreed, stating that the third-party complaint should not be dismissed because it was possible that the negligence of both the primary defendants and the appellant contributed to the plaintiff's injury.

In *Rutnik v. Colonie Center Court Club, Inc.*,[19] a 47-year-old man collapsed and died while participating in a racquetball tournament sponsored by the American Amateur Racquetball Association (AARA) and Colonie Center Court Club, Inc. CPR was immediately performed by a physician who was also participating in the tournament and by a bystander. In addition, EMS was called with a unit arriving within five minutes that took him to the hospital. The cause of death was determined to be cardiac arrest related to atherosclerotic heart disease. The estate of the decedent brought a wrongful death action against the defendants claiming that "(1) defendant failed to ensure that the decedent was in good health before permitting his participation in the tournament, (2) defendants failed to have proper procedures, personnel and equipment (i.e., defibrillator) ready to respond to medical emergencies at their tournament, and (3) defendants failed to warn decedent of the risks of his participation."[20]

The defendants moved for summary judgment contending they did not owe a duty to the decedent because he assumed the risks when he volunteered to participate in the tournament. The trial court did not grant the motion for summary judgment and the defendants appealed. On appeal, the appellate court reversed the trial court's decision and ruled in favor of the defendants stating, "It is well-settled law that voluntary participants in sporting events assume the risk of injuries normally associated with the sport."[20] In addition, because the decedent was an experienced racquetball player and had participated in similar tournaments previously, the court concluded that the decedent should have known there was an apparent and foreseeable risk of cardiac arrest while participating in a strenuous sport such as racquetball. The court also stated that "relieving an owner or operator of a sporting facility from liability for the inherent risk of engaging in sports is justified when the consenting participant is aware of the risk, has appreciation of the nature of the risk and voluntarily assumes the risk."[20]

This is an excellent case to demonstrate how the assumption of risk defense can work in favor of defendants when participants are clearly aware of inherent risks, have an appreciation for them, and voluntarily assume them. With regard to the claim that the defendants were negligent in failing to have a defibrillator present, the courts stated that this lacked merit, stating "the entire staff at the Court Club was trained in CPR, that emergency 911 was called shortly after decedent collapsed and that a rescue squad arrived at the facility within five minutes,"[20] which, according to this court, demonstrated performance of their duties in a reasonable manner.

In *Chai v. Sports & Fitness Clubs of America Inc.*,[21,22] the plaintiff member suffered a cardiopulmonary arrest while exercising at the defendant's club ("Q" The Sports Club) and consequently was left in a vegetative state. He was 40 years of age at the time of the event, a husband and father of three children. Many of the allegations of negligence in this case were provided in Chapter 5, but the following specifically pertained to pre-activity health screening: "Negligently failed to require prescreening of members, including . . . [the member], to assess his fitness and health, prior to his use of the Defendant's exercise facilities."[21]

Interestingly in this case, there was a pre-verdict settlement between the two parties—if a defense verdict was returned, the plaintiff would receive no less that $2.25 million and if a plaintiff's verdict was returned, the plaintiff would receive no more than $7 million. The jury ruled in favor of the defense, and therefore the plaintiff received $2.25 million. Although the defendant club was not found negligent of any of the allegations just listed, this case may demonstrate that the defendant perhaps was not confident (given the pretrial settlement agreement) it would prevail at trial—perhaps because the jury may have been sympathetic toward the plaintiff and therefore ruled in favor of the plaintiff by finding the defendant liable for conduct inconsistent with the standard of care.

Another interesting factor in *Chai* was that the plaintiff did sign an Assumption of Risk document upon becoming a member of the club, which stated, in part, "I understand that it is my responsibility to seek physician approval concerning any preexisting health risks. I understand that there are some discomforts and risks associated with physical activity, such as muscle soreness, strains and sprains, and very rarely cardiovascular problems including high blood pressure and, very rarely, 'heart attack.'"[21] Although this was clearly an express assumption of risk (written document signed by the plaintiff; see Chapter 4), the defendant did not appear to rely on it as a viable defense, given the pre-verdict settlement agreement. Whereas in *Rutnik*, the assumption of risk defense is what protected the defendant from liability, and based on what is known from this case, it was not in an express written form.

In another case, *Julianna Tringali Mayer v. L.A. Fitness International, LLC*,[23] a Florida court rendered a verdict (sum of $616,650) in favor of the family of Alessio Tringali, who died while working out at the defendant's fitness facility. Many of the claims in this wrongful death complaint addressed issues related to emergency care, including the failure of the fitness facility to have on the premises an automated external defibrillator (AED). However, one of the claims also addressed the failure of the fitness facility to conduct pre-activity health screening. The plaintiff claimed that the defendant acted negligently and carelessly and breached its duty "by failing to properly screen the Plaintiffs Decedent's health condition at or about the time that he joined Defendant's health club."[24]

In the preceding cases, the plaintiffs made various claims of negligence along with the claim that the defendant failed to conduct pre-activity health screening, so it is difficult to conclude how a court might rule on the pre-activity health screening issue by itself. However, *Rostai v. Neste Enterprises*[25] is a recent case that specifically addressed the pre-activity health screening issue. This case is also analyzed in Chapter 4 as an illustrative case that focused on the primary assumption of risk defense. Rostai entered into an agreement with defendants Jared Shoultz and Neste Enterprises (dba Gold's Gym) to provide him with a personalized fitness program. During his *first* training workout with personal trainer Shoultz, Rostai allegedly suffered a heart attack toward the end of his 60-minute session. In his negligent action, Rostai claimed the defendants owed him a duty to investigate his health history, physical condition, and cardiac risk factors. He also claimed that Shoultz knew he was not physically fit and was overweight, but aggressively trained him in his first workout although he complained several times during the workout he needed a break. The defendants moved for summary judgment, asserting primary assumption of risk as their defense.

The trial court granted the defendant's motion for summary judgment and the plaintiff appealed. Upon appeal, the appellate court affirmed the trial court's decision, agreeing with the defendant's defense that the plaintiff assumed the risks. The plaintiff contended in his appeal that the doctrine of primary assumption of risk applied only to sports and not to fitness training. However, the appellate court disagreed with this view, citing previous California cases that have concluded that primary assumption of risk is not limited to sports but also applies to any activities that contain elements of risk or danger. In *Rostai,* the appellate court stated, "Fitness training under the guidance of a personal trainer is such an activity. The obvious purpose of working out with a personal trainer is to improve physical fitness and appearance. In order to accomplish that goal, the participant must engage in strenuous physical activity. The risks inherent in that activity include physical distress in general and in particular muscle strains, sprains, . . . not only in the obvious muscles such as those in the legs and arms, but also of less obvious muscles such as the heart. . . . Eliminating that risk would alter the fundamental nature of the activity."[26] Note: Most health/fitness professionals would disagree with this court's view that a participant "must engage in strenuous physical activity" to improve fitness and appearance.

In response to the plaintiff's claim that Shoultz failed to assess his physical condition and in particular his cardiac risk factors, and challenged him to perform beyond his level of physical ability and fitness, the court stated, "That challenge, however, is the very purpose of fitness training, and is precisely the reason one would pay for the services of a personal trainer. Like the coach in other sports or physical activities, the personal trainer's role in physical fitness training is not only to instruct the participant in proper exercise techniques but also to develop a training program that requires the participant to stretch his or her current abilities in order to become more physically fit. The trainer's function in the training process is, at bottom, to urge and challenge the participant to work muscles to their limits and to overcome physical and psychological barriers to doing so. Inherent in that process is the risk that the trainer will not accurately assess the participant's ability and the participant will be injured as a result."[27] Note: Most health/fitness professionals would again disagree with this court's view that it is the "trainer's function . . . to challenge the participant to work muscles to their limits" and therefore "inherent in that process is the risk that the trainer will not accurately assess the participant's ability."

Rostai was 46 years old, overweight (5 feet 10 inches tall and weighed 228 pounds) and inactive. Given these risk factors, he probably should have had physician clearance prior to starting an exercise program, based on published standards of practice (discussed later). However, it appears that no published standards of practice with regard to pre-activity health screening were introduced into the evidence before the court (through the testimony of an expert witness) as evidence of the standard of care. The trial court sustained (approved) defendants' objection to a portion of a declaration made by expert witness Dr. Girandola (associate professor of exercise science at the University of Southern California) that stated "greater scrutiny should be exercised in monitoring individuals at health and fitness clubs like Gold's Gym" and that "defendant Gold's Gym's acts and omissions also constituted a substantial factor in the cause of the [plaintiffs] heart attack."[28] The appellate court's response to this was that it was not relevant because whether a duty of care exists is an issue for the court to resolve. Note: Yes, the court does determine duty in negligence cases, but most courts allow expert testimony to educate the court as to what the standard of care (or duty) was that the defendant owed to the plaintiff. It appears this court did not do that.

Again, relying on previous California case law to support its decision, the appellate court stated that the doctrine of primary assumption of the risk "embodies a legal conclusion that there is 'no duty' on the part of the defendant to protect the plaintiff from a particular risk."[29] Interestingly, the appellate court did state that the evidence showed that defendant Shoultz did not accurately assess plaintiff's level of fitness and he may have interpreted plaintiff's complaints (e.g., tiredness, shortness of breath, profuse sweating) as usual signs of physical exertion rather than symptoms of a heart attack. However, because no evidence indicated that Shoultz's conduct was intentional or reckless, which would have increased the risks to Rostai, the court concluded there was no evidence that Shoultz breached any duty owed to the plaintiff. Note: As discussed in Chapter 4, primary assumption of risk is a defense that generally applies only to injuries due to "inherent" risks—not those caused by negligence (e.g., where the defendant, via his or her conduct, has increased the risks on the plaintiff above and beyond those that are inherent). However, this court expands this defense in this case to include the failure of the personal trainer to assess health risks and to properly train (given the health/fitness status of an individual) and monitor for signs/symptoms of overexertion when training a sedentary individual. Other courts are more likely to view all of these failures as negligent omissions and acts of the personal trainer, especially if expert witnesses were allowed to educate the court through their testimony as to the standard of care in this regard, and because of such, not apply the assumption of risk defense.

Rostai is the first case to focus clearly on the question of whether or not personal trainers have a duty to conduct pre-activity health screening. Although the outcome of the *Rostai* case (i.e., personal trainers do not have a duty to conduct pre-activity health screening) may set a precedent in a portion of California (Fourth District), it is not an outcome in which personal trainers and health/fitness facilities should rely. Primary assumption of risk did apply in *Rutnik*, but the plaintiff was an experienced racquetball player and therefore the court believed he was fully informed, understood, and appreciated the risks. Whereas in *Chai*, even with an assumption of risk document signed by the plaintiff prior to participation, assumption of risk did not appear to be a viable defense for the defendant. However, in *Rostai*, the primary assumption of risk defense did protect the defendants from liability, but the court's application of this defense is questionable given the conduct of the personal trainer and the fact that the plaintiff was a "novice" exerciser and therefore unlikely perhaps to fully understand and appreciate the risks associated with exercise. It is not known in this case if the plaintiff signed any type of assumption of risk document prior to participation.

Signed assumption of risk documents help strengthen the assumption of risk defense for defendants (see Chapter 4) for injuries due to inherent causes but do not protect defendants for injuries related to their negligence. As discussed in Chapter 3, published standards of practice can be introduced into a court of law (through expert testimony) as evidence of the standard of care owed to the plaintiff. Therefore, instead of relying on the outcome in *Rostai*, health/fitness professionals should review the published standards of practice related to pre-activity health screening and develop procedures consistent with them.

THE PUBLISHED STANDARDS OF PRACTICE

Of the ten published standards of practice identified in Chapter 3, pre-activity health screening is addressed in nine of them—all except the ACSM/AHA Joint PP-AEDs, which only deals with AEDs. A summary of these published statements is presented next. It is also important to point out that some of these are stated verbatim (direct quotes) and others are paraphrased. In some cases, an interpretation is neither given nor possible to make.

IHRSA Standards, Canadian Standards, and MFA Standards

IHRSA Standard #1 states, "The club will open its membership to persons of all races, creeds, places of national origin, and physical abilities,"[30] and Standard #8 states, "The club will offer each adult member a pre-activity screening appropriate to the physical activities to be performed by the member.[31] Standard #1 addresses "a minimum level of conduct, and does not supercede [sic] local, state, or federal discrimination laws, which may be more comprehensive."[30] Standard #8 "requires clubs to offer a pre-activity screening device to adult members that will allow them to determine whether they have medical conditions or risk factors that would require particular actions to be taken

Although the plaintiff admitted that the signature on the membership application containing the captioned clause just cited was his, he contended he could not specifically recall reading the application. He also stated because the facility was located in a hospital complex that he believed trained personnel would see to it he could safely exercise and would receive help if needed. He also contended that he did not intend to release any of the defendants for not following their own first aid and safety rules.

An affidavit from a medical doctor was also submitted by the plaintiff. This affidavit indicated that the delay in providing appropriate treatment to the plaintiff for some six hours caused the plaintiff to suffer extensive and irreversible heart damage *"that in all probability would have been avoided if appropriate treatment would have been rendered within the first one to two hours of his collapse."*

The plaintiff also apparently signed an "Informed Consent for Exercise Participation" form when he joined the facility. The form disclosed the *"risk of certain changes that might occur during or following . . . exercise . . . [including] abnormalities of blood pressure or heart rate."* However, no disclosure of the risk of a heart attack (MI) or death were identified within the risk disclosure section of the consent form (although the risks of "injury" and "death" were mentioned in the assumption of risk (indemnification section of the form).

The trial court granted the defendant's motion for summary judgment finding that:

> *The consequence of the waiver provisions contained in the membership agreement expressly relieves the defendants from liability for "acts of active or passive negligence" on the part of the defendants. Thus, the waiver expressed a clear and unambiguous intent by plaintiff to relieve defendants from liability for their negligence.*

The plaintiffs filed a request for reconsideration of this ruling, but the trial court denied the motion. The plaintiffs then appealed (Case N0.95 APE 12–1633), contending that the trial court erred in granting the defendants' motion. Specifically, the plaintiff contended that the release in question was subject to strict scrutiny and violated public policy. The trial court's decision was affirmed on appeal in June of 1996.

Despite the appeal (and the substantial questions it contains, including questions related to the validity of a release in the setting where this occurred when compared with the disclosure document the plaintiff signed, what the plaintiff intended and didn't intend, what the employee did and didn't do, etc.), health and fitness facilities should be very mindful of the insurance coverage issues raised in this case. If the court had determined that insurance coverage for the events that occurred and for the persons involved was excluded under the insurance policy, the facility and perhaps its employee could have been exposed to large out-of-pocket defense costs and potentially horrendous damages in the event the plaintiff prevailed (extensive heart damage to a 47-year-old plaintiff in need of a heart transplant, if the plaintiff's case was meritorious, could be the subject of a substantial award).

What is important for health and fitness facilities to realize in this regard is that the defendants in the case apparently (according to the insurance company's brief) made a conscious decision to obtain only a commercial general liability insurance policy rather than one that provided coverage for professional services—coverage for fitness-related services. Although the defendants were afforded coverage owing to the court's construction of the phrase "professional services" in this case, a different result could have been, as previously noted, very costly. Facilities should review their insurance coverage and any relevant exclusions before untoward events like this one ever occur, to ensure they have appropriate insurance coverage in place that will not be the subject of extensive litigation as occurred in this case.

York Insurance Company v. Houston Wellness Center, Inc.

In this case from Georgia,[34] a fitness center member filed suit when she was injured due to alleged improper instructions on how to use an exercise machine. When the facility turned the suit over to their liability insurance company, the company denied liability

Physical Activity Readiness
Questionnaire - PAR-Q
(revised 2002)

PAR-Q & YOU

(A Questionnarire for People Aged 15 to 69)

Regular physical activity is fun and healthy, and increasingly more people are starting to become more active every day. Being more active is very safe for most people. Howerver, some people should check with their doctor before they start becoming much more physically active.

If you are planning to become much more physically active then you are now, start by answering the seven questions in the box below. If you are between the ages of 15 and 69, the PAR-Q will tell you if you should check with your doctor before you start. If you are over 69 years of age, and you are not used to being every active, check with your doctor.

Common sense is your best guide when you answer these questions. Please read the questions carefully and answer each one honestly: check YES or NO.

YES	NO		
☐	☐	1.	Has your doctor ever said that you have a heart condition <u>and</u> that you should only do physical activity recommended by a doctor?
☐	☐	2.	Do you feel pain in your chest when you do physical activity?
☐	☐	3.	In the past month, have you had chest pain when you were not doing physical activity?
☐	☐	4.	Do you lose your balance because of dizziness or do you ever lose consciousness?
☐	☐	5.	Do you have a bone or joint problem (for example, back, knee or hip) that could be made worse by a change in your physical activity?
☐	☐	6.	Is your doctor currently prescribing drugs (for example, water pills) for your blood pressure or heart condition?
☐	☐	7.	Do you know if <u>any other reason</u> why you should not do physical activity?

If **you** **answered**

YES to one or more questions

Talk with your doctor by phone or in person BEFORE you start becoming much more physically active or BEFORE you have a fitness appraisal. Tell your doctor about the PAR-Q and which questions you answered YES.

- You may be able to do any activity you want—as long as you start slowly and build up gradually. Or, you may need to restrict your activities to those which are safe for you. Talk with your doctor about the kinds of activities you wish to participate in and follow his/her advice.
- Find out which community programs are safe and helpful for you.

NO to all questions

If you answered NO honestly to <u>all</u> PAR-Q questions, you can be reasonably sure that you can:
- Start becoming much more physically active—begin slowly and build up gradually. This is the safest and easiest way to go.
- Take part in a fitness appraisal—this is an excellent way to determine your basic fitness so that you can plan the best way for you to live actively. It is also highly recommended that you have your blood pressure evaluated. If your reading is over 144/94, talk with your doctor before you start becoming much more physically active.

DELAY BECOMING MUCH MORE ACTIVE:
- If you are not feeling well because of a temporary illness such as a cold or a fever—wait unitl you feel better; or
- if you are or may be pregnant—talk to your doctor before you start becoming more active

PLEASE NOTE: If your health changes so that you then answer YES to any of the abvoe questins, tell your fitness or health professional. Ask whether you should change your physical activity plan.

<u>Informed Use of the PAR-Q:</u> The Canadian Society for Exercise Physiology. Health Canada, and their agents assume no liability for persons who undertake physical activity, and if in doubt after completing this questionnaire, consult your doctor prior to physical activity.

No changes permitted. You are encouraged to photocopy the PAR-Q but only if you use the entire form.

NOTE: If the PAR-Q is beign given to a person before he or she participates in a physical activity program or a fitness appraisal, this section may be used for legal or administrative purposes.

"I have read, understood and completed this questionnaire. Any questions i had were answered to my ful satisfaction."

NAME _____

SIGNATURE _____   DATE _____

SIGNATURE OF PARENT _____   WITNESS _____
or GUARDIAN (for participants under the age of majority)

Note: This physical activity clearance is valid for a maximum of 12 months from the date it is completed and becomes invalid if your condition changes so that you would answer YES to any of the seven questions.

CSEP / SCPE   © Canadian Society for Exercise Physiology   Supported by: 🍁 Health Canada   Santé Canada   continued on othe side.....

FIGURE 6-1 PAR-Q & YOU. (Source: Physical Activity Readiness Questionnaire (PAR-Q) (©)2002. Used with permission from the Canadian Society for Exercise Physiology, www.csep.ca.)

(e.g., physician approval, fitness testing, program modification) before they would be permitted to engage in physical activity."[31] It also states that clubs could comply by "including a pre-activity screening device such as the PAR-Q" (Physical Activity Readiness Questionnaire) "with each new member's contract . . . and as part of the membership renewal procedure."[31] See Figure 6-1 for the PAR-Q. If a participant answers "yes" to one or more questions on the PAR-Q, they are directed to talk with their physician before they start becoming much more physically active. To comply, clubs could also "post the pre-activity screening device in appropriate areas within the club, and/or have copies available for members to read prior to participating in an activity."[31]

In the Canadian Standards, Standard #1 under Pre-Screening & Informed Consent states, "Fitness service providers shall provide or require a pre-activity screening procedure (e.g., PAR-Q or appropriate signage)" and Standard #2 states, "Facility operators and other fitness service providers shall inform participants of the risks inherent in physical activity participation and fitness facility usage."[32] In addition, Standards #1 and #2 under Special Exercising Populations state that fitness providers shall recommend that "pregnant women obtain medical advice regarding their participation in physical activity" and "individuals 70 years and over receive medical advice before initiating a physical activity program or becoming more physically active,"[32] respectively.

Under Medical Oversight in the MFA Standards, Standard #2 states, "The Medical Fitness Centers must offer each member an appropriate pre-activity screening process, and refer moderate to high-risk individuals to their respective physician for medical clearance prior to participation."[33] Under Accessibility and Safety, Standard #12 states, "A Medical Fitness Center must meet all current local code, ADA and other accessibility and safety requirements."[34]

YMCA Recommendations, AFAA Standards, ACSM's H/F Standards, and NSCA Standards

The YMCA Recommendations[35] and AFAA Standards[36] are similar in that they both refer to the ACSM/AHA Joint PP[37] and the ACSM's Guidelines[2]—discussed later—with regard to pre-activity health screening and medical clearance procedures. They also state that the PAR-Q be used as a minimum screening procedure. The YMCA Recommendations also state that "YMCA executives and health fitness staff review these publications, become knowledgeable about their content for potential application in their operations, and determine their procedures for pre-activity screening and medical evaluation according to these guidelines."[38] For overweight participants, the AFAA Standards state, "It is discriminatory to require medical clearance based solely on size of the individual" and that everyone "beginning an exercise program, regardless of size, should complete a risk factor profile."[39] For participants in prenatal programs, AFAA recommends that written physician approval be obtained and that instructors obtain health histories on prospective students to learn of any limitations or the need for more extensive screening.[36] For senior fitness programs, AFAA recommends that participants complete a comprehensive health history questionnaire and have written physician approval.[36] Regarding fitness programs for children, the AFAA Standards state, "Because children are not able to give legal consent, parents must sign a permission or consent form before children are allowed to participate in youth fitness classes" and that instructors should "verify that medical clearance has been obtained."[40]

In addition to the AFAA Standards,[36] the YMCA Recommendations[41] and the NSCA Standards[42] provide recommendations regarding pre-activity health screening for children. The YMCA encourages parents of youth to have their children screened by a physician or other qualified health care professional for purposes of "(1) determining the general health of the child; (2) detecting medical or musculoskeletal conditions that may predispose a child to injury or illness during competition; and (3) detecting potentially life-threatening or disabling conditions that may limit a child's participation."[43] In addition, the YMCA Recommendations suggest "that on the registration form for each youth sports program there should be a statement requiring a parent's/guardian's signature that indicates that the child has been properly screened and that there are no medical conditions or injuries that preclude his or her participation in that sport."[43] See Chapter 4 that describes "agreements to participate," which are often recommended for children and their parents/guardians to sign that include such statements. In addition, the YMCA recommends that members (children or adults) who have asthma or experience symptoms of exercise-induced asthma (EIA) be referred to their physician for a thorough medical evaluation.[41]

The ACSM's H/F Standards[44] contain the following three standards:

1. All facilities offering exercise equipment or services must offer a general pre-activity cardiovascular risk screening, e.g., Physical Activity Readiness Questionnaire (PAR-Q) and/or a specific pre-activity screening tool, e.g., health risk appraisal (HRA), health history questionnaire (HHQ), to all new members and prospective users. 2. All specific pre-activity screening tools (e.g., HRA, HHQ) must be interpreted by qualified staff and the results of the screening must be documented. 3. If a facility becomes aware that a member or user has known cardiovascular, metabolic, or pulmonary disease, or two or more major cardiovascular risk factors, or any other major self-disclosed medical concern, as a result of pre-activity screening, that person must be advised to consult with a qualified health-care provider before beginning a physical activity program.[45] (From American College of Sports Medicine, 2007, *ACSM's Health/Fitness Facility Standards and Guidelines*, 3rd ed., pp. 1–2. (c) 2007 by American College of Sports Medicine. Reprinted with permission from Human Kinetics, Champaign, IL.)

The NSCA Standards[42] establish standards and guidelines for strength and conditioning professionals who work in both athletic and recreational settings. Under Preparticipation Screening & Clearance, Standard #1.1 states, "Strength & Conditioning professionals must require athletes to undergo health care provider screening and clearance prior to participation" and in recreational activity programs, "strength & conditioning professionals must require participants to undergo preparticipation screening and clearance."[46] Screening for athletes should follow instructions published by the Preparticipation Physical Evaluation Task Force[47] as well as other governing bodies such as NCAA for collegiate athletes, state legislatures, and high school athletic associations for scholastic athletes. Applicable to health/fitness professionals and recreational physical activity programs, this standard requires participants to undergo pre-participation screening and clearance in accordance with published statements such as the ACSM/AHA Joint PP.[37]

NSCA Guideline #8.1 (under Participation in Strength & Conditioning Activities by Children) specifies that children participating in strength and conditioning activities should be cleared as specified in NCSA's Standard #1. In addition, Guideline #6.1 under Records & Record Keeping recommends that "preparticipation medical clearance, and return to participation clearance documents . . . be preserved and maintained for a period of time determined by professional legal advice and consultation."[48] Standard #7.1 states, "Strength & Conditioning professionals . . . must provide facilities, training, programs, services, and related opportunities in accordance with all laws, regulations and requirements mandating equal opportunity, access and non-discrimination."[48]

ACSM/AHA Joint PP

The ACSM/AHA Joint PP,[37] which is often referred to by several of the organizations cited earlier, is quite complex with regard to pre-activity health screening and medical clearance. This position paper states, "All facilities offering exercise equipment should conduct cardiovascular screening of all new members and/or prospective users."[49] Two practical tools are suggested as cost-effective approaches for identifying high-risk individuals for cardiovascular disease risk factors prior to exercise versus clinical or diagnostic testing: the PAR-Q (see Figure 6-1) and the AHA/ACSM Health/Fitness Facility Preparticipation Screening Questionnaire (see Figure 6-2). The ACSM/AHA questionnaire is slightly more complex than the PAR-Q. Depending on the participant's responses, it directs participants to the type of facility that would be best (e.g., facility with medically qualified staff or a facility with professionally qualified staff), as well as whether or not they should consult their health care provider prior to engaging in exercise. This position paper does not discuss how health/fitness facilities with professional staff should use these forms (e.g., if staff members should review them and then require

AHA/ACSM Health/Fitness Facility Preparticipation Screening Questionnaire

Assess your health needs by marking all *true* statements.

History
You have had:
___ a heart attack
___ heart surgery
___ cardiac catheterization
___ coronary angioplasty (PTCA)
___ pacemaker/implantable cardiac defibrillator/rhythm disturbance
___ heart valve disease
___ heart failure
___ heart transplantation
___ congenital heart disease

*If you marked any of the statements in this section, consult your healthcare provider before engaging in exercise. You may need to use a facility with a **medically qualified staff**.*

Symptoms
___ You experience chest discomfort with exertion.
___ You experience unreasonable breathlessness.
___ You experience dizziness, fainting, blackouts.
___ You take heart medications.

Other health issues:
___ You have musculoskeletal problems.
___ You have concerns about the safety of exercise.
___ You take prescription medication(s).
___ You are pregnant.

Cardiovascular risk factors
___ You are a man older than 45 years.
___ You are a woman older than 55 years or you have had a hysterectomy or you are postmenopausal.
___ You smoke.
___ Your blood pressure is greater than 140/90.
___ You don't know your blood pressure.
___ You take blood pressure medication.
___ Your blood cholesterol level is >240 mg/dL.
___ You don't know your cholesterol level.
___ You have a close blood relative who had a heart attack before age 55 (father or brother) or age 65 (mother or sister).
___ You are diabetic or take medicine to control your blood sugar.
___ You are physically inactive (i.e., you get less than 30 minutes of physical activity on at least 3 days per week).
___ You are more than 20 pounds overweight.

*If you marked two or more of the statements in this section, you should consult your healthcare provider before engaging in exercise. You might benefit by using a facility with a **professionally qualified exercise staff** to guide your exercise program.*

___ None of the above is true.

You should be able to exercise safely without consulting your healthcare provider in almost any facility that meets your exercise program needs.

AHA/ACSM indicates American Heart Association/American College of Sports Medicine.

FIGURE 6-2   AHA/ACSM Health/Fitness Facility Preparticipation Screening Questionnaire. (Reprinted with permission from AHA/ACSM Scientific Statement: Recommendations for Cardiovascular Screening, Staffing, and Emergency Policies at Health/Fitness Facilities (*Circulation*. 1998;97:2283–2293) (©)1998 American Heart Association.[37])

physician clearance based on the criteria stated on the forms). However, it does state that both of these forms should be prominently displayed (posted) in unsupervised or nonstaffed fitness facilities, (e.g., hotels, apartment complexes) so that participants can self-administer them.

If health/fitness facilities use "health appraisal questionnaires," qualified staff should interpret them to make decisions with regard to the need for medical evaluation.[37] The statement does not include any examples of health appraisal questionnaires, but it is probably referring to screening tools such as a Health Risk Appraisal (HRA) or a Health History Questionnaire (HHQ) as described in the ACSM's H/F Standards.[44] It is recommended that results of screening be documented for facilities that provide staff supervision. However, because of the potential costs associated with screening procedures that would involve physician clearance, each facility should determine the most cost-effective way to conduct and document pre-participation screening procedures. In addition, it is recommended that all prospective participants be educated about the importance of obtaining a health appraisal (and the potential risks of not obtaining a health appraisal) and, if indicated, medical evaluation/recommendation prior to participation in exercise testing/training.

The ACSM/AHA Joint PP also states, "Due to safety concerns, persons with known cardiovascular disease who do not obtain recommended medical evaluations and those who fail to complete the health appraisal questionnaire upon request may be excluded from participation in a health/fitness facility exercise program to the extent permitted by law."[50] This statement does not refer to any particular law(s), but it is probably referring to the ADA (or other similar laws) that prohibits any discrimination against persons with disabilities with regard to programs and services offered by places of public accommodation. As mentioned earlier, health/fitness facilities are considered places of public accommodation under the ADA. Therefore, before adopting such an "exclusion" policy, health/fitness facilities should review the ADA and any other similar laws to help ensure they are not being discriminatory; that is, treating persons with disabilities any differently than anyone else in their pre-activity health screening procedures.

The ACSM/AHA Joint PP also states, "Persons without symptoms or a known history of cardiovascular disease who do not obtain the recommended medical evaluation after completing a health appraisal should be required to sign an assumption of risk or release/waiver."[51] In addition, those who do not sign a release/waiver upon request may be excluded from participation to the extent permitted by law, but those who do sign the release/waiver may be permitted to participate—but "encouraged to participate in only moderate- or lower-intensity physical activities and counseled about the warning symptoms and signs of an impending cardiovascular event."[51] It may be difficult to interpret these recommendations. First, *all* participants should sign some type of an assumption of risk statement prior to participation informing them of the inherent risks associated with exercise (see Chapter 4), not just those who refuse to obtain medical evaluation/recommendation. Regarding signing a waiver, health/fitness facilities that have participants sign a waiver as a matter of policy have *all* participants read and sign it prior to participation, not just those who refuse to complete a health appraisal or obtain medical evaluation/recommendation. Perhaps the ACSM/AHA Joint PP here is recommending a waiver that specifically addresses the refusal to complete a health appraisal and/or obtain medical evaluation/recommendation. Releases/waivers should be used in all facilities for all adults except where prohibited by state law (see Chapter 4). In those latter situations, express assumption of risk documents should be used.

The ACSM/AHA Joint PP[37] strongly recommends that written and active communication with an individual's physician should occur when a medical evaluation/ recommendation is either advised or required. Example forms for "physician referral" and "authorization for release of medical information" are provided in this position paper. If health/fitness professionals use these (or some modification of them), they should be aware that the patient must sign a medical release form before records can be obtained from the individual's physician.

According to the ACSM/AHA Joint PP,[37] the screening results can be used for **risk stratification:** placing individuals into certain risk categories that then can be used to make a recommendation about the type of facility (levels 1 to 5) that would be best, given the risk category assigned to the individual (see Table 6-2). As stated in Chapter 1, the information in this book is designed for health/fitness facilities classified as levels 2 to 4 in the table. Note that in Table 6-2 both children and adolescents are included, suggesting these age groups should also be screened and categorized into one of the risk categories as described. The ACSM/AHA Joint PP also describes how screening results can be used for exercise prescription, which is discussed in Chapter 7.

Note: Direct quotes that appeared above in this section have been reprinted with permission from AHA/ACSM Scientific Statement: Recommendations for Cardiovascular Screening, Staffing, and Emergency Policies at Health/Fitness Facilities (*Circulation.* 1998;97:2283–2293) (c)1998 American Heart Association.[37]

ACSM's Guidelines

Finally, we discuss the ACSM's Guidelines.[2] This book presents an algorithm with regard to pre-participation screening for both self-guided physical activity and for professionally guided exercise testing/prescription (see Table 6-3). Pre-activity health screening devices such as the PAR-Q (Figure 6-1) and the AHA/ACSM Questionnaire (Figure 6-2) are suggested for self-guided physical activity, whereas a more complex approach that involves classifying participants into low, moderate, and high categories is recommended for professionally guided exercise testing/prescription. Definitions of "self-guided" and "professionally guided" are provided at the bottom of Table 6-3. Based on these definitions, it appears that individuals who participate on their own (e.g., at home) or in an unsupervised facility are in "self-guided" programs, and those who participate at a facility that provides exercise testing/prescription and supervision by qualified health/fitness staff members are in "professionally guided" programs.

Table 6-3 indicates that the ACSM/AHA Questionnaire (Figure 6-2) could be used for professionally guided programs. However, this device does not contain the necessary information to classify individuals into low, moderate, and high categories using the criteria established in the ACSM Guidelines.[2] However, a similar device, called the Pre-Activity Screening Questionnaire (PASQ), described later, was designed for this purpose. The ACSM Guidelines[2] also indicate that many health/fitness facilities use a more elaborate health/medical history questionnaire to obtain additional information regarding health habits and medical history. In addition, the ACSM Guidelines state that "regardless of the scope of preparticipation screening employed, information should be interpreted by qualified professionals and the results should be documented."[52]

As indicated in Table 6-3, for professionally guided exercise testing/prescription programs, health/fitness professionals should identify coronary artery disease (CAD) risk factors, major signs or symptoms suggestive of cardiovascular, pulmonary, and metabolic diseases, and any known cardiovascular, pulmonary, and metabolic diseases to classify individuals into low-, moderate-, and high-risk categories (see Table 6-4). The ACSM Guidelines[2] list seven positive CAD risk factors and one negative CAD risk factor as follows:

- Family history
- Cigarette smoking
- Hypertension
- Dyslipidemia
- Impaired fasting glucose
- Obesity
- Sedentary lifestyle
- High-serum HDL cholesterol (negative risk factor)

TABLE 6-2 Participant Health/Fitness Facility Chart

Participant Characteristics	Risk Class A-1	Risk Class A-2	Risk Class A-3	Risk Class B	Risk Class C	Risk Class D
Age/gender	Children Adolescents Men ≤45 yr Women ≤55 yr	Men >45 yr Women >55 yr	Men >45yr Women >55 yr	Children[a] Adolescents[a] Men Women	Children[a] Adolescents[a] Men Women	Children[a] Adolescents[a] Men Women
Cardiovascular risk factors	None	None	≥2	May be present	May be present	May be present
Known CVD	None	None	None	Yes	Yes	Yes
CVD features (see text for details)	Class A apparently healthy	Class A apparently healthy	Class A apparently healthy	Class B known CVD: low risk	Class C known CVD: moderate risk	Class D known CVD: high risk
Low intensity	Facility 1–4	Facility 1–4	Facility 1–4	Facility 1–5	Facility 4–5	Not recommended
Moderate intensity	Facility 1–4	Facility 1–4	Facility 1–4	Facility 4–5	Facility 5	Not recommended
Vigorous intensity	Facility 1–4	Facility 1–4	Facility 1–4	Facility 4–5	Facility 5	Not recommended

Facility Characteristics

	Level 1	Level 2	Level 3	Level 4	Level 5
Type of facility	Unsupervised exercise room	Single exercise leader	Fitness center for healthy clients	Fitness center serving clinical populations	Medically supervised clinical exercise program
Personnel	None	Exercise leader *Recommended: medical liaison*	General manager Health/fitness instructor Exercise leader *Recommended: medical liaison*	General manager Exercise specialist Health/fitness instructor Medical liaison	General manager Exercise specialist Health/fitness instructor Medical liaison
Emergency plan	Present	Present	Present	Present	Present
Emergency equipment	Telephone in room Signs	Telephone Signs *Recommended: blood pressure kit Stethoscope*	Telephone Signs *Recommended: blood pressure kit Stethoscope*	Telephone Signs Blood pressure kit Stethoscope	Telephone Signs Blood pressure kit Stethoscope Oxygen Crash cart Defibrillator

[a] Risk stratification for patients with congenital heart disease should be guided by recommendations of the 26th Bethesda Conference. CVD indicates cardiovascular disease.

Reprinted with permission from AHA/ACSM Scientific Statement: Recommendations for Cardiovascular Screening, Staffing, and Emergency Policies at Health/Fitness Facilities (*Circulation.* 1998;97:2283–2293) ©1998 American Heart Association.[37]

TABLE 6-3 ACSM Pre-Participation Screening Algorithm

	Screening Recommended Prior to Self-Guided[a] Physical Activity	Screening Recommended Prior to Professionally-Guided[b] Exercise Testing/Prescription		
Level-1 Risk Stratification & Medical Clearance (Chapter 2)	1. Complete ACSM/AHA Questionnaire or PAR-Q (Figures 2-1 & 2-2) 2. Determine need for medical clearance and obtain recommended 3. Proceed to Level 2	1. Identify presence of major CAD risk factors (Table 2-2) and major signs/symptoms suggestive of cardiovascular, pulmonary or metabolic disease (Table 2-3). This process could include the use of the ACSM/AHA Questionnaire (Figure 2-1)(2). This process may also include a more elaborate, facility-specific medical/health history questionnaire. 2. Determine ACSM risk category from Table 2-4 for use in Levels 2 and 3. 3. Determine need for medical clearance prior to testing and/or participation and obtain if recommended. 4. Proceed to Level 2 and follow recommendations based on ACSM risk category.		
		Low Risk	**Moderate Risk**	**High Risk**
Level-2 Additional Pre-Participation Assessment (Chapters 3-4)	• Initiate general physical activity recommendations as outlined by the United States Surgeon General.[6] • For a specific self-guided exercise assessment and examples of both aerobic and resistance training regimens see Chapters 4–6 of the ACSM Fitness Book.[10] • Individuals identified as needing medical clearance in Level 1 may benefit from participation in a professionally-guided pre-exercise assessment and prescription.	• Perform informed consent for testing (sample Figure 3-1) and/or training[c] • Complete appropriate assessment procedures outlined in Chapters 3-4 • Medical history, physical examination, laboratory tests, body composition, etc.	• Perform informed consent for testing (sample Figure 3-1) and/or training[c] *Both the depth and breadth of pre-exercise test assessment should increase as a function of risk category. Refer to Chapters 3 & 4 for advanced assessment procedure.*	
Level-3 Exercise Test Considerations (Chapters 4-5)		• Further medical examination and exercise testing not necessary[d] prior to initiation of exercise training • Medical supervision for sub-maximal or maximal exercise testing not necessary	• Medical examination and exercise testing recommended prior to initiation of vigorous exercise training • Medical supervision[e] recommended for maximal exercise testing	• Medical examination and exercise testing recommended prior to initiation of moderate or vigorous exercise training • Medical supervision[e] recommended for maximal or sub-maximal exercise testing

Moderate exercise intensity = 40.59% VO_2R; Vigorous exercise intensity = > 60% VO_2R (See Table 1-1)

[a] Physical activity regimen that is initiated and guided by the individual with little or no input or supervision from an exercise program professional.

[b] Professionally-guided implies that the fitness/clinical assessment is conducted by—and exercise program designed and supervised by—appropriately trained personnel that possess academic training and practical/clinical knowledge, skills and abilities commensurate with the credentials defined in Appendix F, or the ACSM Program Director or Health/Fitness Director.

[c] Published samples of appropriate consent forms for participation in preventive and rehabilitative exercise programs are found in references 3 & 9.

[d] The designation of not necessary reflects the notion that a medical examination, exercise test, and medical supervision of exercise testing would not be essential in the pre-activity screening; however, they should not be viewed as inappropriate.

[e] When medical supervision of exercise testing is "recommended," the physician should be in proximity and readily available should there be an emergent need.

Reprinted with permission from *ACSM's Guidelines for Exercise Testing and Prescription.* 7th ed. Philadelphia: Lippincott Williams & Wilkins, 2006.

TABLE 6-4	ACSM Risk Stratification Categories
1. Low risk	Men <45 years of age and women <55 years of age who are asymptomatic and meet no more than one risk factor threshold from Table 2-2
2. Moderate risk	Men ≥45 years and women ≥55 years *or* those who meet the threshold for two or more risk factors from Table 2-2
3. High risk	Individuals with one or more signs and symptoms listed in Table 2-3 *or* known cardiovascular,* pulmonary,[†] or metabolic [‡]disease

*Cardiac peripheral vascular, or cerebrovascular disease.
[†]Chronic obstructive pulmonary disease, asthma, interstitial lung disease, or cystic fibrosis (see Reference 24: American Association of Cardiovascular and Pulmonary Rehabilitation, Guidelines for pulmonary rehabilitation programs. 2nd ed. Champaign, IL: Human Kinetics, 1998:97–112.)
[‡]Diabetes mellitus (IDDM, NIDDM), thyroid disorders, renal, or liver disease.
Reprinted with permission from *ACSM's Guidelines for Exercise Testing and Prescription.* 7th ed. Philadelphia: Lippincott Williams & Wilkins; 2006.

The major signs or symptoms suggestive of cardiovascular, pulmonary, or metabolic diseases include the following:

- Pain, discomfort (or anginal equivalent) in the chest, neck, jaw, arms, or other areas that may result from ischemia
- Shortness of breath at rest or with mild exertion
- Dizziness or syncope
- Orthopnea or paroxysmal nocturnal dyspnea
- Ankle edema
- Palpitations or tachycardia
- Intermittent claudication
- Known heart murmur
- Unusual fatigue or shortness of breath with usual activities[53]

The ACSM Guidelines suggest that when using screening devices such as those in Figures 6-1 and 6-2, medical clearance should be obtained as indicated on the device. If a device is used that can classify individuals into low-, moderate-, or high-risk categories, then health/fitness professionals can follow the guidelines provided in Table 6-3 to determine whether or not medical examination and exercise testing are recommended prior to initiation of exercise training. Most health/fitness professionals would interpret "medical examination and exercise testing" in this context to mean physician/medical clearance. The individual's physician then would decide the need for a medical examination and what it would entail (e.g., a diagnostic or clinical graded exercise test).

For high-risk individuals, medical examination and exercise testing are recommended for both moderate and vigorous exercise. However, for moderate-risk individuals, medical examination and exercise testing are recommended for participants who will be involved in vigorous exercise but not moderate exercise. When following these recommendations, health/fitness professionals and their risk management advisory committees need to consider the criteria they will use to recommend/require physician clearance (e.g., if all moderate-risk individuals should obtain physician clearance because it will be difficult to ensure that these individuals will only be participating in moderate-only exercise). For low-risk individuals, medical examination and exercise testing is not necessary. Lastly, the ACSM Guidelines recommend that all low-, moderate-, and high-risk participants complete an informed consent for testing and/or training (see Table 6-3). This process informs participants of the inherent risks associated with physical activity. Note: Tables 6-3 and 6-4 above are Tables 2-1 and 2-4, respectively, in the ACSM's Guidelines.[2] Figures and tables referred to within these tables can be found in the ACSM's Guidelines.[2]

STEP 2 DEVELOPMENT OF RISK MANAGEMENT STRATEGIES

The preceding section presented relevant administrative and statutory laws such as HIPAA and the ADA that can apply to the pre-activity health screening process. In addition, case law examples were described in which the failure to conduct pre-activity health screening procedures was a claim that plaintiffs made in negligence lawsuits against health/fitness professionals and the organizations they represent. Several professional organizations have also published standards of practice associated with the pre-activity health screening process. This section describes how health/fitness professionals and their risk management advisory committees can develop risk management strategies that will apply the law and published standards of practice and thus help minimize legal liability associated with the pre-activity screening process.

The forms listed here appear in Appendix 6 and are referred to when describing some of the risk management strategies listed. These were designed to incorporate the pre-activity health screening recommendations as established in the ACSM's Guidelines. Of the published standards of practice described earlier, we believe these are the most authoritative to consider when establishing pre-activity health screening procedures.

> Form 6-1: Instructions: Pre-Activity Health Screening Process
> Form 6-2: Pre-Activity Screening Questionnaire (PASQ)
> Form 6-3: PASQ: Detailed Interpretive Guidelines
> Form 6-4: PASQ Interpretive Guidelines: Abbreviated Version
> Form 6-5: Physician Clearance Form

These forms have been successfully used with the pre-activity health screening process in the exercise science program at the University of South Florida (USF) for the last three years. They have been used with students as well as employees at USF prior to participation in exercise testing and/or training. Research is currently underway at USF to establish the reliability and validity of these forms. Once this research is completed, any changes made to the forms as a result of the study will be available on the LWW website (http://thePoint.lww.com/Eickhoff), where the many forms/documents contained in this book are provided. As stated previously, these forms/documents are provided on this website in an electronic version so that health/fitness professionals and risk management advisory committees can easily review them.

Risk Management Strategy 1: Comply with federal HIPAA and ADA laws as well as any similar state and local laws.

As the pre-activity health screening process is being developed, all aspects of the process should be consistent with HIPAA, ADA, and any other similar state and local laws. To determine if any similar state or local laws apply to the pre-activity health screening process, health/fitness professionals can consult with the legal expert(s) on their risk management advisory committees.

As stated earlier, health/fitness facilities may or may not be subject to HIPAA's provisions. However, it is good idea to comply with these provisions in case they (or provisions in other similar laws) do apply and as a matter of professionalism. Compliance can be met by developing procedures that would keep protected health information (obtained in the pre-activity health screening process) private, confidential, and secure. Privacy procedures help ensure that participant health information is not shared with anyone without the written authorization of the participant. See Figure 6-3 for a sample Authorization Form for Release of Medical Information. If requesting health information from a participant's physician or other health care provider, the participant would need to first sign such a form. Procedures involving confidentiality would involve designating authorized individuals within the health/fitness facility who would have access to the health information. This may be only those who have a "need to know," such as the staff

Release of Information Form

TO WHOM IT MAY CONCERN:

Please furnish to _____
(hereinafter "Facility") and/or any or all of its personnel, information, copies of any and all hospital and medical records or reports of any sort, charts, notes, x-rays, lab reports and prescription information, including the right to inspect and copy such records. Facility is to be furnished any and all other information without limitation pertaining to any confinement, examination, treatment or condition of myself, including medical, dental, psychological or other treatment, examinations, or counseling for any condition, medical, dental or psychological.

This AUTHORIZATION shall be considered as continuing and you may rely upon it in all respects unless you have previously been advised by me in writing to the contrary. It is expressly understood by the undersigned and you are hereby authorized to accept a copy or photocopy of this medical authorization with the same validity as though an original had been presented to you.

Dated this _____ day of _____, 20__.

Signature: _____

Name: _____

Address: _____

_____

Phone: _____

FIGURE 6-3 Sample Authorization Form for Release of Medical Information. (Reproduced with permission from Herbert & Herbert, *Legal Aspects of Preventive, Rehabilitative and Recreational Exercise Programs*. 4th ed. PRC Publishing, Inc. Canton, Ohio 2002. All other rights reserved.)

member(s) who will be working directly with that participant. Security procedures would entail having a system in place where health information, whether it is in paper and/or electronic form, is stored to control access. For facilities subject to HIPAA's provisions, a HIPAA compliant Authorization to Disclose Health Information form may be required (see Figure 6-4).

Title III of the ADA prohibits discrimination of those with defined disabilities with regard to programs and services offered by health/fitness facilities. Therefore, it is essential that any aspect of the pre-activity health screening process does not violate any of the provisions within the ADA. For example, the criteria used to determine whether or not physician clearance is necessary should be preestablished and analyzed in the same fashion for all participants. In addition, any policies that might exclude participation, for example, participants who do not complete the pre-activity screening process or those who do not sign a waiver when refusing to complete the pre-activity health screening process will not be allowed to participate, need to be carefully considered.

AUTHORIZATION TO DISCLOSE HEALTH INFORMATION

1. Patient Name:_____

   Address: _____

   _____

   Date of Birth:_____

   Social Security No. (last four digits): _____

2. I hereby authorize the disclosure/use of the above named individual's health information as described below. The following individual or organization is authorized to make the disclosure:

3. Name: _____

   Address: _____

   _____

   _____

   The type and amount of information to be used or disclosed is as follows:
   (Include dates where appropriate)

4. ____ entire record   _____ problem list   _____ medication list

   ____ list of allergies   _____ immunization record   _____ most recent history and physical

   ____ most recent discharge summary

   ____ most recent admission documents

   ____ emergency department records

   ____ laboratory results   from (date) _____ to (date)_____

   ____ x-ray and imaging reports   from (date) _____ to (date)_____

   ____ consultation reports   from (doctor's names) _____

   ____ other: _____

   a) I understand that the information in my health record may include information relating to sexually transmitted disease, acquired immunodeficiency syndrome (AIDS), or human immunodeficiency virus (HIV). It may also include information about behavioral or mental health services, and treatment for alcohol and drug abuse.

   b) This information may be disclosed to and used by the following organization and individuals for the purposes of ___

   _____:

   _____

   _____

   _____

   c) I understand that I have the right to revoke this authorization at any time. I understand that if I revoke this authorization I must do so in writing and present my written revocation to the health information management department of the health services organization or individual listed in Section 3 above. I understand that the revocation will not apply to information that has already been released in response to this authorization. I understand that the revocation will not apply to my insurance company when the law provides my Insurer with the right to contest a claim under my policy. Unless otherwise revoked, this authorization will expire on the following date, event, or condition: 60 days.

   d) I understand that authorizing the disclosure of this health information is voluntary. I acknowledge that I can refuse to sign this authorization. I need not sign this form in order to assure treatment. I understand that I may inspect or copy the information to be used or disclosed, as provided in 45 C.F.R. 164.524. I understand that any disclosure of information carries with it the potential for an unauthorized re-disclosure and the information may not be protected by federal confidentiality rules.

   _____   _____

   Signature of Patient or Legal Representative   Date

   _____

   If signed by Legal Representative, Relationship to Patient

   _____   _____

   Signature of Witness   Date

This authorization complies with the Federal HIPAA Privacy Rules of 45 C.F.R. Parts 160 and 164, entitled Standards for Privacy of Individually Identifiable Health Information as promulgated by the United States Department of Health and Human Services. ** Photocopy of this signed authorization will serve as original**

FIGURE 6-4 HIPAA Compliant Authorization to Disclose Health Information Form

Risk Management Strategy 2: Select a pre-activity health screening device that participants would complete.

Many health/fitness facilities have opted to use the PAR-Q (Figure 6-1) or the AHA/ACSM Health/Fitness Facility Preparticipation Screening Questionnaire (AHA/ACSM Questionnaire) (Figure 6-2) as their pre-activity health screening device. These health history questionnaires (HHQs) are considered "general" screening devices, and follow-up procedures (e.g., consulting your physician prior to engaging in exercise) are stated directly on the form. If using these questionnaires, it would be best to implement the follow-up procedures as indicated. Some health/fitness professionals may opt to delete these recommended follow-up procedures on these HHQs so they are not visible to participants but still use them when establishing the follow-up procedures.

Other health/fitness facilities, and perhaps personal fitness trainers who prescribe individualized exercise programs for their clients, may opt to use a more detailed HHQ such as a Health Risk Appraisal (HRA) or a HHQ that solicits more health information than the PAR-Q or the AHA/ACSM Questionnaire. In all cases, health/fitness professionals who interpret the health information on any HHQ should understand the health information obtained and any implications it may have regarding exercise.

The PAR-Q and AHA/ACSM Questionnaire do not provide the necessary information to classify participants into low-, moderate-, or high-risk categories, as indicated in the ACSM's Guidelines.[2] For an HHQ that incorporates these guidelines, see the PASQ (Form 6-2 in the appendix). This HHQ is similar to the PAR-Q and AHA/ACSM Questionnaire in that it is easy and quick for participants to complete. It is also simple for health/fitness professionals to interpret and then classify participants into low-, moderate-, and high-risk categories. Prior to using the PASQ, health/fitness professionals should review the PASQ's Detailed Interpretive Guidelines (Form 6-3), which explains and interprets how the PASQ incorporates the ACSM's Guidelines for pre-activity health screening. Once this is done, they can use the PASQ Interpretive Guidelines: Abbreviated Version (Form 6-4) for easy and quick interpretation of the PASQ and classification of participants into low-, moderate-, and high-risk categories.

In addition to obtaining health history information, health/fitness facilities should also obtain the names and contact information of at least two individuals to serve as the participant's emergency contacts. If this information is not obtained in the membership application form or other documents, it could be included on the pre-activity health screening device that is used.

Risk Management Strategy 3: Provide instructions for participants that describe the pre-activity health screening process and purpose as well as develop related communication strategies.

All prospective participants should receive instructions regarding the pre-activity screening process. Instructions such as those described in Form 6-1 will help participants understand the steps involved in the pre-activity screening process and why it can improve their safety. They will learn that all information obtained will be kept private, confidential, and secure as provided by law. Health/fitness professionals should view and communicate the pre-activity health screening process positively rather than negatively because it provides a professional service that is in the best interest of the participant. It is not administered just to minimize legal liability on part of the health/fitness facility.

Health/fitness professionals should consider all the potential objections or perceived barriers that participants (and parents of youth participants) may express, especially regarding obtaining physician clearance (e.g., it will cost money, it will take too much time, the family does not have a physician, or the person has not seen a physician lately). Strategies should be developed that can be used positively to overcome some of these types of comments when communicating with participants. It will be essential to train all staff members who will be dealing with this process (e.g., front desk staff, professional staff) on these communication strategies.

Risk Management Strategy 4: Establish criteria that will be used to determine whether or not participants need to obtain physician clearance.

With regard to the pre-activity health screening process, several of the published standards of practice described earlier indicate that certain individuals (e.g., those who indicate health conditions and/or medical risks on a HHQ) should seek physician/medical clearance or consultation or obtain a medical evaluation and exercise testing prior to starting an exercise program. The best and most practical approach is to have these individuals obtain physician/medical clearance. An individual's physician will determine the need or extent of a medical evaluation and whether of not a diagnostic/clinical exercise test is needed before initiating exercise training.

When establishing criteria to determine the need for physician clearance, it is important that the same criteria be used for all participants, as stated earlier (Risk Management Strategy 1). Those health/fitness facilities that opt to use the PAR-Q or the AHA/ACSM Questionnaire could follow the recommendations in this regard as stated on these HHQs. Health/fitness facilities and personal fitness trainers who opt to use an HRA or a more in-depth HHQ will need to establish their own criteria using the information obtained. Those who choose to use the PASQ that solicits health information to classify participants as low, moderate, or high risk should have all moderate- and high-risk participants obtain physician clearance. The rationale for this is contained in the PASQ Detailed Interpretive Guidelines (see Form 6-3).

Risk Management Strategy 5: Have qualified health/fitness professionals interpret data from the pre-activity health screening device and determine the need for physician clearance.

Although a health/fitness facility may opt to have front desk staff members distribute a pre-activity health screening device to participants, a qualified health/fitness professional should conduct interpretation and any follow-up procedures (e.g., determining need for physician clearance). Qualified health/fitness professional should have the knowledge, skills, and abilities to complete these tasks properly (i.e., a degree, certification, and experience in the field). Procedures need to be developed so that front desk staff members know how to handle and communicate this process properly (see Risk Management Strategy 3). Also, to better serve a prospective participant, it is recommended that a qualified health/fitness professional be on duty at all times so this process is not delayed.

Risk Management Strategy 6: Create a physician clearance form that includes its purpose and instructions for the physician to complete.

A physician clearance form, such as the example provided (Form 6-5), informs the physician, in a succinct manner, the purpose of the form and how to complete it. It also includes the name and contact information of the health/fitness professional responsible for the physician clearance process. If the physician has any questions regarding the form, he or she can easily contact this professional. It may be best to make a copy of the participant's completed pre-activity health screening device and staple it to the physician clearance form so the physician can review the patient's response(s) that indicated the need for clearance.

To accomplish this task, perhaps the most time efficient and easiest way is to have the participant take full responsibility for obtaining physician clearance because of the relationship that already exists between the participant and his or her physician. If health/fitness facilities opt to mail and/or fax the physician clearance form directly to the physician, a written authorization to release such information may need to be considered. In addition, if the physician clearance form is faxed back to the health/fitness facility, the facility must use a secure fax machine. It will be difficult to obtain physician clearance electronically over the Internet because physicians rarely disclose their e-mail addresses. Lastly, if the physician clears the participant with restrictions and/or limitations (see Form 6-5), these restrictions/limitations must be fully understood and incorporated into the participant's exercise program by the health/fitness professionals who will be working with that participant. Perhaps the health/fitness professional who processed the physician clearance would have this responsibility.

Risk Management Strategy 7: Inform participants of the potential inherent risks associated with fitness and exercise activities provided at the health/fitness facility.

Once the first two steps of the pre-activity health screening process is complete, participants should be informed, via a written and signed document, of the many inherent risks associated with fitness and exercise activities (step 3 in the pre-activity health screening process). Various documents can achieve this objective (see Chapter 4). These documents can help strengthen the assumption of risk defense for defendant health/fitness facilities and their personnel. Once all three steps have been completed (and any other procedures the facility may require), the participant is now ready to participate in the programs and services offered by the facility.

Risk Management Strategy 8: Establish a pre-activity health screening process for youth.

The pre-activity health screening procedures just discussed would apply to all adults: those who are 18 years (age of majority in most states) or older. However, what procedures should youth and their parents/guardians follow? Several of the published standards of practice already described recommend that youth (minors who are 17 years or younger) be medically cleared prior to participation in sports and/or physical activities. This may involve the parent and/or guardian signing a form that indicates the child has been properly screened and that there are no existing medical conditions that would preclude participation in the sport or physical activities. Forms such as "agreements to participate" can be used for this purpose (see Form 4-5 in Chapter 4). Health/fitness professionals, in consultation with their risk management advisory committees, need to decide if this approach is adequate, or if further steps should be implemented. Because of the increased prevalence of health problems among youth, such as obesity, type 2 diabetes, and hypertension, additional steps may be warranted.

Risk Management Strategy 9: Establish a pre-activity health screening process for guests.

Some of the published standards of practice described earlier indicate that prospective users as well as members need to complete a pre-activity health screening device. These prospective users could be guests that perhaps only want to use the health/fitness facility once, or they may be prospective members using a short "trial" period/membership. A formal pre-activity health screening process involving the completion of an HHQ that also may include obtaining physician clearance might not be practical or reasonable. And it may not be appropriate to exclude guests from participation. Perhaps having guests sign a waiver and assumption of risk document (see Chapter 4 for examples) may be a good alternative, but waivers are not valid in all states. Perhaps in these states, guests should sign an express assumption of risk as a minimum requirement in order to participate. Health/fitness professionals and their risk management advisory committees need to consider what steps in the pre-activity health screening process would be best for their guests to complete.

Risk Management Strategy 10: Create a system to keep all documents obtained in the pre-activity health screening process, private, confidential, and secure.

As described in Risk Management Strategy 1, all health information needs to be kept private, confidential, and secure. This includes the pre-activity health screening device and the physician clearance form that contain protected health information. A system that includes written procedures on how these documents will be kept private, confidential, and secure should be in place. Staff members should be well trained with regard to these procedures. In addition, all documents obtained in the pre-activity health screening process should be kept for the length of time that would be commensurate with the statute of limitations.

Risk Management Strategy 11: Determine how often participants complete the pre-activity health screening process.

Most of the published standards of practice described here do not provide any information about how often the pre-activity health screening process should occur. The ACSM's Health/Fitness Standards under Standard 1 state that "pre-activity screening may be repeated at appropriate intervals."[54] At the bottom of the PAR-Q (Figure 6-1), it states, "This physical activity clearance is valid for a maximum of 12 months from the date it is completed and becomes invalid if your condition changes so that you would answer YES to any of the above questions." Health/fitness facilities need to determine their own policy as to how often the process is repeated. Perhaps annually when most participants are renewing their membership would be considered a reasonable time period. However, one's health status can change overnight. To address this issue for health/fitness professionals who use the PASQ, a statement has been included on the PASQ (see Form 6-2, Section 4) that says, "If my health status changes at any time, I understand that I am responsible to inform this health/fitness facility of any such changes." This puts the responsibility on the participant; however, the health/fitness facility needs to decide what procedures to follow when this occurs (e.g., having the participant repeat the pre-activity health screening process).

Risk Management Strategy 12: Establish procedures for those who refuse to complete the pre-activity health screening process.

Health/fitness facilities that, as a matter of policy, allow participants to have the option to refuse to complete the pre-activity health screening process or some aspect of it (e.g., obtaining physician clearance), need to establish procedures to help minimize any potential liability associated with this policy. For example, a participant who does not complete the pre-activity screening process and then experiences a cardiac arrest while exercising at the facility could subsequently bring a negligence claim and/or lawsuit against the facility, claiming the health/fitness facility failed to conduct pre-activity health screening. In this situation, the facility may want to have participants sign a refusal form. See Figure 6-5 for a sample refusal form, which is a waiver. However, waivers are not valid in all states. Therefore, in these situations, health/fitness professionals and their legal expert(s) on their risk management advisory committees should carefully review such a policy. When using forms such as the one in Figure 6-5, language should be included that indicates the participant is fully aware of the benefits of completing the pre-activity health screening process, as well as the potential risks of not completing it. These benefits and risks can be provided in writing or explained verbally to the participant.

Health/fitness professionals and their risk management advisory committees can use the following Put into Practice Checklist to assess their phase of development for each of the risk management strategies just described.

Refusal to Participate in the Pre-Activity Health Screening Process

To help ensure safe participation in health/fitness activities, most major professional fitness organizations have published standards and/or guidelines that require or recommend that health/fitness facilities and personnel have all participants complete a pre-activity health screening process prior to their beginning a fitness program. Therefore, to comply with these national standards and guidelines, _____ (name of health/fitness facility) ("Facility") has established a policy that requires all participants to complete its pre-activity health screening process. However, though not recommended, participants may refuse to participate in this process by reading and signing the following:

I _____ (name of participant) understand that Facility requires all participants to complete a pre-activity health screening process that includes: a) completing the Facility's health history questionnaire (HHQ), and if indicated based upon the completion of that document, b) obtaining medical clearance from my physician if deemed necessary by a qualified staff member of the Facility.

However, I have chosen not to participate in:
_____ Completing the Facility's HHQ
_____ Obtaining medical clearance from my physician

Risks associated with refusal to participate in the Pre-Activity Screening Process

The purpose of a Pre-Activity Screening is to determine if an individual may participate in exercise testing and/or activity without examination and clearance by a health care provider. I understand and appreciate that there exists the possibility of adverse effects during exercise testing and exercise. I have been informed that these potential adverse effects, though remote, include abnormal blood pressure, fainting, disorders of heart rhythm, stroke, and very rare instances of heart attack or even death. In addition, I understand that during participation in testing and/or exercise, participants may experience musculoskeletal conditions or injuries such as fractured bones, muscle strains, muscle sprains, muscular fatigue, contusions, muscle soreness, joint injuries, torn muscles, heat-related illnesses, and back injuries. I also understand that other risks not listed here, both minor and major, can also occur. I understand that the benefits of participating in the Pre-Activity Screening Process are to reduce the chances of those risks occurring while I participate in exercise testing and/or exercise activity and that screening is to help enhance my safety. I assert that my participation without screening is voluntary and that I knowingly assume all risks.

Waiver/Release

**My signature below indicates that I have been fully informed of, understand, and appreciate the benefits of completing the pre-activity health screening process as well as the potential risks of not completing the pre-activity screening process. In addition, my signature also indicates that I have executed a release and waiver document with the Facility which, among other things, contractually binds me and my estate not to bring any type of legal claim and/or lawsuit against the Facility and/or its staff members for among other things, the failure of the Facility and/or its staff to conduct any aspect of the pre-activity health screening process including Facility's request that I obtain medical clearance prior to participation. I also understand that this release/waiver gives up and relinquishes my right to institute a claim or lawsuit against the Facility and/or its staff members for a number of other acts and/or omissions related to the ordinary negligence of those released.
I hereby reaffirm my understanding and agreement to that release and waiver documents and to this statement.**

_____   _____
Signature of Participant   **Date**

_____   _____
Signature of Staff Member   Date

FIGURE 6-5 Refusal to Participate in the Pre-Activity Health Screening Process.

PUT INTO PRACTICE CHECKLIST 6-1

Rate your phase of development for each of following risk management strategies related to pre-activity health screening process:

	Developed	Partially Developed	Not Developed
1. Complying with federal HIPAA and ADA laws as well as any similar state and local laws.			
2. Selecting a pre-activity health screening device that participants would complete.			
3. Providing instructions for participants that describe the pre-activity health screening process and purpose as well as developing related communication strategies.			
4. Establishing criteria that will be used to determine whether or not participants need to obtain physician clearance.			
5. Having qualified health/fitness professionals interpret data from the pre-activity health screening device and determine the need for physician clearance.			
6. Creating a physician clearance form that includes its purpose and instructions for the physician to complete.			
7. Informing participants of the potential inherent risks associated with fitness and exercise activities provided at the health/fitness facility.			
8. Establishing a pre-activity health screening process for youth.			
9. Establishing a pre-activity health screening process for guests.			
10. Creating a system to keep all documents obtained in the pre-activity health screening process, private, confidential, and secure.			
11. Determining how often participants complete the pre-activity health screening process.			
12. Establishing procedures for those who refuse to complete the pre-activity health screening process.			

SUMMARY

As health/fitness professionals and their risk management committees consider the development of their risk management strategies with regard to the pre-activity health screening process, they must review relevant laws (e.g., HIPAA and ADA), as well as the many published standards of practice that have addressed pre-activity health screening procedures. Although there is not a lot of case law that clearly establishes that pre-activity health screening and obtaining physician clearance is a legal duty of health/fitness facilities, it is likely there will be in the future, given all the professional organizations that have published standards of practice in this area that at any time could be introduced into a court of law (via expert witness testimony) as evidence of the standard of care in this area.

In addition, the knowledge, attitudes, and beliefs among health/fitness professionals regarding these procedures may also need to change. Sometimes they view the pre-activity health screening process negatively and find it is an inconvenience to conduct such procedures or a barrier to getting people physically active. Some often ask, "Isn't inactivity more risky than being active" so why create barriers for inactive individuals who want to become active? Yes, inactivity is more risky than being active, but this does not have anything to do with carrying out a potential legal duty to conduct pre-activity health screening. It is even more important for those who have been sedentary than those who have been physically active to complete a pre-activity health screening process because inactivity is a major independent risk factor for CAD. In addition, any of these reasons for not conducting pre-activity screening will probably not hold up in a court of law as a viable defense. If health/fitness professionals approach this process with their participants as a step that is in the best interest of the participant and what professional facilities do to adhere to published standards of practice, it will likely be well received by the participants.

Pre-activity health screening may also help prevent an untoward event such as a heart attack or sudden death owing to CAD if the process works properly. For example, what if the plaintiff in *Rostai* had been required to obtain physician clearance? And then when he went to his doctor with the physician clearance form (and the pre-activity screening questionnaire attached), his physician decided a medical evaluation was needed before participation in physical activity. The physician might have then prescribed a diagnostic stress test (determined to be positive) and a follow-up test such as a coronary angiogram that would have showed significant occlusion in the coronary arteries. The patient would then have received treatment, perhaps coronary bypass surgery, which reduces the likelihood of a heart attack or sudden death. If the pre-activity health screening process works as it is designed to and leads to saving a life—even in one case—it is well worth any perceived inconvenience.

RISK MANAGEMENT ASSIGNMENTS

1. Develop a PowerPoint presentation to use in staff training that addresses the major components of the HIPAA and ADA laws.

   _____

   _____

   _____

   _____

2. Develop a written procedure that describes the steps in the entire pre-activity health screening process that could be included in a health/fitness facility's Risk Management Policies and Procedures Manual.

   _____

   _____

   _____

   _____

3. Describe and list all the perceived objections/barriers that health/fitness staff members and participants may have with regard to a pre-activity health screening process. Then develop a sound rationale to refute each one, as well as a way staff members can address these when communicating with participants.

   _____

   _____

   _____

   _____

4. Develop written pre-activity health screening procedures to be followed by all youth and their parents/guardians.

_____

_____

_____

_____

5. Develop a written procedure on how health/fitness professionals will keep all pre-activity health screening documents private, confidential, and secure.

_____

_____

_____

_____

KEY TERMS

Injunction   Pre-activity health screening process   Risk stratification

REFERENCES

1. Heart Disease and Stroke Statistics—2007 Update at-a-Glance, American Heart Association. Available at: http://www.americanheart.org/presenter.jhtml?identifier=3037327 - 391 - cached. Accessed October 15, 2007.
2. Whaley MH, ed. *ACSM's Guidelines for Exercise Testing and Prescription*. 7th ed. Philadelphia: Lippincott Williams & Wilkins; 2006.
3. American College of Sports Medicine and American Heart Association Joint Position Statement. Exercise and acute cardiovascular events: Placing the risks into perspective. *Med Sci Sports Exerc*. 2007;39:866–897.
4. Whaley MH, ed. *ACSM's Guidelines for Exercise Testing and Prescription*. 7th ed. Philadelphia: Lippincott Williams & Wilkins; 2006:19.
5. HIPAA Administrative Simplification, *Regulation Text*: 45 CFR Parts 160, 162, and 164, U.S. Department of Health and Human Services Office for Civil Rights. Available at: http://dhhs.gov/ocr/hipaa. Accessed February 16, 2006.
6. Blair SA. Implementing HIPAA. *ACSM's Health Fitness J*. 2003;7:25–27.
7. OCR Privacy Brief: Summary of the HIPAA Privacy Rule, U.S. Department of Health and Human Services Office for Civil Rights. Available at: http://dhhs.gov/ocr/hipaa. Accessed October 15, 2007:4.
8. Blair SA. Implementing HIPAA. *ACSM's Health Fitness J*. 2003;7:25–27, 25.
9. Herbert DL, Herbert WH. *Legal Aspects of Preventive, Rehabilitative and Recreational Exercise Programs*. 4th ed. Canton, Ohio: PRC; 2002.
10. Herbert DL, Herbert WH. *Legal Aspects of Preventive, Rehabilitative and Recreational Exercise Programs*. 4th ed. Canton, Ohio: PRC; 2002:297.
11. Americans with Disabilities Act, 42 U.S.C. § 12101 et. seq.
12. O'Hara M. Please wait to be seated: Recognizing obesity as a disability to prevent discrimination in public accommodations. *Whittier Law Rev*. 1996;17:895–954.
13. Moorman AM, Eickhoff-Shemek JM. Is obesity a disability under the ADA? *ACSM's Health Fitness J*. 2005;9:29–31.
14. ADA Title III Part 36: Nondiscrimination on the Basis of Disability by Public Accommodation and Commercial Facilities. Available at: http://www.ada.gov/reg3a.html. Accessed June 26, 2006:7.

15. Herbert DL. May health/fitness facilities exclude individuals form participation based upon a participants' health status? *Exercise Science Standards and Malpractice Reporter.* 2007;21(3):33, 36–40.

16. Herbert DL. May health/fitness facilities exclude individuals form participation based upon a participants' health status? *Exercise Science Standards and Malpractice Reporter.* 2007;21:33, 36–40, 40.

17. ADA Title III Part 36: Nondiscrimination on the Basis of Disability by Public Accommodation and Commercial Facilities. Available at: http://www.ada.gov/reg3a.html. Accessed June 26, 2006.

18. *Contino v. Lucille Roberts Health Spa,* 509 N.Y.S 2d 369 (N.Y. App. Div. 2d 1986).

19. *Rutnik v. Colonie Center Court Club, Inc.,* 672 N.Y.S 2d 451 (1998 N.Y. App. Div. LEXIS 4845).

20. *Rutnik v. Colonie Center Court Club, Inc.,* 672 N.Y.S 2d 451 (1998 N.Y. App. Div. LEXIS 4845), 452.

21. *Chai v. Sports and Fitness Clubs of America, Inc.* Analyzed in: Failure to defibrillate results in new litigation. *Exercise Standards and Malpractice Reporter.* 1999;13:55–56.

22. *Chai v. Sports and Fitness Clubs of America, Inc.* Analyzed in: Herbert DL. Alleged failure to have AED litigation in Florida results in another defense verdict—but the plaintiff receives $2.25 million. *Exercise Standards and Malpractice Reporter.* 2000;14:54–55.

23. Herbert DL. Large verdict against AED deficient health and fitness facility. *Exercise Standards and Malpractice Reporter.* 2006;20:49, 52–54.

24. Herbert DL. Large verdict against AED deficient health and fitness facility. *Exercise Standards and Malpractice Reporter.* 2006;20:49, 52–54, 52.

25. *Rostai v. Neste Enterprises,* 41 Cal. Reptr.3rd 411 (Cal. Ct. App., 4th Dist. 2006).

26. *Rostai v. Neste Enterprises,* 41 Cal. Reptr.3rd 411 (Cal. Ct. App., 4th Dist. 2006): 415–416.

27. *Rostai v. Neste Enterprises,* 41 Cal. Reptr.3rd 411 (Cal. Ct. App., 4th Dist. 2006): 416–417.

28. *Rostai v. Neste Enterprises,* 41 Cal. Reptr.3rd 411 (Cal. Ct. App., 4th Dist. 2006): 418–419.

29. *Rostai v. Neste Enterprises,* 41 Cal. Reptr.3rd 411 (Cal. Ct. App., 4th Dist. 2006): 419.

30. IHRSA Club Membership Standards. In: *IHRSA's Guide to Club Membership & Conduct.* 3rd ed. Boston: International Health, Racquet & Sportsclub Association (IHRSA); 2005.

31. IHRSA Club Membership Standards. In: *IHRSA's Guide to Club Membership & Conduct.* 3rd ed. Boston: International Health, Racquet & Sportsclub Association (IHRSA); 2005:4.

32. *Canadian Fitness Safety Standards & Recommended Guidelines.* 3rd ed. 2004. Available at: http://www.oases.on.ca/safety/safetyStdsCurrent.htm. Ontario, Canada: Ontario Association of Sport and Exercise Sciences (OASES). Accessed September 2, 2007:5.

33. *The Medical Fitness Model: Facility Standards and Guidelines.* Richmond, Va: Medical Fitness Association (MFA); May 2006:8.

34. *The Medical Fitness Model: Facility Standards and Guidelines.* Richmond, Va: Medical Fitness Association (MFA); May 2006:13.

35. *Medical Advisory Committee Recommendations: A Resource Guide for YMCAs.* Chicago: YMCA of the USA; February 2007.

36. *Exercise Standards & Guidelines Reference Manual.* 4th ed. Sherman Oaks, Calif: Aerobics and Fitness Association of America (AFAA); 2005.

37. American College of Sports Medicine and American Heart Association Joint Position Statement. Recommendations for cardiovascular screening, staffing, and emergency policies at health/fitness facilities. *Med Sci Sports Exerc.* 1998;30:1009–1018.

38. *Medical Advisory Committee Recommendations: A Resource Guide for YMCAs.* Chicago: YMCA of the USA; February 2007:66.

39. *Exercise Standards & Guidelines Reference Manual.* 4th ed. Sherman Oaks, Calif: Aerobics and Fitness Association of America (AFAA); 2005:41.

40. *Exercise Standards & Guidelines Reference Manual.* 4th ed. Sherman Oaks, Calif: Aerobics and Fitness Association of America (AFAA); 2005:83–84.

41. *Medical Advisory Committee Recommendations: A Resource Guide for YMCAs.* Chicago: YMCA of the USA; February 2007.

42. *NSCA Strength & Conditioning Professional Standards & Guidelines.* May 2001. Available at: http://www.nscalift.org/Publications/standards.shtml. Colorado Springs: National Strength and Conditioning Association (NSCA). Accessed September 2, 2007.

43. *Medical Advisory Committee Recommendations: A Resource Guide for YMCAs.* Chicago: YMCA of the USA; February 2007:107.

44. Tharrett SJ, McInnis KJ, Peterson JA, eds. *ACSM's Health/Fitness Facility Standards and Guidelines.* 3rd ed. Champaign, Ill: Human Kinetics; 2007.

45. Tharrett SJ, McInnis KJ, Peterson JA, eds. *ACSM's Health/Fitness Facility Standards and Guidelines.* 3rd ed. Champaign, Ill: Human Kinetics; 2007:1.

46. *NSCA Strength & Conditioning Professional Standards & Guidelines.* May 2001. Available at: http://www.nscalift.org/Publications/standards.shtml. Colorado Springs: National Strength and Conditioning Association (NSCA). Accessed September 2, 2007:12–13.

47. Preparticipation Physical Evaluation Task Force: American Academy of Family Physicians, American Academy of Pediatrics, American Medical Society for Sports Medicine, American Orthopaedic Society for Sports Medicine and American Osteopathic Academy of Sports Medicine. *Preparticipation Physical Evaluation.* 2nd ed. Minneapolis: McGraw-Hill; 1996.

48. *NSCA Strength & Conditioning Professional Standards & Guidelines.* May 2001. Available at: http://www.nscalift.org/Publications/standards.shtml. Colorado Springs: National Strength and Conditioning Association (NSCA). Accessed September 2, 2007:15.

49. American College of Sports Medicine and American Heart Association Joint Position Statement. Recommendations for cardiovascular screening, staffing, and emergency policies at health/fitness facilities. *Med Sci Sports Exerc.* 1998;30:1009–1018, 1010.

50. American College of Sports Medicine and American Heart Association Joint Position Statement. Recommendations for cardiovascular screening, staffing, and emergency policies at health/fitness facilities. *Med Sci Sports Exerc.* 1998;30:1009–1018, 1011–1012.

51. American College of Sports Medicine and American Heart Association Joint Position Statement. Recommendations for cardiovascular screening, staffing, and emergency policies at health/fitness facilities. *Med Sci Sports Exerc.* 1998;30:1009–1018, 1012.

52. *ACSM's Guidelines for Exercise Testing and Prescription.* 7th ed. Philadelphia: Lippincott Williams & Wilkins; 2006:21.

53. *ACSM's Guidelines for Exercise Testing and Prescription.* 7th ed. Philadelphia: Lippincott Williams & Wilkins; 2006:23–24.

54. Tharrett SJ, McInnis KJ, Peterson JA, eds. *ACSM's Health/Fitness Facility Standards and Guidelines.* 3rd ed. Champaign, Ill: Human Kinetics; 2007:9.

APPENDIX 6

FORM 6-1
Instructions: Pre-Activity Health Screening Process

Dear Participant:

To help improve your safety in our health/fitness programs and services as well as to comply with standards and/or guidelines established by most major professional exercise/fitness organizations, we have all participants complete our Pre-Activity Health Screening Process prior to participation in our programs and services. **Step 1** in this process is to complete the attached PASQ, our health history questionnaire that will take you about 5 minutes to complete. The major purpose of obtaining this information is to help us identify individuals who may be at risk for an adverse event during exercise and who have any medical conditions that may require physician clearance prior to participation in health/fitness activities.

Once completed, it will be reviewed by one of our qualified staff members who will determine (using pre-established criteria) whether or not **Step 2** (obtaining physician clearance) is necessary prior to your participation in our programs and services. We realize that obtaining clearance from your physician may be a slight inconvenience and may delay your participation, but we feel this is an important step to help improve your safety while participating in our programs/services.

Physician Clearance

If necessary, you will receive our Physician Clearance Form. Attached to it will be a copy of your completed PASQ. Please take this form to your physician and ask him/her to complete and sign it. If you have recently seen your physician, he/she may complete/sign the form without seeing you for a medical evaluation. However, if is been a while (or for other reasons), your physician may want you to make an appointment for a medical evaluation. We believe that regular medical evaluations are important for a variety of reasons such as having certain medical screenings/tests (e.g., cholesterol, blood pressure, cancer) that may detect an underlying health problem or disease. Early detection can save your life.

Privacy-Confidentiality-Security

All information obtained in our Pre-Activity Health Screening Process will be kept private, confidential, and secure. At no time will any of this information be shared with any unauthorized individuals and it will be stored in a secure location.

Thank you for your participation in our Pre-Activity Health Screening Process. We appreciate your understanding as to why this is an important process prior to participation in our health/fitness activities, which is to help improve your safety.

Sincerely,

The Management at _____ (Name of health/fitness facility)

FORM 6-2
Pre-Activity Screening Questionnaire (PASQ)

Section 1-Diagnosed Medical Conditions

Please mark either Y (Yes) or N (No) *for* **each the items below that you have had diagnosed by a physician.**

Cardiovascular (Heart) Disease	*Pulmonary (Lung) Disease*	*Metabolic Disease*
Y☐ N☐ Heart attack	Y☐ N☐ Emphysema	Y☐ N☐ Liver disease
Y☐ N☐ Heart surgery	Y☐ N☐ Chronic bronchitis	Y☐ N☐ Diabetes
Y☐ N☐ Coronary angioplasty	Y☐ N☐ Interstitial lung disease	Y☐ N☐ Thyroid disorders
Y☐ N☐ Heart valve disease	Y☐ N☐ Cystic fibrosis	Y☐ N☐ Kidney disease
Y☐ N☐ Heart failure	Y☐ N☐ Asthma	
Y☐ N☐ Heart transplantation	➡ If Yes to asthma, is this a current condition Y☐ N☐	
Y☐ N☐ Congenital heart disease		
Y☐ N☐ Abnormal heart rhythm		
Y☐ N☐ (Cardiac defibrillator) Pacemaker or implantable device		
Y☐ N☐ Heart murmur		

➡ If Yes, to heart murmur, is this a current condition Y☐ N☐

Y☐ N☐ Do you have any other medical conditions that are not listed above such as musculoskeletal problems, recent surgery, arthritis, seizures, pregnancy, cancer, etc.?

Y☐ N☐ Do you take any prescription medications?

Section 2- Signs & Symptoms

Please mark either Y (Yes) or N (No) for each item below that you have recently experienced.

Y☐ N☐ Pain, discomfort in the chest, neck, jaw or arms at rest or upon exertion

Y☐ N☐ Shortness of breath at rest or with mild exertion

Y☐ N☐ Dizziness, fainting, or blackouts

Y☐ N☐ Shortness of breath occurring 2–5 hours after the onset of sleep

Y☐ N☐ Ankle edema (swelling)

Y☐ N☐ An unpleasant awareness of forceful or rapid beating of the heart

Y☐ N☐ Pain in the legs while walking; often more severe when walking upstairs/uphill

Y☐ N☐ Unusual fatigue or shortness of breath with usual activities

Section 3- Risk Factors

Please mark Y (Yes) or N (No) for each the following:
Age Risk Factor
Y❑ N❑ I am a man who is 45 years or older.
Y❑ N❑ I am a woman who is 55 years or older.

Other Risk Factors
Y❑ N❑ I have a close blood relative who had a heart attack, coronary (heart) by-pass surgery, or
        who died suddenly before age 55 (father or brother) OR before age 65 (mother or sister).
Y❑ N❑ I am a smoker *or* I have quit smoking in the last 6 months.
Y❑ N❑ I take medication for high blood pressure.
Y❑ N❑ I take medication for high cholesterol.
Y❑ N❑ I have a BMI greater than 30 (see BMI chart on next page).
Y❑ N❑ In the last 6 months, my physical activity level has been less than 30 minutes/day
        most days of the week.

Please mark Y (Yes), N (No), or DK (Don't Know) for each the following:
Y❑ N❑ DK❑ My fasting blood glucose is greater than or equal to 100 mg/dL.
Y❑ N❑ DK❑ My blood pressure is greater than or equal to 140/90 mm Hg.
Y❑ N❑ DK❑ My total blood cholesterol level is greater than 200 mg/dL.
Y❑ N❑ DK❑ My high-density lipoprotein (HDL) cholesterol level is greater than 60 mg/dL.

Section 4- Acknowledgment, Follow-up, and Signature
I acknowledge that I have read this questionnaire in its entirety and have responded accurately, completely, and to the best of my knowledge. Any questions regarding the items on this questionnaire were answered to my satisfaction. Also, if my health status changes at any time, I understand that I am responsible to inform this health/fitness facility of any such changes.

_____   _____   _____
(Participant's Name-Please Print)   (Participant's Signature)   (Date)

Body Mass Index Chart: BMI= Weight (kg)/height (m²)

Instructions:

1. Find the appropriate height in the left-hand column labeled **Height** (in inches).
2. Move across to a given body **weight** (in pounds).*
3. Move up to the top of that column to find the corresponding **BMI**.
4. If your weight (for your height) is greater than the information provided in the chart below, your BMI is greater than 30.

Pounds have been rounded off

BMI	19	20	21	22	23	24	25	26	27	28	29	30	31	32	33	34	35
Height (inches)								Body Weight (pounds)									
58	91	96	100	105	110	115	119	124	129	134	138	143	148	153	158	162	167
59	94	99	104	109	114	119	124	128	133	138	143	148	153	158	163	168	173
60	97	102	107	112	118	123	128	133	138	143	148	153	158	163	168	174	179
61	100	106	111	116	122	127	132	137	143	148	153	158	164	169	174	180	185
62	104	109	115	120	126	131	136	142	147	153	158	164	169	175	180	186	191
63	107	113	118	124	130	135	141	146	152	158	163	169	175	180	186	191	197
64	110	116	122	128	134	140	145	151	157	163	169	174	180	186	192	197	204
65	114	120	126	132	138	144	150	156	162	168	174	180	186	192	198	204	210
66	118	124	130	136	142	148	155	161	167	173	179	186	192	198	204	210	216
67	121	127	134	140	146	153	159	166	172	178	185	191	198	204	211	217	223
68	125	131	138	144	151	158	164	171	177	184	190	197	203	210	216	223	230
69	128	135	142	149	155	162	169	176	182	189	196	203	209	216	223	230	236
70	132	139	146	153	160	167	174	181	188	195	202	209	216	222	229	236	243
71	136	143	150	157	165	172	179	186	193	200	208	215	222	229	236	243	250
72	140	147	154	162	169	177	184	191	199	206	213	221	228	235	242	250	258
73	144	151	159	166	174	182	189	197	204	212	219	227	235	242	250	257	265
74	148	155	163	171	179	186	194	202	210	218	225	233	241	249	256	264	272
75	152	160	168	176	184	192	200	208	216	224	232	240	248	256	264	272	279
76	156	164	172	180	189	197	205	213	221	230	238	246	254	263	271	279	287

Reprinted with permission from the National Heart Lung and Blood Institute (NHLBI).
Available at http://www.nhlbi.nih.gov/guidelines/obesity/bmi_tbl.htm.

FORM 6-3
Pre-Activity Screening Questionnaire (PASQ)
Detailed Interpretive Guidelines for Health/Fitness Professionals

The PASQ was developed to be a user-friendly and time efficient instrument that stream lines the pre-activity health screening process for health/fitness professionals. Unlike similar question-naires, the PASQ incorporates the screening guidelines as established in Chapter 2 of *ACSM's Guidelines for Testing and Exercise Prescription** which we believe are the are the most author-itative with regard to pre-activity health screening procedures. The PASQ allows health/fitness professionals to easily and quickly interpret a prospective participant's health status in order to determine his/her risk category, i.e., low, moderate, or high and whether or not the prospective participant needs to obtain physician clearance prior to participation in fitness activities. It is assumed that health/fitness professionals who interpret the data obtained in the PASQ are famil-iar with *ACSM's Guidelines for Exercise Testing and Prescription (ACSM's Guidelines)* and meet the qualifications to conduct such interpretation as described in the *ACSM's Guidelines*. **It is best to refer Tables 2-1, 2-2, 2-3, 2-4 and Figure 2-1 in the *ACSM's Guidelines* as reading through these interpretive guidelines.**

The information below provides an explanation and interpretation of each of the sections presented on the PASQ (Sections 1-4). An explanation is first given describing the items selected in that section and how they relate to the *ACSM's Guidelines* as well as any modifications that were made to make the items easily understood by prospective participants. The interpretation follows.

Note: It is assumed that health/fitness facilities obtain the contact information (address, phone, e-mail) of prospective participants when completing a facility's membership (or participation) application form. If the pre-activity health screening process is completed prior to a participant filling out an application form, the participant's contact information could be added to the PASQ. Prior to beginning the interpretation, be sure that the participant has properly completed the PASQ. It is best to check for completeness and accuracy right after the participant fills out the PASQ. If the PASQ is not completed properly, the participant should be contacted so he/she can then properly complete it.

Section 1- Diagnosed Medical Conditions

Explanation:
The *ACSM's Guidelines* book indicates that anyone with known cardiovascular, pulmonary, or metabolic disease would be considered high risk (see Table 2-4 in *ACSM's Guidelines*). This section of the PASQ lists major cardiovascular, pulmonary and metabolic diseases. Some terms used by ACSM have been modified (re-worded) so they can be understood by participants (the lay public), e.g., terms such as "heart attack" and "abnormal heart rhythm" are used instead of "myocardial infarction" and "complex ventricular arrhythmias," respectively. This section also includes two additional questions regarding "other medical conditions" and "prescribed medications."

Interpretation:
If there are any boxes marked "Y" in this section, the participant is considered HIGH risk. *Note:* The reason for the follow-up "yes-no" questions for heart murmur and asthma is that these conditions

sometimes are diagnosed in childhood and no longer exist as an adult. If a participant answers "Y" to one of these follow-up questions, he/she would be considered HIGH risk. Also, it was decided to classify participants who marked "Y" to either of the two added questions (other medical conditions and prescription medications) as HIGH risk. In addition to cardiovascular, pulmonary, or metabolic diseases, there are many other medical conditions that warrant physician clearance prior to exercise. This is commensurate with recommendations that appear on the AHA/ACSM Health/Fitness Facility Preparticipation Screening Questionnaire (see Figure 2-1) in the *ACSM's Guidelines*. To keep the PASQ easy and quick to interpret, it was decided *not* to list numerous other medical conditions here or to have participants list prescribed medications they take so that health/fitness professionals would not need to make any judgments here that are not only difficult to make but difficult to make on a consistent basis.

Section 2- Signs & Symptoms

Explanation:
The *ACSM's Guidelines* book lists nine major signs and symptoms suggestive of cardiovascular, pulmonary, or metabolic disease (see Table 2-3). This section of the PASQ contains eight of these nine. One of the nine (known heart murmur) was listed in Section 1 under Cardiovascular Disease on the PASQ because this is a condition diagnosed by a physician, versus a sign or symptom that a participant would likely recognize. Almost all of the eight signs and symptoms listed in Section 2 have been modified with phrases that participants would understand, e.g., "shortness of breath occurring 2-5 hours after the onset of sleep" (versus "paroxysmal nocturnal dyspnea") and "pain in the legs while walking; often more severe when walking upstairs/uphill" (versus "intermittent claudication"). It is also important to recognize that the modified phrases do not reflect all of the information under Clarification/Significance in Table 2-3, again to make the PASQ easy and quick to complete.

Interpretation:
If there are any boxes marked "Y" in this section, the participant is considered HIGH risk.

Section 3- Risk Factors

Explanation:
In addition to age, the *ACSM's Guidelines* book lists seven positive risk factors and one negative risk factor for coronary artery disease (see Table 2-2). Please note the following for each of these risk factors as they are listed in Section 3 on the PASQ and how some of these have been modified so they can be easily understood by a participant:

Age risk factor
Age—In Table 2-4 (*ACSM's Guidelines*), age is included as a criterion to determine if the participant is low risk (men < 45 years and women < 55 years) or moderate risk (men ≥ 45 years and women ≥ 55 years). The two items related to age are listed first in this Section.

Positive Risk Factors
Family history—modified by using terms such as heart attack (versus myocardial infarction) and coronary (heart) by pass surgery (versus coronary revascularization) as well as using the terms brother and sister for male and female first-degree relative.

Cigarette smoking—slightly modified.

Hypertension—modified by using two items to address this risk factor: a) "I take medication for high blood pressure" (included in first list with Y and N boxes), and b) "My blood pressure is greater than or equal to 140/90 mm Hg" (included in second list with Y, N, and DK boxes).

Dyslipidemia—modified by using two items to address this risk factor: a) "I take medication for high cholesterol" (included in first list with Y and N boxes), and b) "My blood cholesterol is greater than 200 mg/dL" (included in second list with Y, N, and DK boxes). *Note:* It was decided to not list items related to HDL and LDL levels to keep the PASQ easy/quick for participants to complete and because many participants will not know these values.

Impaired fasting glucose—slightly modified (included in second list with Y, N, and DK boxes).

Obesity—modified by using BMI only (waist girth and waist/hip ratio not included) to keep this form easy/quick for participants to complete. Participants are instructed to the next page (attached to PASQ) for a chart to calculate their own BMI.

Sedentary lifestyle—slightly modified by specifying (quantifying) the recommendations from the U.S. Surgeon General's Report. *Note:* "6" months was selected to be consistent with the cigarette smoking timeframe.

Negative Risk Factor
High-serum HDL cholesterol—slightly modified. Though many participants will not know this value, it was included because it can be subtracted from the sum of positive risk factors according to *ACSM's Guidelines*.

Interpretation:
This interpretation involves counting the total number of "positive" risk factors that the participant has. If a participant does not know (indicates DK) for his/her Blood Pressure, Cholesterol, or Blood Glucose, then for each DK indicated, it would count as one positive risk factor, until determined otherwise. *Note:* Some health/fitness facilities provide screening tests to obtain these values or some participants can obtain these values from their physician or elsewhere. Once these values are obtained, the responses on the PASQ can be changed accordingly.

If the participant indicated "Y" for the age risk factor (male ≥45 years or female ≥55 years), they are considered MODERATE risk OR if the participant indicated "Y" for two or more of the other (other than age) positive risk factors, the participant is considered MODERATE risk. However, because there are two items each to assess hypertension and dyslipidemia as described above, it will be important to not count these twice, if they are both marked "Y." For example, a participant may indicate "Y" to the statement "I take medication for high blood pressure" and then also indicate "Y" for "My blood pressure is greater than or equal to 140/90 mm Hg." In this situation, the "hypertension" risk factor would be counted once. If one of these statements is marked "Y," then this also counts as a positive risk factor. The same also applies to the two similar cholesterol items.

If the participant indicates "Y" to "My high-density lipoprotein (HDL) cholesterol level is greater than 60 mg/dL," then subtract one "positive" risk factor from the total. If marked "N" or "DK," do not use this item when counting the total number of positive risk factors.

To assist in the accurate counting of "positive" risk factors and determination of "low" or moderate" risk, see gray box (Staff Use Only) on the PASQ Interpretive Guidelines—Abbreviated Version.

Note: If the participant provides his/her LDL, HDL, waist girth, or waist/girth ratio (e.g., these values are obtained at the health/fitness facility or elsewhere), then these values could be used in addition to the above to count the total number of positive risk factors. The following would be considered positive risk factors:

For Dyslipidemia:
LDL > 130 mg/dL
HDL < 40 mg/dL

For Obesity:
Waist girth: > 102 cm for men and > 88 cm for women
Waist/girth ratio: ≥ 0.95 for men and ≥ 0.86 for women

Section 4- Acknowledgement, Follow-up, and Signature

Explanation and Interpretation:
Be sure that each blank (signature and date) is completed in a legible manner. The *ACSM's Guidelines* book does not provide any recommendations on how often pre-activity health screening should occur. A reasonable time period would perhaps be at least yearly. Because one's health status can change overnight, the statement "if my health status changes at anytime . . ." has been included so that the participant understands that it is his/her responsibility to inform the health/fitness facility of any such changes. Health/fitness facilities should have procedures to follow when this occurs such as having the participant complete the pre-activity screening process again.

To continue, see the Gray Box on the PASQ Interpretive Guidelines—Abbreviated Version

Explanation:
In the gray box, for Risk Category, indicate "HIGH" risk for any "Y" responses in Sections 1 and 2. If there are no "Y" responses in Sections 1 and 2, indicate MODERATE risk for anyone with "age" as a risk factor OR for anyone with two more positive risk factors. *Note:* In the gray box, check (√) the risk factors that apply and add these up. If the negative risk factor applies (HDL > 60), then subtract one positive risk factor from the total. Indicate in the gray box the number of "positive" risk factors for "total positive risk factors." If a participant: (a) did not mark any items "Y" in Sections 1 and 2, (b) did not mark "Y" for the age risk factor item, and (c) marked none or only one "Y" for the positive risk factor items in Section 3, indicate LOW risk. Complete the remaining information requested in the gray box as described below under Interpretation.

Interpretation:
The *ACSM's Guidelines* book indicates (see Table 2-1) that anyone classified as HIGH risk should obtain medical examination and exercise testing (meaning diagnostic/clinical exercise testing) prior

to initiating moderate (40–59% VO_2R) and vigorous (>60% VO_2R) exercise training. Health/fitness professionals do not determine if a participant needs a medical examination or exercise testing, but should require physician clearance for HIGH and MODERATE risk individuals. It will be the physician's decision if a medical evaluation is needed and what tests, if any, are needed prior to exercise.

The *ACSM's Guidelines* book indicates (see Table 2-1) that anyone classified as MODERATE risk should have a medical examination and exercise testing (or for the purposes herein, obtain physician clearance) prior to initiating vigorous (>60% VO_2R) exercise training. It is assumed from the *ACSM's Guidelines* that an individual who will be exercising at moderate levels and is classified as MODERATE risk that a medical evaluation and exercise testing is not recommended. However, all individuals classified as MODERATE risk should obtain physician clearance, because it will be difficult to know if a participant will be exercising at moderate or vigorous levels while using the health/fitness facility. For individuals classified as LOW risk, it is indicated in the *ACSM's Guidelines* that a medical evaluation and exercise testing is not necessary prior to initiation of exercise training. (It is assumed that "exercise training" means both moderate and vigorous exercise). Therefore, they do not need to obtain physician clearance. Indicate "Y" or "N" in the gray box as to whether or not physician clearance is needed.

Obtaining physician clearance

Once it is determined that physician clearance is needed, we recommend making a copy of the PASQ and giving it to the participant along with the health/fitness facility's physician clearance form. (See example Physician Clearance Form). Ask the participant to take these documents to his/her physician for completion and signature. Indicate the date in the gray box when this was done. *Note:* Some health/fitness facilities may opt to fax (or mail) these documents to the physician, but we believe it may be more efficient if the participant takes these documents directly to his/her physician due to the relationship that exists between the participant and physician and at the same time, protect the privacy of the information obtained. If the PASQ is faxed to the physician, the participant should first complete and sign a medical release. If the Physician Clearance Form is faxed back to the health/fitness facility, be sure it is faxed to a "secure" fax machine to comply with privacy laws. For participants that do not have a physician, it may be a good idea to provide participants a list of physicians (that are taking new patients) who have offices in the geographical area of the health/fitness facility.

Once the physician clearance form is completed and returned, indicate the date in the gray box. Also, the staff member who processed the PASQ should include his/her name in the gray box. Health/fitness facilities should have procedures in place that describe how to properly file the: (a) PASQ (original), (b) PASQ Interpretive Guidelines—Abbreviated Version, and (c) Physician Clearance Form (these forms should be stapled together) as well as how this information is used and by whom.

The PASQ Detailed Interpretive Guidelines: Developed by the authors of the PASQ—Aaron C. Craig and JoAnn M. Eickhoff-Shemek. Copyright © 2007. All rights reserved.
ACSM's Guidelines for Exercise Testing and Prescription. 7th Ed. Philadelphia, PA: Lippincott Williams & Wilkins; 2006.

FORM 6-4
Pre-Activity Screening Questionnaire (PASQ) Interpretive Guidelines:
Abbreviated Version

Once the "Detailed Interpretive Guidelines" are used to train health/fitness professionals who will be interpreting the PASQ, the following can then be used for easy and quick interpretation.

Step 1: If any items are marked "Y" in Sections 1 or 2, indicate HIGH risk in the gray box.

Step 2: If no items are marked "Y" in Sections 1 and 2, but the age risk factor item is marked "Y" in Section 3, then indicate MODERATE risk in the gray box.

Step 3: If no items are marked "Y" in Sections 1 and 2 and the age risk factor item is marked "N" in Section 3, but there is a total of 2 or more positive risk factors, then indicate MODERATE risk in the gray box. *Note:* Check (√) the risk factors that apply in the gray box and then total the number of positive risk factors.

Step 4: If no items are marked "Y" in Sections 1 and 2, the age risk factor item is marked "N" in Section 3, and there is a total of only one (or none) for positive risk factors, then indicate LOW risk in the gray box.

Step 5: All participants classified as LOW risk do not need to obtain physician clearance. All participants classified as MODERATE or HIGH risk do need to obtain physician clearance. Make a copy of the PASQ to give to the participant along with the Physician Clearance Form and ask them to take these documents to his/her physician for completion and signature. Indicate the date this occurred in the gray box. Once the Physician Clearance Form is returned to the health/fitness facility, indicate this date in the gray box. Also, the staff member who processed the PASQ needs to include his/her name in the gray box.

Step 6: Follow the health/fitness facility's procedures regarding proper filing of these documents and how this information will be used and by whom.

Staff Use Only

Positive (+) Risk Factors: ❏ Fam. Hist. ❏ Cig. Smoking ❏ BP ❏ Chol. ❏ Glucose
❏ Obesity ❏ Sedentary

Negative (−) Risk Factor: ❏ High HDL (>60mg/dL)

Total Positive (+) Risk Factors: _____   **Risk Category:** ❏ Low ❏ Mod. ❏ High

Physician Clearance Needed: ❏ Yes ❏ No

PASQ and Physician Clearance form given to participant on: _____
                                                              (Date)

Physician Clearance received: _____
                                   (Date)

Processed by: _____
            (Staff Member's Name)

FORM 6–5
Physician Clearance Form

Your patient _____ (Name of Participant) would like to participate in the exercise/fitness programs and services at _____ (Facility Name). _____ (Facility Name) is a **non-clinical health/fitness facility** that provides a variety of low, moderate, and high intensity exercise/fitness activities. To comply with recommendations established by the American College of Sports Medicine, we have all participants complete the PASQ, a brief health history questionnaire that is used to classify them into low, moderate, or high risk categories. Based on the responses to the PASQ (see attached), your patient has been classified as either "moderate" or "high" risk and therefore needs to obtain physician clearance prior to participating in our exercise/fitness programs and services. Once completed and signed by you, your patient can return this form to us. Or, you can fax this form back to me at _____ (secure fax number of health/fitness facility). If you have any questions, please feel free to contact me _____ .
(phone, e-mail address of staff member responsible for processing pre-activity health screening).

Thank you,

_____
(Name and title of staff member responsible for processing pre-activity health screening)

Please check (√) one of the following:
☐ Cleared to exercise at this facility
☐ Not cleared to exercise at this facility
☐ Not cleared to exercise at this facility—should be referred to a clinically-supervised exercise program
☐ Cleared to exercise at this facility with the following restrictions and/or limitations:

_____
_____
_____

_____
Physician's Name (printed)

_____   _____
Physician's Signature   Date

_____
Mailing address   City   State   Zip
(_____)_____
Phone

7

Health/Fitness Assessment and Prescription

After reading this chapter, health/fitness students and professionals will be able to:

1. Identify applicable laws related to health/fitness assessments and prescriptions.

2. Describe the various published standards of practice that address health/fitness assessments and prescriptions.

3. Understand the different roles of varoius levels of health/fitness professionals with regard to health/fitness assessments and prescriptions and the potential legal implications of practicing outside scopes of practice.

4. Develop risk management strategies that will help minimize legal liability associated with health/fitness assessments and prescriptions.

This chapter describes statutory, administrative, and case law as well as various standards of practice published by professional organizations relevant to health/fitness assessment and prescription. Specific risk management strategies are also presented so that health/fitness professionals and their risk management committees can consider the steps they can take to help minimize any criminal charges and civil liability that can potentially arise when providing health/fitness assessment and prescription programs/services.

Once an individual completes a facility's pre-activity health screening process (see Chapter 6), he or she may opt to participate in various health/fitness assessments provided by the professionals who work at the facility. Health/fitness assessments may include: (a) biometric screening tests such as blood pressure, cholesterol, and glucose; (b) body composition; and (c) fitness variables such as cardiovascular endurance, muscle strength/endurance, and flexibility. Once a participant completes certain health/fitness tests, an individualized exercise prescription is often prepared by a health/fitness professional for that individual. Although various health/fitness professionals may be involved in the delivery of these types of programs/services, they must be qualified to do so. This is especially important when providing these types of services for participants who represent special populations, such as those with certain medical conditions.

STEP 1 ASSESSMENT OF LEGAL LIABILITY EXPOSURES

This section presents laws and published standards of practice related to health/fitness assessments and prescriptions. However, it is important to first distinguish the terms *health-related physical fitness testing* and *clinical exercise testing*.[1] These are the purposes of health-related fitness testing:

- "Educating participants about their present health-related fitness status relative to health-related standards and age- and sex-matched norms
- Providing data that are helpful in development of exercise prescriptions to address all fitness components
- Collecting baseline and follow-up data that allow evaluation of progress by exercise program participants
- Motivating participants by establishing reasonable and attainable fitness goals
- Stratifying cardiovascular risk."[2]

Health-related fitness tests are commonly conducted in health/fitness facilities. Clinical exercise tests prescribed by physicians are primarily conducted in hospitals or medical clinics with the major purpose of "diagnosing" or ruling out coronary artery disease (CAD). It would be rare for health/fitness facilities to conduct clinical testing because of the need for medical supervision during such testing.[1] Therefore, discussing the law (and related published standards of practice) related to clinical exercise testing is not the focus of this section. However, regarding clinical testing, it is interesting to note that according to Herbert and Herbert,[3] negligence claims/lawsuits have been filed against physicians, exercise technicians, and the health care organizations they represent for alleged failure to (a) conduct such a test for a moderate- or high-risk individual, (b) give proper informed consent prior to testing, (c) stop the test when the patient's signs/symptoms indicated a need to do so, (d) monitor the patient immediately after the test, and (e) follow published standards of practice addressing clinical testing such as those established by ACSM,[1] AHA,[4,5] ACC (American College of Cardiology)/AHA,[6] and ACC/ACP (American College of Physicians).[7] Health/fitness facilities that opt to offer clinical exercise testing should follow these published standards of practice.

THE LAW

Health/fitness professionals need to be aware of federal and state laws that apply to health/fitness assessments and prescriptions. These include the Health Insurance Portability and Accountability Act (HIPAA), Americans with Disabilities Act (ADA), Occupational Safety and Health Administration's (OSHA's) Bloodborne Pathogens Standard, Clinical Laboratory Improvement Amendments (CLIA), and state statutes that govern the practice of medicine or other licensed health care professions. In addition, this section addresses several interesting legal cases involving some nonlicensed individuals whose conduct crossed over into a licensed profession, as well as personal fitness trainers whose conduct with regard to health/fitness assessments and prescriptions resulted in harm to their clients.

Federal Laws

Because virtually all types of health/fitness assessments involve the collection of individual health information, laws such as HIPAA and state/local privacy laws may apply. See Chapter 6 for additional information on these laws. However, to be compliant with these laws, health/fitness professionals need to ensure that individual health/fitness assessment and prescription data are kept private, confidential, and secure. And, as also discussed in Chapter 6, failure to keep individual health information private, confidential, and secure can also result in civil claims and lawsuits due to unintended uses or disclosure to individuals who do not have a need or requirement to know.[3] In addition, for health/fitness professionals who work in employer-sponsored health and fitness programs, they must understand that the ADA requires the maintenance of confidentiality with regard to any employee's individual health information obtained in the program.[3] ADA regulations would also apply, as described in Chapter 6, regarding any policies that would possibly exclude individuals from participation in health/fitness assessments and prescriptions. To help achieve compliance with the Title III of the ADA, it may be a good idea for health/fitness facilities to have qualified staff members who can conduct health/fitness assessments and prescriptions (as well as other programs/services) appropriately for individuals with disabilities. Health/fitness facilities may want to consider having staff members obtain the new Specialty Certification that was developed as a collaborative effort between the ACSM and the National Center on Physical Activity and Disability (NCPAD). For more information, see the ACSM or NCAPD websites: www.acsm.org and www.ncpad.org.

Health/fitness facilities that conduct health screenings requiring a blood test (e.g., a fingerstick to determine cholesterol and glucose values) need to comply with the requirements of OSHA's Bloodborne Pathogens Standard (see Chapter 11). In addition to this federal law, they should review the Clinical Laboratory Improvement Amendments (CLIA) passed by Congress in 1998. For more information on the CLIA, visit www.fda.gov/cdrh/clia. This law established quality standards for all laboratory testing including testing for the assessment of health regardless of where the test is performed. This regulation requires obtaining CLIA certification, which is quite complex and costly. In some cases, such as performing fingerstick testing, a Certificate of Waiver can be obtained. In most cases, it would be best for health/fitness facilities to collaborate with a local hospital or clinic that already possesses the CLIA certification to provide such screenings. Health/fitness professionals and their risk management advisory committees should also research any applicable state or local laws regarding the qualification/credential requirements of individuals who can conduct these types of tests as well as any other related legal requirements.

As mentioned earlier, negligence cases exist where physicians have failed to conduct proper informed consent procedures prior to clinical exercise testing.[3] Because clinical exercise testing is considered a medical procedure, informed consent is a legal requirement as it is prior to other medical procedures. The failure to do so can result in either breach of contract or negligence/malpractice claims and lawsuits, and in some cases, battery—an intentional tort.[3] For more information on informed consent, see Chapter 4. Although informed consent is perhaps not a legal requirement prior to health-related fitness tests or prescription in health/fitness facilities, it is highly recommended.

However, if health/fitness facilities are conducting research involving human subjects or collaborating with another organization to conduct research that involves health-related fitness testing, prescription, or participation, informed consent is required by administrative law, 45 C.F.R. §46—Protection of Human Subjects. This law is quite complex and contains many parts. In general, this law requires institutional review boards (IRBs) to approve the procedures of any study involving human subjects, including obtaining informed consent. Because many types of risks exist with participation in fitness testing and exercise programs, a written informed consent (versus implied consent) would most likely be required and would need to be approved by an IRB. Although obtaining IRB approval of the research procedures and informed consent is the responsibility of the principal investigator (PI)—the person overseeing the research project—health/fitness professionals involved in the research need to understand the importance of their legal requirement to carry out the informed consent and other procedures properly. See the Development of Risk Management Strategies section later in this chapter.

State Laws

When obtaining or interpreting health/fitness data collected during health/fitness assessments or when prescribing an individual health/fitness program, health/fitness professionals should do so within their own **scope of practice.** It is critical that they do not "diagnose," "prescribe," "treat," or cross over into the practice of a licensed profession because this can lead to criminal charges for practicing medicine (or some allied health profession) without a license or the unauthorized practice of medicine (or some allied health profession). Because these statutes can vary from state to state, health/fitness professionals and their risk management advisory committees should research these statutes in their respective states. For example, in Florida the title of this statute is "Unlicensed Practice of a Health Care Profession"[8] and covers all licensed health care professions. In Ohio, a statute governs the practice of dietetics called the "Unauthorized Practice of Dietetics"[9] and another statute is titled "Practice of Medicine and Surgery without Certificate."[10]

These state statutes often describe the licensed practice by listing what a person with such a license does. Ohio's "Unauthorized Practice of Dietetics" statute states that the practice of dietetics means any of the following:

(1) *Nutritional assessment to determine nutritional needs and to recommend appropriate nutritional intake, including enteral and parenteral nutrition;*

(2) *Nutritional counseling or education as components of preventive, curative, and restorative health care;*

(3) *Development, administration, evaluation, and consultation regarding nutritional care Standards.*[11]

Statutes like this one are of particular importance because health/fitness professionals often provide nutrition and weight management information and advice to their clients and participants. This statute distinguishes "nutrition education" (which only licensed dieticians can do) and "general nonmedical nutrition information" which defines what nonlicensed dieticians can do. "Nutritional education" means a planned program based on learning objectives with expected outcomes designed to modify nutrition-related behaviors.[12] "General nonmedical nutrition information" is defined as follows:

1. *principles of good nutrition and food preparation;*
2. *foods to be included in the normal daily diet;*
3. *the essential nutrients needed by the body;*
4. *recommended amounts of the essential nutrients;*
5. *the actions of nutrients on the body;*
6. *the effects of deficiencies or excesses of nutrients; or*
7. *food and supplements that are good sources of essential nutrients."*[13]

Therefore, health/fitness professionals in Ohio whose conduct goes beyond providing general nonmedical nutrition information would be violating this state statute and potentially subject to criminal charges. Although other similar state statues governing the practice of dietetics may not be as specific as Ohio's, which provides a definition of general nonmedical nutrition education, this definition can provide some direction for the development of a risk management procedure in this area for all health/fitness professionals to consider.

Health/fitness professionals need to be careful not to violate other similar statutes, (e.g., practicing medicine without a license) when conducting health/fitness assessments and/or providing exercise prescriptions. This is especially important when dealing with individuals who would be classified as moderate or high risk. For example, when working with a participant with arthritis, saying something to a participant like "this exercise will help *treat* your arthritis" goes beyond the scope of practice of a health/fitness professional and could be violating a state statute that specifies only physicians can treat arthritis and other medical conditions.

Health/fitness professionals should avoid *diagnosing, treating, prescribing,* and *counseling*. These terms describe behaviors that often reflect the practices of licensed health care professionals. Health/fitness professionals may ask about the use of the term *exercise prescription*—a term used often and included in competencies such as those published by ACSM for Health/Fitness Instructors.[1] Unless specified in a state licensing statute, a term used by an individual (e.g., the term *exercise prescription* used by a health/fitness professional) alone does not violate the parameters within that statute. Most often, a violation is determined by the "conduct" of the individual. For example, if a health/fitness professional "prescribed" exercise to *treat* a medical condition, he or she likely would be violating a state statute versus prescribing exercise for general improvement of health and fitness, which would be within the scope of practice of health/fitness professionals. More on this topic is covered later.

Depending on the state, penalties can include both misdemeanor and felony charges against an individual whose conduct violates state statute(s). For example, the Florida statute[8] includes the following penalties:

a. *A **cease and desist notice**, which requires the individual to stop the practice. This violation can result in a fine between $500 and $5,000. Each day the unlicensed practice continues after the notice is given, another separate violation can be charged. In addition to this administrative remedy, the state licensing board or department can seek civil penalties.*
b. *3rd-degree felony: Minimum penalty is a fine of $1,000 and mandatory period of incarceration of 1 year.*
c. *2nd-degree felony: Practice results in serious bodily injury; minimum penalty is the same as 3rd-degree felony.*
d. *1st-degree misdemeanor: Minimum penalty is a fine of $500 and imprisonment for 30 days.*

Health/fitness professionals must recognize that the violation of a state statute does not require that "harm" occurred to the plaintiff as it does in negligence claims and lawsuits. Therefore, a health/fitness professional can suffer the penalties just listed even though no harm or injury occurred to the participant or client.

In additional to criminal charges, **negligence per se** may also apply when the conduct of a health/fitness professional violates these types of state statutes. In these cases, a finding of negligence is not automatic; however, the plaintiff will *not* have to prove the defendant had a duty, breached the duty, and that the breach caused the harm as in ordinary negligence, but he or she will have to show that the violation of a state statue caused the harm.[14]

In a negligence claim or lawsuit, if the conduct of a health/fitness professional crossed over into that of a licensed health care provider, the health/fitness professional can also be held to the standard of care commensurate with that licensed health care professional. Obviously, health/fitness professionals will not be able to meet this standard of care because they do not have the necessary credentials and license to do so.

Case Law

Although there are no known cases in which health/fitness professionals have been criminally charged with violating state statutes that govern the practice (or unauthorized practice) of medicine or some other allied health profession, there are cases in which individuals have violated state statutes with regard to the practice of medicine and dietetics. In *Stetina v. State Medical Licensing Board,*[15] the defendant Janice Stetina was using questionnaires and examining eyes to assess and determine various health problems (e.g., nutritional and abdominal problems) and then recommending colonic irrigation, mineral water, kelp, amelade, progestin, and more raw food. The appellate court upheld the trial court's decision that:

1. *The Defendant, Janice R. Stetina, is hereby permanently enjoined from practicing medicine in Indiana until she is issued a license by the state of Indiana.*
2. *The Defendant, Janice R Stetina, is not enjoined from lecturing or educating members of the public on her view of the value of nutrition or from selling products to members of the public so long as the defendant does not examine the member, diagnose or treat the member, sell the member health products based on the Defendant's assessment of the members' needs or problems or otherwise engage in the practice of medicine . . .[16]*

Stetina argued that the trial court's decision was outside the intended scope of the state of Indiana's Medical Practice Act and that her acts fell within some exceptions to the prohibition of unlicensed medical practice. The appellate court's response to this was that the act "protects people generally in their relationships with professionals to whom they entrust medical judgments . . . and also protects against the well-intentioned but unskilled practices of health care professionals, as well as against those well-intentioned and skilled practices which simply exceed the scope of acceptable health care."[17]

Stetina also claimed that she was not practicing medicine because none of the vitamins she recommended required medical prescription and they can be purchased over the counter.

Quoting a 1978 case, *Norville v. Mississippi State Medical Association* (364 So.2d 1084), the court stated, "We are fully cognizant that any layman can obtain such vitamins and that any retailer can sell vitamins. Purchase of or sale of vitamins is not however the vice which is condemned here. Rather the vice condemned and that which constitutes the unlicensed practice of medicine is prescription of vitamins to cure an ailment or disease for compensation."[18]

In *Ohio Board of Dietetics v. Brown,*[19] the defendant (a) performed nutritional assessments and recommended nutritional supplements to individuals, (b) engaged in nutritional counseling and education for the purpose of treating specific complaints and ailments of individuals, and (c) represented himself as a nutritionist, registered nutritionist, doctor of nutrition, and/or as a Ph.D. or M.D. The appellate court upheld the trial court's ruling allowing the board's (Ohio Board of Dietetics) request for an **injunction** against the defendant because as the trial court stated,

> *(1) the defendant was not licensed to practice dietetics in the state of Ohio; (2) defendant was engaged in the practice of dietetics as defined in R.C. 4759.01(A); (3) defendant's activities were not protected by the Free Exercise Clause of the First Amendment to the United States Constitution, and; (4) until defendant "obtains a license, he is barred from engaging in nutritional counseling or assessments of any other activity set forth in R.C. 4759.02(A)."*[20]

Interestingly, the defendant in this case attempted to excuse his unlawful activities by calling himself a "nutritionist" versus a dietician. However, the appellate court stated "the acts defendant performs are more important than his title and since he does not possess a license to provide nutritional counseling and assessments, defendants acts are in violation of R.C. 4759.02(A)."[21] This ruling has application to health/fitness professionals as well. Although titles of health/fitness professionals should be commensurate with job duties and responsibilities, a title a person gives himself or herself will probably not be a factor when it comes to determining if there was a violation of a state statute (unless titles are clearly defined by statute as to who can use them) or practicing outside one's scope of practice in a civil claim. It will be the acts or conduct of health/fitness professionals that courts will use to make these types of determinations.

No known case law exists where health/fitness professionals have been found liable for improperly conducting health/fitness assessments. However, the issue of failing to assess health and fitness variables has been alleged in some cases. For example, in *Chai v. Sports & Fitness Clubs of America Inc.* (previously described in Chapters 5 and 6), one of the claims was that the defendant failed to assess the plaintiff's fitness and health prior to his use of the facility, and in *Rostai v Neste Enterprises* (also described in Chapter 6), the plaintiff claimed that the defendant owed him a duty to assess his physical condition. Most claims involving health/fitness professionals have involved improper health/fitness prescriptions for clients in personal training programs as described in the following two cases.

In *Capati v. Crunch Fitness International, et al.*[22,23] personal trainer August Casseus allegedly recommended that his client Anne Marie Capati, a 37-year-old woman, take a variety of over-the-counter nutritional and dietary supplements including some that contained ephedra. It was also alleged that Capati had informed the personal trainer that she was taking prescribed medications for hypertension. While performing light squats at the club, Capati became ill, lost consciousness, and several hours later died at the hospital of a brain hemorrhage (stroke). The decedent's family filed a wrongful death claim and sought $320 million in both compensatory and punitive damages.

The personal trainer testified he had given his client suggestions and advice as to certain foods and supplements but that he did not advise Capati there may be negative health consequences for her to do so while on hypertension medication and while working out. Regarding his qualifications, he testified that he (a) had completed high school through a GED, (b) had been in the Air Force, (c) had applied for a correspondence school course to obtain certification in personal training, (d) had not received certification while employed by Crunch Fitness, (e) was not certified in CPR, and (f) was initially hired by Crunch Fitness as a Level I personal trainer and later became a Level II personal trainer.

A consultant who testified for Crunch Fitness and who was in charge of hiring and developing personal trainers at Crunch testified that (a) Crunch Fitness had an unwritten rule for personal trainers not to give out nutritional advice, (b) he would not put a member with high blood pressure on a leg press with a lot of weight because it would elevate her systolic blood pressure, (c) he would not allow somebody on hypertensive medication to take ephedra or work out because such a person might have a stroke, and (d) there was something wrong with the trainer giving Capati a workout that involved a leg press, no matter what the weight, given the hypertensive medication and ephedra.

This case was settled before going to trial for a total aggregate payment of $4,065,000.[24] Crunch Fitness International and August Casseus were liable for $1,750,000 of the total settlement amount. Other defendants named in this case also contributed to the settlement (e.g., Vitamin Shoppe Industries, Inc. was liable for $2 million of the total amount). This case is a good example of how the legal principle *respondeat superior* is applied. That is, employers (Crunch Fitness in this case) can be liable for the alleged negligent acts of their employees (personal trainer August Casseus, in this case).

In *Makris v. Scandinavian Health Spa, Inc.*,[25] Caliope Makris received two free personal training sessions with personal trainer Jeannette Estromirez when she joined the spa. While using a leg press machine during her first training session (March 1, 1994), Makris informed her trainer that she felt a sharp pain in her neck that radiated down her arm. The trainer told her the pain was related to upper body weakness. Makris experienced the same pain during the second training session (March 3, 1994) with the personal trainer while using the leg press machine. Makris went to a physician the day after her second training session, but the physician did not provide any indication of her problem. Toward the end of April, Makris signed up for 10 more personal training sessions with the same personal trainer, in which she continued using the leg press machine. On May 11, 1994, she returned to her physician because her neck pain was so intense and constant. On this visit, the doctor told her she might have multiple sclerosis, but Makris denied any testing because she was leaving on a three-month trip to Greece. In November 1994, magnetic resonance imaging (MRI) revealed that she had three herniated cervical disks. In August 1995, a former employee of the spa told Makris that her slipped disks were probably caused by the leg press and the personal trainer should have never allowed her to use the machine.

In April 1996, Makris filed a personal injury suit against Ms. Estromirez (her trainer), Scandinavian, and Bally's Total Fitness Corporation, alleging the defendants "rendered negligent training, monitoring, instruction, supervision, and advice"[26] during the time period of the 10 training sessions. The defendants filed a motion for summary judgment, claiming the suit was not filed within the two-year statute of limitations since Makris first experienced her pain on March 1 and 3, 1994. The trial court granted summary judgment in favor of the defendants. However, the appellate court's response was that no evidence indicated the plaintiff should have discovered by March 3 that her neck pain was due to an actual injury caused by the leg press, especially because the trainer told her at that time that the pain related to upper body weakness and it would subside as she got stronger. The appellate court stated, "Before a statute of limitations begins to run, not only must the plaintiff discover that they have an injury, but the plaintiff must also discover with reasonable diligence that the defendant's wrongful conduct caused that injury."[27] According to the appellate court, it was undisputed that the allegedly negligent conduct of the defendants occurred 10 more times starting on April 29, 1994, and thus held that the April 24, 1996, complaint was filed in a timely manner. They reversed the trial court's decision and remanded to the trial court for further proceedings.

This is an excellent case to demonstrate that the personal fitness trainer in this case may not have had the knowledge, skills, and abilities necessary for training clients. It appears that the trainer may not have known how to distinguish different types of "pain," that is, the general pain or discomfort associated with training versus pain associated with a possible injury or problem. Sharp pain in the neck that radiates down the arm is not consistent with the type of pain or discomfort associated with training—even for a deconditioned person. And then the trainer actually "diagnosed" this pain, stating to the plaintiff that it was due to weakness and would go away as she became stronger. This conduct is clearly outside of the scope of practice of personal fitness trainers. This is also a good case to demonstrate how the statute of limitations works in personal injury cases. Often, the time period does not begin until the plaintiff discovers he or she has an injury likely caused by the defendant. With personal injuries involving health/fitness participants, this can sometimes occur after they are no longer a member or participant at the facility. Lastly, this is a good case to show that health/fitness facilities should inform all employees that they should never talk about the conduct of other employees when communicating with participants. It was the suggestion of a former employee in this case that triggered Makris's lawsuit against the defendants.

It appears the personal fitness trainers in the cases just cited may not have had the necessary knowledge, skill, and abilities to safely prescribe health/fitness activities to meet the individual needs of their clients. With programs like personal fitness training, it is likely that the professional standard of care will be applied when determining whether or not a health/fitness professional was negligent.

It is important to understand that the professional standard of care does not vary given the credentials or experience of the person in charge.[14] According to van der Smissen, "if one accepts responsibility for giving leadership to an activity or providing a service, one's performance is measured against the standard of care of a qualified professional *for that situation*."[28] In other words, the professional standard of care in such a situation is determined by (a) the nature of the activity (e.g., the professional must be aware of the skills and abilities the participant needs to participate safely in the activity; if these are complex, the professional must have knowledge to apply these skills and abilities, and if simple, the knowledge and skill level required of the professional is less); (b) the type of participants (e.g., the professional must be aware of individual factors related to the participant such as any health conditions that impose increased risks and then how to minimize those risks); and (c) the environmental conditions (e.g., the professional must be aware of any conditions such as heat and humidity or slippery floor surfaces within a facility and how to minimize risks associated with these conditions).[14]

In addition, as described in Chapter 3, a **fiduciary relationship** is potentially formed between a health/fitness professional and the participant or client when providing health/fitness assessments and prescriptions. These types of relationships require additional duties of the health/fitness professional, including acting in good faith, trust, special confidence, and candor.[29] Any health/fitness information, advice, or prescription given to a participant or client must be appropriate given her or his individual needs because the person will rely on it. For example, if a client is harmed or injured by following the information, advice, and/or prescription provided by the personal fitness trainer, the trainer may be liable for the harm or injury.

Because it is likely a professional standard of care will be applied to health/fitness professionals who provide programs like individual health/fitness assessments and prescriptions, and because of the added duties associated with the potential fiduciary relationship formed when providing such services, it is critical that only "qualified" health/fitness professionals be assigned to provide health/fitness assessments and prescriptions. Generally, the knowledge, skills, and abilities of health/fitness professionals working with low-risk individuals would be less than those health/fitness professionals working with moderate- or high-risk individuals.

THE PUBLISHED STANDARDS OF PRACTICE

Before describing published standards of practice that address health/fitness assessments and prescriptions, it is important to review the scope of practice of professionals that provide such services. Of the ten published standards of practice identified in Chapter 3, four of the organizations that published these standards of practice offer certification programs for professionals who provide health/fitness assessments and prescriptions. Two of the four specifically define the scope of practice of these professionals (ACSM and NSCA); the other two (YMCA and AFAA) describe these roles in a more general way. As presented in Chapter 1, ACSM has defined the scope of practice of a Health/Fitness Instructor as follows:

The ACSM Health/Fitness Instructor® (HFI) is a degreed health and fitness professional qualified for career pursuits in the university, corporate, commercial, hospital, and community settings. The HFI has knowledge and skills in management and administration and training and supervising entry level personnel. The HFI is skilled in conducting risk stratification, conducting physical fitness assessments and interpreting results, constructing appropriate exercise prescriptions in motivating apparently healthy individuals with medically controlled diseases to adopt and maintain health lifestyle behaviors.[30]

The scope of practice for an ACSM Certified Personal Trainer is defined as follows:

An ACSM Certified Personal Trainer[SM] is a fitness professional involved in developing and implementing an individualized approach to exercise leadership in healthy populations and/or those individuals with medical clearance to exercise. Using a variety of teaching techniques, the Certified Personal Trainer[SM] is proficient in leading and demonstrating safe and effective methods of exercise by applying the fundamental principles of exercise science. The Certified Personal Trainer[SM] is proficient in writing appropriate exercise recommendations, leading and demonstrating safe and effective methods of exercise, and motivating individuals to begin and to continue with their healthy behaviors.[31]

The scope of practice for the NSCA-Certified Personal Trainer (CPT) credential is defined as follows:

Personal trainers are health/fitness professionals who, using an individualized approach, assess, motivate, educate, and train clients regarding their health and fitness needs. They design safe and effective exercise programs, provide the guidance to help clients achieve their personal health/fitness goals, and respond appropriately in emergency situations. Recognizing their own area of expertise, personal trainers refer clients to other health care professionals when appropriate.[32]

The scope of practice for the NSCA Certified Strength and Conditioning Specialist (CSCS) credential is defined as follows:

Certified Strength and Conditioning Specialists (CSCSs) are professionals who apply scientific knowledge to train athletes for the primary goal of improving athletic performance. They conduct sport-specific testing sessions, design and implement safe and effective strength training and conditioning programs and provide guidance regarding nutrition and injury prevention. Recognizing that their area of expertise is separate and distinct, CSCSs consult with and refer athletes to other professionals when appropriate.[33]

YMCA Recommendations[34] state that "only appropriately credentialed staff members employed by the YMCA should provide personal training and other wellness services "and that these staff be trained to carry out their duties safely and responsibly, certified as YMCA of the USA Personal Training Instructors (or similarly credentialed in their field)."[35] In addition, YMCA staff involved in health and fitness programs "should ideally include an opportunity for a health assessment; recommendations on safe and effective exercise participation; and education related to a variety of health and wellness issues such as nutrition, and weight management."[35]

AFAA[36] specifies that their personal trainer certification is designed for the experienced fitness professional working one-on-one with clients and their three-day certification workshop includes content such as fitness assessment testing procedures (3-minute step test, sit-and-reach, push-up, abdominal crunch, body composition screening with skin-fold caliper measurement), nutrition fundamentals and weight management, special populations and medical considerations, and wellness programming and screening guidelines.

Although all of the four organizations just listed that offer personal training certifications do not require a degree in the field, the scope of practice varies. For example, NSCA, YMCA, and AFAA indicate (or at least allude to the fact) that personal trainers should be able to conduct health/fitness assessments and design exercise programs for individuals. The ACSM Personal Trainer's scope of practice does not include conducting any types of health/fitness assessments (as does the HFI scope of practice), but it does include implementing an individual program for healthy populations and/or those medically cleared. The HFI's scope of practice includes conducting health/fitness assessments and prescriptions for apparently healthy individuals and those with controlled disease.

IHRSA Standards, NSCA Standards, ACSM's H/F Standards, and ACSM/AHA Joint PP

The IHRSA Standards[37] do not include any standards with regard to health/fitness assessments and/or prescriptions. The NSCA Standards[38] also do not provide specific standards in this area. However, Guideline #1.1 under Participation Screening & Clearance states that "[P]rofessionals should cooperate with a training participant's health care providers at all times, and . . . provide service . . . according to instructions specified by such providers."[39] The following three NSCA guidelines (listed, in part) relate to participation in strength and conditioning activities for children. Guideline #8.1 under Participation in Strength & Conditioning Activities by Children states that youth "under seven (7) years of age should not be permitted to engage in Strength & Conditioning activities with free weights or exercise devices/machines . . . and should be denied access to such training areas."[40] Guideline #8.2 states that youth "between seven (7) and fourteen (14) . . . should be individually assessed by the Strength & Conditioning professional in conjunction with the child's parent(s)/custodian(s) and health care provider(s) to determine if such children may engage in such activities."[41] Guideline #8.3 states that youth "fourteen (14) years of age and older who . . . have reached a level of maturity . . . may engage in such activities . . . with a greater degree of instruction and supervision than that applied to adult populations."[41] In addition, NSCA Standard #9.1 regarding supplements, ergogenic aids, and drugs states that "professionals must not prescribe, recommend, or provide drugs, controlled substances or supplements that are illegal, prohibited, or harmful to athletes for any purpose."[41]

The ACSM H/F Standards[42] include the following two standards with regard to health/fitness assessments and prescription: (a) Standard #9 states that "fitness and healthcare professionals who serve in counseling, instructional, and physical activity supervision roles for the facility must have an appropriate level of professional education, certification, or experience," and (b) Standard #10 states that "fitness and healthcare professionals engaged in pre-activity screening, instructing, monitoring or supervising physical activity programs for facility members or users must have current automated external defibrillation and cardiopulmonary resuscitation (AED/CPR) certification from an organization qualified to provide such certification."[43] (From American College of Sports Medicine, 2007, *ACSM's Health/Fitness Facility Standards and Guidelines*,

3rd ed., pp. 1–2. © 2007 by American College of Sports Medicine. Reprinted with permission from Human Kinetics (Champaign, IL.) In addition, the ACSM H/F Standards[42] provide some related guidelines that address qualifications for those staff members who provide services such as health/fitness assessments and personal instruction, as well as the provision of a medical adviser or medical advisory committee when prescribing physical activity programs for individuals considered at an elevated risk.

The ACSM/AHA Joint PP[44] indicates that submaximal exercise tests are conducted in health/fitness facilities for nondiagnostic purposes such as physical fitness assessment and exercise prescription. This publication also states that "nondiagnostic testing should be conducted only for persons in Class A and only by appropriately qualified, well-trained personnel . . . who are knowledgeable about the indications and contraindications for exercise testing, indications for test termination and test interpretation."[45] Persons in Risk Class A are "apparently healthy" individuals (see Table 6-2 in Chapter 6). Additional recommendations are provided regarding exercise prescription for persons in Risk Class B and Risk Class C. Fitness directors of health/fitness facilities who have responsibility for exercise program design and staff supervision "must have a degree in exercise science, another health-related field or equivalent experience . . . and must hold a professional certification . . . In level 3 facilities, this certification should be comparable to ACSM's health fitness instructor certification . . . In level 4 and 5 facilities, the fitness director should be certified at a level that correlates to ACSM exercise specialist certification . . . The exercise specialist typically holds a master's degree in exercise science or related field and has extensive experience in exercise testing and leadership in clinical populations."[46] See Table 6-2 for a description of facility characteristics for facilities categorized as levels 1 through 5. Direct quotes that appear in this paragraph have been Reprinted with permission. AHA/ACSM Scientific Statement: Recommendations for Cardiovascular Screening, Staffing, and Emergency Policies at Health/Fitness Facilities (Circulation.1998;97:2283-2293.) © 1998 American Heart Association (44).

Canadian Standards, MFA Standards, and AFAA Standards

Canadian Standard #3 under Special Exercising Populations states that "maximal testing of individuals who (a) are not accustomed to regular strenuous exercise, or (b) are males over 40 years of age, or (c) are females over 50 years of age shall be conducted under the supervision of either a physician or personnel with current appraisal certification and ACLS (Advance Cardiac Life Support)."[47] In addition, under Fitness Related Personnel, Standard #2 states that "fitness personnel shall be certified in the area with which they are providing program services (e.g., fitness appraisal, personal training, aerobic classes, aqua fitness classes etc.)."[48]

The MFA Standards, under Standard #2 that addresses pre-activity screening (stated in Chapter 6), provide the following two guidelines (Guidelines #2 and #3) related to health/fitness assessment and prescription: "2. The facility should employ accepted methods to assess functional capacity, body composition, strength and flexibility and other components of physical fitness. 3. The facility should be able to offer exercise testing for fitness assessment as well as exercise prescription purposes."[49] In addition, Standard #6 states that Medical Fitness Centers "must have programs and services for: a. A transition between clinical interventions/rehabilitation and fitness programming according to generally accepted guidelines. b. Prevention, health risk reduction and therapeutic lifestyle programming."[50] Regarding staff qualifications, Standard #9 states that Medical Fitness Centers "must employ one or more professional(s) who hold degrees(s), certification(s), and/or license(s) appropriate to the program(s) offered and populations served."[51] The guidelines underneath this standard describe the specific recommended credentials for fitness directors, personal trainers, group fitness instructors, fitness staff members that provide programming for special populations, and aquatic staff members.

AFAA Standards[52] include a chapter on each of the following: Basic Exercise Standards and Guidelines, Large-Sized Participants, Prenatal Fitness, Youth Fitness, Senior Fitness—Healthy Sedentary Older Adults, and Senior Fitness—Frail Elderly.

These standards and guidelines primarily address "group" exercise for these special populations. However, these could also apply to health/fitness professionals who provide individual health/fitness assessment and prescription programs.[52]

Regarding large-sized participants, the AFAA Standards state that "any kind of fitness testing . . . , unless specifically recommended by a physician, should be optional for the participant."[53] For prenatal participants, the AFAA standards state that "only qualified specialists may assess the safety of exercise, administer an exercise stress test and write an exercise program for the prospective prenatal exercise class participant."[54] In addition, fitness instructors should maintain a close alliance with the participant's physician. Regarding youth programs, a variety of recommendations are provided for safe and effective design. In addition, it is recommended that instructors design an activity questionnaire to determine the appropriate activities for a beginner. For older adults, the AFAA Standards state that "only qualified specialists (e.g., physicians with the assistance of exercise test technologists or clinical exercise physiologists) may assess the safety of exercise and administer an exercise stress test. Individual exercise programs may be developed by senior fitness specialists of AFAA Fitness Practitioners based on information received from the physician and from a comprehensive health questionnaire filled out by the participant."[55] In addition, certain chapters in the AFAA Standards[52] refer to published position statements such as those from the American Academy of Pediatrics and the American College of Obstetricians and Gynecologists.

Because of the many ethical, professional, and legal concerns related to nutritional supplements, AFAA first published a Policy Statement on the Sale, Provision or Recommendation of Nutritional Supplements (http://pdfs.afaa.com) in 1999. This statement has 10 principles that should be considered by health/fitness professionals, three of which (numbers 1, 3, and 5) are briefly described as follows:

1. *Health and fitness facilities and fitness professionals should not sell, recommend or provide ('provide') nutritional supplement products . . . to their employees and/or members/guests/clients unless the sale, recommendation, or provision of such products is justified by scientific and medical research . . .*
3. *Nutritional supplements which have been determined by the FDA to be harmful or those which have been associated with certain adverse effects should not be provided by fitness professionals to clients . . .*
5. *[F]itness professionals who decide to provide nutritional supplement products while also providing information related to those products must be aware of and fully comply with . . . the Dietary Supplement Health and Education Act of 1994 (DSHEA) . . . to determine what is permissible and what is not permissible in that regard. . . . It may also be helpful for such professionals to review Federal Trade Commission (FTC) requirements dealing with claims in advertising . . . and even state/local/regulations which may impact the provision of such products and information.[56]*

YMCA Recommendations and ACSM's Guidelines

For health/fitness assessment and prescription, the YMCA Recommendations[34] refer to ACSM's 1998 position statement—The Recommended Quantity and Quality of Exercise for Developing and Maintaining Cardiorespiratory and Muscular Fitness, and ACSM's and the Centers for Disease Control and Prevention (CDC's) 1995 joint position stand—Physical Activity and Public Health: A Recommendation. The ACSM/CDC joint position stand has recently been updated.[57] The YMCA Recommendations also cover several special populations, including those with chronic health conditions; selected examples are categorized and briefly summarized (see Table 7-1). The YMCA Recommendations[34] also include guidelines for YMCAs to follow with regard to the use of bioelectrical impedance analysis (a method of assessing body composition) that support the National Institutes of Health (NIH) position paper based on an independent review of the literature on the same subject. In addition, guidelines are provided for cholesterol and diabetes screening, which refer to the laws such as the CLIA and OSHA's Bloodborne Pathogens Standard.

TABLE 7-1	Summary of "Selected" YMCA Recommendations[34]

Special Populations and/or Those with Chronic Illnesses
- Exercise and Asthma—general guidelines are provided with reference to the American Academy of Allergy, Asthma, and Immunology regarding Exercise-Induced Asthma (EIA).
- Cardiac Rehabilitation Programs in YMCAs—general recommendations are provided with reference to published guidelines from the American Association of Cardiovascular and Pulmonary Rehabilitation (AACVPR).
- Exercise and Type 2 Diabetes—general guidelines are provided with reference to ACSM's position stand—Exercise and Type 2 Diabetes and to organizations such as the American Diabetes Association.
- Prevention and Control of High Blood Pressure for Adults in YMCAs—general recommendations are provided with a special focus on the guidelines released by the National Heart, Lung, and Blood Institute (NHLBI).
- HIV/AIDS: Operating Guidelines for YMCAs—provides brief summary of OSHA's Bloodborne Pathogens Standard and the ADA as stated that "Persons with HIV/AIDS should be permitted to full participation in YMCA programs. Exceptions to this practice should be made in accordance with the guidelines established by the Federal Centers for Disease Control" (p. 74).
- Prenatal and Postpartum Exercise Guidelines—ACOG's publication entitled *Guidelines for Exercise During Pregnancy and the Postnatal Period* is provided.

Overweight/Obesity, Weight Loss, Diet, Eating Disorders, and Supplements
- Preventing and Decreasing Overweight and Obesity—provides general recommendations with special reference to the U.S. Surgeon General's—*Call to Action to Prevent and Decrease Overweight and Obesity*.
- Guidelines for Adult Weight-Loss Programs—general guidelines are provided and reference is made to ACSM's position stand "Appropriate Intervention Strategies for Weight Loss and Prevention of Weight Regain for Adults" and YMCA of the USA's "YMCA Healthy Lifestyle Principles."
- Dietary Guidelines—the recommendations of the U.S. Department of Agriculture and the Department of Health and Human Services are listed and local YMCAs are encouraged to use them to educate members and the community.
- Eating Disorders—provides recommendations on how to handle members who may be suspected of having an eating disorder and refers to position papers of the American Academy of Pediatrics (Identifying and Treating Eating Disorders), the American Dietetic Association (Nutrition Intervention in the Treatment of Anorexia Nervosa, Bulimia Nervosa, and Eating Disorders Not Otherwise Specified [EDNOS]), and ACSM (The Female Athlete Triad and Current Comment titled "Eating Disorders: Anorexia and Bulimia").
- Vitamin and Mineral Supplementation—refers to the position papers of the American Dietetics Association (ADA) "Food Fortification and Dietary Supplements" and "Dietary Guidance for Healthy Children Ages 2 to 11 Years" and a statement from the American Academy of Pediatrics.
- Use of Alleged Performance Enhancing Supplements—states that "the use of supplements that claim to enhance athletic and/or exercise performance for non-medical purposes should not be recommended, encouraged, or sold by YMCAs" (p. 100) and refers to the joint position paper of the ACSM, ADA, and the Dietitians of Canada on "Nutrition and Athletic Performance" (2000).
- Anabolic Steroids and Anabolic Precursors for Non-Medical Purposes—supports that position of the International and U.S. Olympic Committees that prohibit use of these substances.

Youth
- Aquatic Program Guidelines for Children Under the Age of Three—10 guidelines are presented addressing issues such as parent/guardian involvement and responsibilities, activities that are prohibited, appropriate title for the program, water temperatures, and compliance with any applicable state and local laws.
- Boxing Involving Children and Adolescents—recommends, as do the American Medical Association and the American Academy of Pediatrics, that YMCAs have a complete ban on boxing for children/adolescents.
- Participation by Children in Organized Youth Sports Programs—recommends that these programs be developmentally appropriate to meet the needs of children; eight guidelines are presented for varying ages (e.g., up to 5, 5–8, 8–12, and 12 and up); reference is also made to the policy of the American Academy of Pediatrics "Organized Sports for Children and Preadolescents."
- Heading in YMCA Youth Soccer Programs—recommends that the skill of "heading" not be introduced until age 12.
- Promoting Healthy Nutrition for Youth in YMCA Programs—encourages YMCAs to use the U.S. Department of Agriculture and the Department of Health and Human Services Dietary Guidelines when planning food and/or snacks for youth in YMCA programs; also provides four additional recommendations.

(Continued)

TABLE 7-1	Summary of "Selected" YMCA Recommendations [34] (*Continued*)

- Physical Activity Guidelines for Children (Birth to Five years)—provides the guidelines for infants (0–12 months), toddlers (1–3 years), and preschoolers (3–5 years) established by the National Association for Sport and Physical Education (NASPE).
- Promoting Physical Activity Among Youth—refers to the Centers for Disease Control and Prevention (CDC) guidelines entitled *Guidelines for School and Community Programs to Promote Lifelong Physical Activity Among Young People (2000)* and also provides four additional recommendations.
- Youth Strength Training—refers to the American Academy of Pediatrics' policy statement "Strength Training by Children and Adolescents" and NSCA's position paper "Participation in Strength & Conditioning Activities by Children."

The ACSM's Guidelines[1] provide numerous recommendations regarding exercise testing and prescription for both general and special populations. Regarding supervision of exercise testing (see Table 6-3), medical supervision is not necessary for low-risk individuals for either maximal or submaximal exercise testing, whereas medical supervision is recommended for high-risk individuals for both maximal and submaximal exercise testing. Medical supervision is recommended for maximal testing of moderate-risk individuals, but it is not indicated if it is needed for submaximal testing. Regarding the qualifications of personnel who perform the tests, it is stated, "Whenever possible, testing should be performed by ACSM-credentialed personnel because these credentials document the individual's knowledge, skills and abilities directly related to testing,"[72] and in all situations where testing is performed, site personnel should at least be certified at the basic life support level.

For health-related physical fitness testing, the ACSM Guidelines recommend at a minimum that individuals complete a pre-activity screening device such as the AHA/ACSM Questionnaire (see Figure 6-2) and that other guidelines regarding pre-participation screening (see Table 6-3) also be implemented (e.g., determining whether or not a medical evaluation is needed prior to exercise testing). In addition, participants should receive pretest instructions (see Table 7-2) and sign an informed consent. The pretest instructions can vary depending on the purpose and type of test. A sample informed consent, used at the University of South Florida (USF) in the USF FIT program, is provided in Figure 7-1.

TABLE 7-2	Participant Instructions Prior to Exercise Testing

- Participants should refrain from ingesting food, alcohol, or caffeine or using tobacco products within 3 hours of testing.
- Participants should be rested for the assessment, avoiding significant exertion or exercise on the day of the assessment.
- Clothing should permit freedom of movement and include walking or running shoes. Women should bring a loose-fitting, short-sleeved blouse that buttons down the front and should avoid restrictive undergarments.
- If the evaluation is on an outpatient basis, participants should be made aware that the evaluation may be fatiguing and that they may wish to have someone accompany them to the assessment to drive home afterward.
- If the test is for diagnostic purposes, it may be helpful for patients to discontinue prescribed cardiovascular medications, but only with physician approval. Currently prescribed antianginal agents alter the hemodynamic response to exercise and significantly reduce the sensitivity of ECG changes for ischemia. Patients taking intermediate- or high-dose β-blocking agents may be asked to taper their medication over a 2- to 4-day period to minimize hyperadrenergic withdrawal responses.
- If the test is for functional purposes, *patients should continue their medication regimen* on their usual schedule so that the exercise responses will be consistent with responses expected during exercise training.
- Participants should bring a list of their medications, including dosage and frequency of administration, to the assessment and should report the last actual dose taken. As an alternative, participants may wish to bring their medications with them for the exercise testing staff to record.
- Drink ample fluids over the 24-hour period preceding the test to ensure normal hydration before testing.

USF FIT Program -- Informed Consent for Exercise Testing

1. Purpose and Explanation of Tests

I hereby consent to voluntarily engage in various exercise tests to estimate my cardiovascular (aerobic) endurance, muscle strength/endurance, flexibility, and body composition. It is my understanding that the information obtained will help me evaluate future physical activities and sport activities in which I may engage. The tests will include:

- **Cardiovascular Endurance**: Submaximal Bike Test
- **Muscle Strength/Endurance:** Abdominal Curl-up (Crunch) Test; 1 RM for Upper Body Strength, 1 RM for Leg Strength
- **Flexibility**: Sit and Reach
- **Body Composition**: Bioelectrical Impedance Analysis (BIA); 3-site skin fold test; Waist-to-Hip Ratio; Body Weight and Height

Before I undergo the tests, I certify to the *USF Exercise Science FIT Program* that I am in good health and/or have had a physician's clearance if required by the FIT program. Further, I hereby represent and inform the program that I have completed the health history questionnaire presented to me by the instructor of the course and have provided correct responses to the questions as indicated on the history form. It is my understanding that I will be interviewed by my FIT student personal trainer prior to my undergoing the tests who will in the course of interviewing me determine if there are any reasons which would make it undesirable or unsafe for me to take the tests. Consequently, I understand that it is important that I provide complete and accurate responses to the interviewer and recognize that my failure to do so could lead to possible unnecessary injury to myself during the tests.

The cardiovascular endurance test I will undergo will be performed on a bicycle ergometer with the amount of effort gradually increasing. I understand that this test will not continue beyond 85% of my age-predicted maximal heart rate. As I understand it, the gradual increase in effort will continue until I feel and verbally report to my student personal trainer(s) any symptoms such as fatigue, shortness of breath, or chest discomfort which may appear. It is my understanding and I have been clearly advised that it is my right to request that a test be stopped at any point if I feel unusual discomfort or fatigue. I have been advised that I should immediately upon experiencing any such symptoms, or if I so choose, inform my student personal trainer(s) that I wish to stop the test at that or any other point. My wishes in this regard shall be absolutely carried out. It is further my understanding that during the test itself, my student personal trainer(s) will monitor my responses continuously and take frequent readings of blood pressure and my expressed feelings of effort.

The muscular strength tests I will undergo will assess dynamic muscular strength by means of a 1-Repetition Maximum bench press for upper body strength and 1-Repetition Maximum leg press for lower body strength (1). As I understand it, the 1-Repetition Maximum will be determined within four trials with rest periods of 3 to 5 minutes between trials. I have been advised that the test will begin with approximately 50%-70% of my perceived capacity and resistance will progressively increase by 2.5 to 20 kg until I have reached the maximum amount of resistance I can perform with correct speed and range of motion. An abdominal Curl-Up (Crunch) test (1) will also be performed to measure muscular endurance. I understand in this test I will perform as many curl-ups as I can in 1 minute.

The flexibility test that I will undergo will assess low back and hip joint flexibility. I have been advised that this test may be a better predictor of hamstring flexibility than low back flexibility and is limited in its ability to predict incidence of low back pain. I understand that the results of this test have relative importance to activities of daily living and sports performance. It is my understanding that I will perform two trials of this test, after a mild warm-up, and the highest score will be recorded.

The body composition tests that I will undergo will estimate my percentage of body mass that is fat tissue using a low-level electric current, calipers, height/weight, and circumference measures. I have been advised that the low-level electric current is low risk, noninvasive, and measures the impedance or resistance to the flow through the body fluids contained mainly in the lean and fat tissue. I understand that the calipers measure subcutaneous fat and the skinfold sites for men are chest, abdomen, and thigh. The skinfold sites for women are triceps, suprailiac, and thigh (1). I understand that my risk(s) for disease will be estimated by circumference measurements to be taken at the waist and hip and height and weight measurements that will be used to determine my body mass index.

FIGURE 7–1 USF FIT Program: Informed Consent for Exercise Testing

Once the tests have been completed, but before I am released from the test area, I will be given special instructions about recognition of certain symptoms that may appear within 24 hours after the test. I agree to follow these instructions and promptly contact the program personnel or medical providers if such symptoms develop.

2. Risks

I understand and have been informed that there exists the possibility of adverse changes during the actual tests. I have been informed that these changes, though remote, include abnormal blood pressure, fainting, disorders of heart rhythm, stroke, and very rare instances of heart attack or even death. In addition, I understand that I may experience musculoskeletal conditions or injuries such as muscle strains, muscle sprains, muscular fatigue, contusions, post-testing muscle soreness, joint injuries, torn muscles, heat-related illnesses, and back injuries. I have been told that every effort will be made to minimize these occurrences by precautions and observations taken during the tests. I have also been informed that emergency equipment (First-Aid/AED) and personnel (AED/CPR/First-Aid certified) are readily available to deal with these unusual situations should they occur. Even though, I understand that there is a risk of injury, heart attack, stroke, or even death as a result of my performance of these tests, but knowing those risks, it is my desire to proceed to take the test as herein indicated.

3. Benefits to be Expected and Available Alternatives to the Exercise Testing Procedures

The results of these tests may or may not benefit me. Potential benefits relate mainly to my personal motives for taking the tests, that is, knowing my exercise capacity in relation to the general population, understanding my fitness for certain physical, recreational, and sport activities, planning my physical conditioning program, or evaluation of the effects of my recent physical activity habits. Although my cardiovascular endurance test might also be evaluated by alternative means, for example, a bench step test or an outdoor running test, such tests do not provide as accurate a fitness assessment as the bike test nor do these options allow equally effective monitoring of my responses. In addition, although the muscle strength/endurance, flexibility, and body composition tests might also be evaluated by other means, the above tests were selected because they are common tests approved by the American College of Sports Medicine that can be completed within a reasonable amount of time.

4. Confidentiality and Use of Information

I have been informed that the information obtained in this exercise test will be treated as privileged and confidential to the extent possible by FIT and in accordance with permissible law and will consequently not be released or revealed to any person without my express written consent or pursuant to subpoena or court order. I do, however, agree to the use of any information for emergency medical treatment if needed. I also agree to the use for research or statistical purposes so long as the same does not provide facts that could lead to my identification. Any other information obtained, however, will be used only by the FIT program to evaluate my exercise status or needs.

5. Inquiries and Freedom of Consent

I have been given an opportunity to ask certain questions as to the procedures. Generally these requests, which have been noted by my FIT student personal trainer and his /her response, are as follows:

_____

_____

_____

_____

_____

I further understand that there are also other remote risks that may be associated with this procedure. Despite the fact that a complete accounting of all these remote risks has not been provided to me, I still desire to proceed with the test. I acknowledge that I have read this document in its entirety or that it has been read to me if I have been unable to read same. I consent to the rendition of all services and procedures as explained herein by all program personnel.

FIGURE 7–1 *(Continued)*

_____   _____
Participant's Signature   Date

_____   _____
Test Supervisor's (Student) Signature   Date

_____   _____
Course Professor's Signature   Date

FIGURE 7–1 *(Continued)*
(Reproduced and adapted with permission from Herbert & Herbert, *Legal Aspects of Preventive, Rehabilitative and Recreational Exercise Programs,* 4th ed.[3] All other rights reserved. No form should be adopted without individualized legal advice and consultation. Descriptions of some of the tests in Section 1 have been briefly summarized from the ACSM's Guidelines.[1])

The ACSM Guidelines provide recommendations on contraindications to testing, test order, and test environment, and they describe various protocols for all types of health-related testing. Pros and cons are given for both maximal and submaximal cardiorespiratory (CR) testing. It is explained that health/fitness practitioners should rely on submaximal exercise tests to assess CR fitness. Maximal testing is not always feasible in health/fitness facilities because it requires participants to exercise to the point of volitional fatigue, may require physician supervision, and may be inappropriate for certain individuals. In addition, maximal testing may increase the risk of an untoward event in some individuals. Various CR tests, including field tests, are described with the advantages and disadvantages of each. Health/fitness professionals need to select CR tests carefully based on the participant's age, health status, and physical activity history. Field tests, step tests, and sometimes even submaximal tests can quickly result in maximal or near maximal heart rate levels in certain individuals. For safety reasons, most submaximal protocols establish a maximal heart rate that should not be exceeded during the test, (e.g., 85% of an age-predicted formula). In addition, all health/fitness professionals conducting tests should be aware of the indications for stopping a test (see Table 7–3). Once an individual has completed the health-related fitness tests, the ACSM Guidelines recommend the results be interpreted by a competent professional and conveyed to the client.

The ACSM Guidelines also provide numerous recommendations regarding exercise prescription (e.g., general principles of safe and effective training are presented along with guidelines for exercise testing, prescription, and special considerations) for the following clinical conditions:

- Cardiovascular disease
- Arthritis
- Diabetes mellitus
- Dyslipidemia
- Hypertension
- Obesity
- Metabolic syndrome
- Immunology
- Osteoporosis
- Peripheral arterial disease
- Pulmonary disease
- Pregnancy

In addition, guidelines for children and the elderly are provided. Similar to the YMCA Recommendations,[34] reference is made to various position papers/stands published by

TABLE 7-3	General Indications for Stopping an Exercise Test in Low-Risk Adults*

- Onset of angina or angina-like symptoms
- Drop in systolic blood pressure of >10 mm Hg from baseline blood pressure despite an increase in workload
- Excessive rise in blood pressure: systolic pressure >250 mm Hg or diastolic pressure >115 mm Hg
- Shortness of breath, wheezing, leg cramps, or claudication
- Signs of poor perfusion: light-headedness, confusion, ataxia, pallor, cyanosis, nausea, or cold and clammy skin
- Failure of heart rate to increase with increased exercise intensity
- Noticeable change in heart rhythm
- Subject requests to stop
- Physical or verbal manifestations of severe fatigue
- Failure of the testing equipment

*Assumes that testing is nondiagnostic and is being performed without direct physician involvement or ECG monitoring. For clinical testing, Box 5-2 provides more definitive and specific termination criteria. (Box 5-2 can be found in the ACSM's Guidelines.[1])

Reprinted with permission from *ACSM's Guidelines for Exercise Testing and Prescription.* 7th ed. Philadelphia: Lippincott Williams & Wilkins; 2006:78.

government or professional organizations for many of the conditions just listed. See Table 7-4 for a selected list of these position papers. It goes beyond the scope of this book to discuss all of these exercise testing/prescription guidelines, but health/fitness professionals should refer to these guidelines when conducting exercise testing/prescription for individuals with any of the conditions listed to help ensure a reasonably safe program for them. However, to not exceed one's scope of practice, health/fitness professionals would need to have the knowledge, skills, and abilities to understand and properly apply these guidelines prior to providing exercise testing and prescription for individuals with various medical conditions.

STEP 2 DEVELOPMENT OF RISK MANAGEMENT STRATEGIES

The preceding section presented the relevant law and published standards of practice related to health/fitness assessment and prescription services that health/fitness professionals provide for individual participants or clients. This section describes how health/fitness professionals and their risk management advisory committees can develop risk management strategies that address the law and published standards of practice, which will lead to minimizing legal liability associated with these types of programs/services. The minimum qualifications that health/fitness professionals who provide these types of programs should possess are described in some of these risk management strategies. However, as mentioned earlier, the professional standard of care is determined by the situation. Therefore, just because a health/fitness professional has met the desired minimum qualifications as described, it does not necessarily mean that he or she is qualified to provide health/fitness assessments and prescriptions. Not only do health/fitness professionals need to have the necessary knowledge, skills, and abilities (as perhaps demonstrated through a degree in exercise science or related area, certification, and experience), but they must know how to *apply* the appropriate knowledge, skills, and abilities to safely address the individual's unique characteristics (e.g., age, gender, health status, and fitness level).

> **Risk Management Strategy 1:** Comply with federal laws such as HIPAA, ADA, OSHA's Bloodborne Pathogens Standard, and CLIA as well as other applicable state and local laws.

TABLE 7-4	"Selected" List of Policy and Position Stands Published by Professional Organizations Regarding Exercise Testing and Prescription for General and Special Populations*

General Populations

1. ACSM position stand—1998: The Recommended Quantity and Quality of Exercise for Developing and Maintaining Cardiorespiratory and Muscular Fitness, and Flexibility in Healthy Adults[58]
2. ACSM position stand—2001: Appropriate Intervention Strategies for Weight Loss and Prevention of Weight Regain for Adults[59]
3. ACSM position stand—2002: Progression Models in Resistance Training for Healthy Adults[60]

Special Populations and/or Medical Conditions

Youth

4. American Academy of Pediatrics policy statement—2001: Strength Training by Children and Adolescents[61]
5. NSCA position paper—2001: Participation in Strength & Conditioning Activities by Children[62]

Diabetes

6. American Diabetes position statement—2002: Diabetes Mellitus and Exercise[63]
7. ACSM position stand—2000: Exercise and Type II Diabetes[64]

Osteoporosis/Bone Health

8. ACSM position stand—2004: Physical Activity & Bone Health[65]
9. ACSM position stand—1995: Osteoporosis and Exercise[66]

Hypertension

10. ACSM position stand—2004: Exercise & Hypertension[67]

Pregnancy and Postpartum

11. American College of Obstetricians and Gynecologists (ACOG) opinion no. 257–2002: Exercise During Pregnancy and the Postpartum Period[68]

Elderly

12. ACSM position stand—1998: Exercise and Physical Activity for Older Adults[69]

Athletes

13. NSCA position statement—n.d: Basic Guidelines for the Resistance Training of Athletes[70]
14. ACSM position stand—2007: The Female Athlete Triad[71]

*Numerous other "guidelines" regarding safe and effective exercise for various medical conditions, age groups, and so on, have been published by various private and government groups that may or may not be in the form of a policy or position stand.

As procedures are being developed that address health/fitness assessments and prescriptions, these procedures must reflect HIPAA, ADA, and any other similar state and local laws. As stated in Chapter 6, to determine if there are any similar state and/or local laws, health/fitness professionals should consult with their legal expert(s) on their risk management advisory committee. To be compliant with HIPAA and/or state privacy laws, all data/records obtained and documented from health/fitness assessments and prescriptions need to be kept private, confidential, and secure. To be compliant with Title III of the ADA, health/fitness professionals should consider carefully any potential violations of this law when adopting any kind of an exclusion policy. See Risk Management Strategy 1 in Chapter 6 for more information on how to comply with HIPAA and ADA laws.

For health/fitness facilities that provide health screenings that involve a blood sample (e.g., cholesterol and glucose), it will be important to adhere to OSHA's Bloodborne Pathogens (BBP) Standard. See Chapter 11 for a description of the many requirements of this law and how to implement them. The Clinical Laboratory Improvement Amendments (CLIA) established standards for all laboratory testing regardless of where the test is performed. Although health/fitness facilities may obtain a Certificate of Waiver (versus obtaining CLIA certification) for fingerstick testing, it may be best to collaborate with a local hospital or clinic that already possesses the CLIA certification to provide such screenings.

Risk Management Strategy 2: Have only qualified health/fitness professionals conduct and interpret health/fitness assessments.

As recommended in Chapter 6 with regard to interpreting health history questionnaires (HHQs), only health/fitness professionals who are qualified should conduct and interpret health/fitness assessments. A "qualified" health/fitness professional may be one who possesses the following minimum qualifications: BS/BA in exercise science or related field, professional certification commensurate with ACSM's HFI or NSCA's CSCS, current CPR/AED and first-aid certifications, and professional work experience. Note: The term "qualified health/fitness professional" used hereafter means someone with these credentials. Conducting and interpreting health/fitness assessments can be quite complex and should probably *not* be done by health/fitness professionals who have only a high school diploma and perhaps a personal training certification. Health/fitness professionals with a bachelor's degree in exercise science (or related area) usually have at least one entire college course that addresses knowledge, skills, and abilities associated with health/fitness assessments. It is more likely, for example, that qualified health/fitness professionals will select the appropriate health-related fitness testing protocols given the individual's needs, follow the protocol properly to provide as much safety and accuracy as possible, and will be able to properly interpret the fitness data obtained for follow-up decisions and actions.

Risk Management Strategy 3: Have only qualified health/fitness professionals discuss health/fitness assessment results with participants.

Because participants will likely not understand their health/fitness assessment results, it will be important that only qualified health/fitness professionals explain the results. Regarding health screenings such as cholesterol and blood pressure, it is essential that their values are explained to them, and for any values that are outside the normal range; participants should be referred to their health care provider. Interpretation of results and communication with participants involving any follow-up recommendations need to be complete and accurate. For example, if a health/fitness professional gives a participant inaccurate or improper proper follow-up recommendations, and then that participant takes some action relying on those recommendations that leads to some type of harm/injury, the health/fitness professional could be held liable for that injury or harm. With regard to health-related fitness data, it will be important to explain the amount of error that is often associated with such tests as well as any other limitations. As mentioned before, potential fiduciary relationships are formed with participants when health/fitness professionals provide individual health/fitness assessments and exercise prescriptions. Participants will rely on and trust what the health/fitness professional has told or advised them, and therefore this information must be correct and in the participant's best interest.

Risk Management Strategy 4: Establish safety procedures for health-related fitness testing.

A variety of safety procedures should be in place prior to conducting any health-related fitness testing such as the following: (a) All participants should complete a health history questionnaire (HHQ) such as the PASQ (see Form 6-2 in Chapter 6) or a more detailed HHQ in which the necessary data are obtained to classify participants as low, moderate, or high risk using ACSM Guidelines.[1] Note: Prior to fitness testing, more specific health data are needed (than obtained on a general screening device such as the PAR-Q) to determine which fitness testing protocols would be appropriate and to design a "reasonably safe" exercise program for an individual. For example, if an individual has high blood pressure and is on medication to treat it, certain precautions are necessary when testing and/or prescribing exercise for this individual. (b) Only qualified health/fitness professionals should interpret such data and make determinations for physician clearance prior to testing. (c) Physician clearance is obtained for all participants classified as moderate risk, and high-risk participants should not be tested in health/fitness facilities and should be referred to their physician for appropriate clinical exercise testing. Note: When obtaining physician clearance, a similar procedure can be developed as described in Chapter 6. However, in addition to the HHQ, it may be wise to also attach a description of the health-related fitness tests the participant will be performing for the physician to review. (d) Testing equipment has been calibrated and is in proper working order. (e) Emergency procedures are in place. (f) Appropriate protocols are selected given the characteristics of the participant and only submaximal CR tests are performed. Note: In some cases, maximal tests may be performed with "low" risk participants only; otherwise it is generally not necessary to pose increased risks associated with maximal testing for most adults performing health-related fitness tests. (g) Instructions are provided to participants prior to testing (see Table 7-2). (h) Informed consent is administered prior to testing (see Figure 7-1). (i) Health-related fitness tests are conducted according to protocols (e.g., participants are taught proper execution of tests, any signs/symptoms of overexertion are carefully observed, the test is stopped if necessary, etc.).

Risk Management Strategy 5: Establish written "scope of practice" guidelines for health/fitness professionals who provide health/fitness assessments and prescriptions.

Because there are various types of health/fitness professionals that work in health/fitness facilities, as described in Chapter 1, written guidelines should be established to distinguish the scope of practice among them. For example, health/fitness professionals with a high school diploma and a personal training certification probably do not have the necessary knowledge, skills, and abilities to properly interpret data from a health history questionnaire, conduct health-related fitness testing, and prepare an individualized exercise prescription. However, they could design and lead reasonably safe/effective individual exercise programs for healthy adults. In other words, it is recommended to establish scope of practice guidelines for these professionals that would be consistent with the scope of practice as described earlier for the ACSM's Certified Personal Trainer.

For qualified health/fitness professionals who interpret health/fitness assessments, conduct health-related fitness tests, and prepare individualized exercise prescriptions, it may be wise to develop scope of practice guidelines that would be consistent with ACSM's HFI scope of practice. The ACSM HFI scope of practice states that these professionals are skilled to offer these types of programs/services to apparently healthy individuals with medically controlled disease. Health/fitness facilities may want to define more specifically "apparently healthy individuals with controlled disease" so it is clear the type of participants these professionals can serve.

In addition, and as stated in some of the published standards of practice, ongoing communication with a participant's physician (and/or other health care provider) is recommended, especially if the participant is moderate or high risk. Most qualified health/fitness professionals should also be able communicate with a participant's physician and understand and apply any contraindications or limitations to exercise specified by the physician. One way to perhaps minimize findings related to the unauthorized practice of medicine is to establish an ongoing two-way communication with the client's physician.[73] The qualified health/fitness professional can send reports to the physician on the participant's progress, and the physician can update the professional on the patient's state of health or any modifications to the exercise program. Directly involving the physician in the exercise prescription, especially for participants with risk factors or medical conditions, can help demonstrate that the health/fitness professional is following the advice/prescription of the physician versus doing this on his or her own. Scope of practice guidelines should include procedures regarding communication with physicians.

When establishing scope of practice guidelines for various health/fitness professionals, it is best to first consider the education, training, experience, and certification(s) of each professional. However, it is important to remember that the standard of care is not based on the credentials of the professional. As stated earlier, the professional's performance will be measured against the standard of care of a qualified professional, given the situation.[28] For example, if a participant has high blood pressure and is on medication to treat it, the health/fitness professional who conducts a health/fitness assessment and prepares an exercise prescription for this participant should have the necessary knowledge, skills, and abilities (KSAs) to properly do so because his or her conduct will be judged against someone who does possess these KSAs. Therefore, in this situation, only health/fitness professionals who fully understand the implications of high blood pressure and antihypertensive medication with regard to health/fitness assessment and exercise prescription should work with these types of participants. Once the written scope of practice guidelines are prepared, all health/fitness professionals should be trained so they fully understand and appreciate them.

Risk Management Strategy 6: Establish written "scope of practice" guidelines for health/fitness professionals who provide nutrition and weight management education.

Because health/fitness professionals often provide nutrition and weight management education, it will be important to establish written scope of practice guidelines for them to follow so they do not step over into the practice of dietetics. When developing these guidelines, it may be best to use the "general nonmedical nutrition information" definition provided in Ohio's "unauthorized practice of dietetics" statue (described earlier). Examples that appear to meet this definition include the following:

1. Demonstrating how to prepare and cook food
2. Providing information about food guidance systems (i.e., MyPyramid, USDA Dietary Guidelines), healthy eating out or healthy snacks
3. Talking about carbohydrates, proteins, fats, vitamins, minerals, and water as essential nutrients needed by the body and how nutrient requirements may vary through the life cycle
4. Giving statistical information about the relationship between chronic disease and the excesses or deficiencies of certain nutrients
5. Providing information about nutrients contained in foods or supplements.[74]

When developing these guidelines, it may also be good idea to compare and contrast the competencies under "nutrition and weight management" for ACSM certified personal trainers and health/fitness instructors[1] with those of registered dietitians, as well as incorporate guidelines regarding nutritional supplements based on applicable laws and published standards of practice. Again, once these scope of practice guidelines are in place, all health/fitness professionals should be trained so they understand the importance of following them.

Risk Management Strategy 7: Have only "advanced" qualified health/fitness professionals provide health/fitness assessments and prescriptions for high-risk populations as well as medical oversight of these types of programs/services.

The ACSM/AHA Joint PP[44] recommended that "high risk" participants (those in Risk Class B and C) be referred to a medically or clinically supervised program that has medical oversight (e.g., a medical liaison) and health/fitness professionals who have advanced degrees (e.g., a master's degree in exercise science) and advanced certification (e.g., ACSM exercise specialist certification). In addition, for these participants, medical examination and exercise testing should be completed before initiation of moderate or vigorous exercise and medical supervision is recommended for both submaximal and maximal exercise testing.[1] Health/fitness facilities should have risk management strategies in place that would reflect these recommendations, if they choose to serve participants that would be considered "high" risk (e.g., those with known cardiovascular, pulmonary or metabolic disease). It will also be key to develop "scope of practice" guidelines (as discussed earlier) for these advanced qualified health/fitness professionals who would be working with these populations.

Risk Management Strategy 8: Create a system to keep all documents obtained from health/fitness assessments and prescriptions private, confidential, and secure.

As described in Risk Management Strategy 1, all health information should be kept private, confidential, and secure. This includes data obtained from health/fitness assessments and exercise prescriptions. A system that includes written procedures on how these documents will be kept private, confidential, and secure should be in place. Staff members should be well trained with regard to these procedures. In addition, all documents obtained should be kept for the length of time that would be commensurate with the statutes of limitations.

Risk Management Strategy 9: Provide and document continuing education and training programs for health/fitness professionals.

With regard to health/fitness assessments and prescriptions, it will be important that continuing education and training be provided for health/fitness professionals who provide these services. They should keep abreast of any new literature that may impact the safe design of exercise programs, especially for special populations. Health/fitness professionals should also keep records of courses/workshops/conferences they have attended and professional journals or books they have read. They should also review new and updated published standards of practice. Every effort should be made to properly apply the latest peer-reviewed research to help ensure reasonably safe and effective programs for participants. In a negligence claim or lawsuit, the lawyer for the plaintiff may ask the defendant health/fitness professional about efforts in this area to establish the level of his or her credibility (or lack thereof).

Risk Management Strategy 10: Establish written "scope of practice" guidelines for health/fitness professionals that provide health/wellness coaching services over the Internet.

Lastly, providing personal health/wellness coaching (one-on-one services that educate and motivate clients to adopt healthy behaviors) over the Internet has become quite popular. Many health/fitness professionals are providing these services to clients often over the phone or via e-mail. Health/fitness professionals should be well-trained on how to provide these services properly so they do not go outside their scope of practice and understand the many limitations that exist when there is no visual/personal contact with the participant. Many of the legal liability exposures addressed in this chapter would apply, and therefore appropriate risk management strategies should also be in place prior to offering these types of services. There are, however, additional and potentially substantial concerns relevant to the provision of services via the Internet. Additional care and the application of special risk management strategies have been addressed elsewhere.[75–77]

PUT INTO PRACTICE CHECKLIST 7-1

Rate your phase of development for each of the following risk management strategies related to health/fitness assessment and prescription:

	Developed	Partially Developed	Not Developed
1. Complying with federal laws such as HIPAA, ADA, OSHA's Bloodborne Pathogen standard, and CLIA as well as other applicable state and local laws.			
2. Having only "qualified" health/fitness professionals conduct and interpret health/fitness assessments.			
3. Having only "qualified" health/fitness professionals discuss health/fitness assessment results with participants.			
4. Establishing safety procedures for health-related fitness testing.			
5. Establishing written "scope of practice" guidelines for health/fitness professionals who provide health/fitness assessments and prescriptions.			
6. Establishing written "scope of practice" guidelines for health/fitness professionals who provide nutrition and weight management education.			
7. Having only "advanced" qualified health/fitness professionals provide health/fitness assessments and prescriptions for high-risk populations as well as medical oversight of these types of programs/services.			
8. Creating a system to keep all documents obtained from health/fitness assessments and prescriptions private, confidential, and secure.			
9. Providing and documenting continuing education and training programs for health/fitness professionals.			
10. Establishing written "scope of practice" guidelines for health/fitness professionals that provide health/wellness coaching services over the Internet.			

SUMMARY

As health/fitness professionals and their risk management advisory committees consider the development of their risk management strategies regarding health/fitness assessments and prescriptions, they should first review relevant laws and published standards of practice. Although there is not a lot of case law involving negligent conduct with regard to health/fitness assessments, case law does exist regarding health/fitness prescriptions. This chapter presented a few of these cases, but there are many more cases involving health/fitness professionals in which similar issues have been raised.

The primary legal issue with regard to health/fitness assessments and prescriptions is scope of practice. First, does the health/fitness professional possess the necessary knowledge, skills, and abilities to perform such activities; and second, when working with individuals with special needs (e.g., those with medical conditions, risk factors, etc.), does the health/fitness professional have the additional knowledge, skills, and abilities to do so? Health/fitness professionals and their risk management advisory committees need to answer these questions and then develop written scope of practice procedures that can be clearly communicated to all health/fitness professionals working within the facility to help minimize any potential criminal liability (e.g., violation of statutes such as unauthorized practice of medicine or some allied health care profession) or civil liability (e.g., negligence).

RISK MANAGEMENT ASSIGNMENTS

1. Develop a PowerPoint presentation appropriate for staff training that summarizes the Ohio Board of Dietetics statute on the Unauthorized Practice of Dietetics and includes what happened in the *Ohio Board of Dietetics v. Brown* case.

   _____

   _____

   _____

   _____

2. Using the Ohio statute's definition of "general nonmedical information," develop a draft of guidelines that could be presented to and discussed with all health/fitness professionals that eventually could be adopted as a policy on the scope of practice for health/fitness professionals in the area of nutrition and weight management.

   _____

   _____

   _____

   _____

3. Describe the similarities and differences among the published standards of practice with regard to the type of qualifications needed to perform health/fitness assessments, prescriptions, and personal fitness training.

   _____

   _____

   _____

   _____

4. Using published standards of practice with regard to exercise testing, describe the types of individuals who should not be tested in most health/fitness facilities, and are best referred to clinical settings for exercise testing.

   _____

   _____

   _____

   _____

5. Describe how a facility would help ensure their personal fitness trainers are keeping all health/fitness assessment and prescription records of their clients private, confidential, and secure.

   _____

   _____

   _____

   _____

KEY TERMS

Cease and desist notice   Injunction   *Respondeat superior*
Fiduciary relationship   Negligence *per se*   Scope of practice

REFERENCES

1. Whaley MH, ed. *ACSM's Guidelines for Exercise Testing and Prescription*. 7th ed. Philadelphia: Lippincott Williams & Wilkins; 2006.
2. Whaley MH, ed. *ACSM's Guidelines for Exercise Testing and Prescription*. 7th ed. Philadelphia: Lippincott Williams & Wilkins; 2006:55.
3. Herbert DL, Herbert WH. *Legal Aspects of Preventive, Rehabilitative and Recreational Exercise Programs*. 4th ed. Canton, Ohio: PRC; 2002.
4. Assessment of functional capacity in clinical and research applications: An advisory from the committee on exercise, rehabilitation, and prevention. Council on Clinical Cardiology, American Heart Association. *Circulation*. 2000;102:1591–1597.
5. Guidelines for exercise testing in the pediatric age group. Committee on Atherosclerosis and Hypertension in Children, Council on Clinical Cardiology, American Heart Association. *Circulation*. 1994;90:2166–2179.
6. ACC/AHA guidelines for exercise testing, A report of the American College of Cardiology/American Heart Association Task Force on Practice Guidelines (Committee on Exercise Testing). *J Am Coll Cardiol*. 1997;30:260–311.
7. Stress testing: A report of the American College of Cardiology/American College of Physicians—American Society of Internal Medicine Task Force on Clinical Competence, *J Am Coll Cardiol*. 1990;36:1441–1453.
8. Unlicensed practice of a health care profession. Fla. Stat. § 456.065, 2005.
9. Dietetics. Ohio Rev. Code Ann. § 4759, 2006.
10. Practice of medicine and surgery without a license, Ohio Rev. Code Ann. § 4731.41, 1999.
11. Dietetics. Ohio Rev. Code Ann. § 4759.01(A), 2006.
12. Dietetics. Ohio Rev. Code Ann. § 4759-2-01(C), 2006.
13. Dietetics. Ohio Rev. Code Ann. § 4759-2-01(M), 2006.
14. van der Smissen B. Elements of negligence. In: Cotten DJ, Wolohan JT, eds. *Law for Recreation and Sport Managers*. 4th ed. Dubuque, Iowa: Kendall/Hunt; 2007.
15. *Stetina v. State Medical Licensing Board of Indiana*, 513 N.E.2d 1234 (Ohio Ct. App., 2nd Dist., 1987).
16. *Stetina v. State Medical Licensing Board of Indiana*, 513 N.E.2d 1234 (Ohio Ct. App., 2nd Dist., 1987), 1235–1236.
17. *Stetina v. State Medical Licensing Board of Indiana*, 513 N.E.2d 1234 (Ohio Ct. App., 2nd Dist., 1987), 1238.
18. *Stetina v. State Medical Licensing Board of Indiana*, 513 N.E.2d 1234 (Ohio Ct. App., 2nd Dist., 1987), 1240.
19. *Ohio Board of Dietetics v. Brown*, 83 Ohio App. 3rd 242 (Ohio App. LEXIS 88, 1993).
20. *Ohio Board of Dietetics v. Brown*, 83 Ohio App. 3rd 242 (Ohio App. LEXIS 88, 1993): 246–247.
21. *Ohio Board of Dietetics v. Brown*, 83 Ohio App. 3rd 242 (Ohio App. LEXIS 88, 1993): 248.
22. *Capati v. Crunch Fitness International, et al.* Analyzed in: Herbert DL. $320 million lawsuit filed against health club. *Exercise Standards and Malpractice Reporter*. 1999;13; 33, 36.
23. *Capati v. Crunch Fitness International, et al.* Analyzed in: Herbert DL. Update on litigation—Capati v. Crunch Fitness. *Exercise Standards and Malpractice Reporter*. 2001;15: 56.
24. *Capati v. Crunch Fitness International, et al.* Analyzed in: Wrongful death case of Anne Marie Capati settled for in excess of $4 million. *Exercise Standards and Malpractice Reporter*. 2006;20:36.
25. *Makris v. Scandinavian Health Spa, Inc.,* Ohio App. LEXIS 4416 (Ct. of Appeals, 7th Dist., 1999).
26. *Makris v. Scandinavian Health Spa, Inc.,* Ohio App. LEXIS 4416 (Ct. of Appeals, 7th Dist., 1999.): 3.

27. *Makris v. Scandinavian Health Spa, Inc.,* Ohio App. LEXIS 4416 (Ct. of Appeals, 7th Dist., 1999.), 6.
28. van der Smissen, B. Elements of negligence. In: Cotten DJ, Wolohan JT, eds. *Law for Recreation and Sport Managers.* 4th ed. Dubuque, Iowa: Kendall/Hunt; 2007:40.
29. Black HC. *Black's Law Dictionary.* 6th ed. St. Paul, Minn: West; 1991.
30. American College of Sports Medicine. *ACSM Health/Fitness Instructor(®) Scope of Practice.* Available at: http://www.acsm.org/Content/NavigationMenu/Certification/ACSMCertifications/ACSMHealthFitnessInstructo/Health_Fitness_Instr.htm#scope_of_practice. n.d. Accessed October 24, 2007.
31. American College of Sports Medicine. *ACSM Certified Personal Trainer^SM Scope of Practice.* Available at: http://www.acsm.org/Content/NavigationMenu/Certification/ACSMCertifications/ACSMCertifiedPersonal/Certified_Personl_T.htm. n.d. Accessed October 22, 2007.
32. A National Study of the NSCA-Certified Personal Trainer, NSCA Certification Commission. May 2007.
33. A National Study of the Certified Strength and Conditioning Specialist, NSCA Certification Commission. May 2007.
34. *Medical Advisory Committee Recommendations: A Resource Guide for YMCAs.* Chicago: YMCA of the USA; February 2007.
35. *Medical Advisory Committee Recommendations: A Resource Guide for YMCAs.* Chicago: YMCA of the USA; February 2007:101.
36. Aerobics and Fitness Association of America, Personal Fitness Trainer Certification, Available at: http://www.afaa.com. n.d. Accessed June 10, 2006.
37. IHRSA Club Membership Standards. In: *IHRSA's Guide to Club Membership & Conduct.* 3rd ed. Boston: International Health, Racquet & Sportsclub Association (IHRSA); 2005.
38. *NSCA's Strength & Conditioning Professional Standards & Guidelines.* May 2001. Available at: http://www.nscalift.org/Publications/standards.shtml. Colorado Springs: National Strength and Conditioning Association (NSCA). Accessed September 2, 2007.
39. *NSCA's Strength & Conditioning Professional Standards & Guidelines.* May 2001. Available at: http://www.nscalift.org/Publications/standards.shtml. Colorado Springs: National Strength and Conditioning Association (NSCA). Accessed September 2, 2007:13.
40. *NSCA's Strength & Conditioning Professional Standards & Guidelines.* May 2001. Available at: http://www.nscalift.org/Publications/standards.shtml. Colorado Springs: National Strength and Conditioning Association (NSCA). Accessed September 2, 2007:15.
41. *NSCA's Strength & Conditioning Professional Standards & Guidelines.* May 2001. Available at: http://www.nscalift.org/Publications/standards.shtml. Colorado Springs: National Strength and Conditioning Association (NSCA). Accessed September 2, 2007:16.
42. Tharrett SJ, McInnis KJ, Peterson JA, eds. *ACSM's Health/Fitness Facility Standards and Guidelines.* 3rd ed. Champaign, Ill: Human Kinetics; 2007.
43. Tharrett SJ, McInnis KJ, Peterson JA, eds. *ACSM's Health/Fitness Facility Standards and Guidelines.* 3rd ed. Champaign, Ill: Human Kinetics; 2007:2.
44. American College of Sports Medicine and American Heart Association Joint Position Statement. Recommendations for cardiovascular screening, staffing, and emergency policies at health/fitness facilities. *Med Sci Sports Exerc.* 1998;30:1009–1018.
45. American College of Sports Medicine and American Heart Association Joint Position Statement. Recommendations for cardiovascular screening, staffing, and emergency policies at health/fitness facilities. *Med Sci Sports Exerc.* 1998; 30:1009–1018, 1013.
46. American College of Sports Medicine and American Heart Association Joint Position Statement. Recommendations for cardiovascular screening, staffing, and emergency policies at health/fitness facilities. *Med Sci Sports Exerc.* 1998;30:1009–1018, 1016.
47. *Canadian Fitness Safety Standards & Recommended Guidelines.* 3rd ed. 2004. Available at: http://www.oases.on.ca/safety/safetyStdsCurrent.htm. Ontario, Canada: Ontario Association of Sport and Exercise Sciences (OASES). Accessed September 2, 2007:6.
48. *Canadian Fitness Safety Standards & Recommended Guidelines.* 3rd ed. 2004. Available at: http://www.oases.on.ca/safety/safetyStdsCurrent.htm. Ontario, Canada: Ontario Association of Sport and Exercise Sciences (OASES). Accessed September 2, 2007:1.
49. *The Medical Fitness Model: Facility Standards and Guidelines.* Richmond, Va: Medical Fitness Association (MFA); May 2006:8.
50. *The Medical Fitness Model: Facility Standards and Guidelines.* Richmond, Va: Medical Fitness Association (MFA); May 2006:9.

51. *The Medical Fitness Model: Facility Standards and Guidelines.* Richmond, Va: Medical Fitness Association (MFA); May 2006:10.

52. *Exercise Standards & Guidelines Reference Manual.* 4th ed. Sherman Oaks, Calif: Aerobics and Fitness Association of America (AFAA); 2005.

53. *Exercise Standards & Guidelines Reference Manual.* 4th ed. Sherman Oaks, Calif: Aerobics and Fitness Association of America (AFAA); 2005:41.

54. *Exercise Standards & Guidelines Reference Manual.* 4th ed. Sherman Oaks, Calif: Aerobics and Fitness Association of America (AFAA); 2005:54.

55. *Exercise Standards & Guidelines Reference Manual.* 4th ed. Sherman Oaks, Calif: Aerobics and Fitness Association of America (AFAA); 2005:95.

56. Aerobics and Fitness Association of America. *Policy Statement on the Sale, Provision or Recommendation of Nutritional Supplements.* Available at: http://pdfs.afaa.com. 1999. Accessed July 7, 2006:3–4.

57. American College of Sports Medicine. Updated physical activity guidelines released today. August 1, 2007. Available at: http://www.acsm.org/AM/Template.cfm?Section= ACSM_News_Releases&CONTENTID=7769&TEMPLATE=/CM/ContentDisplay.cfm. Accessed October 26, 2007.

58. American College of Sports Medicine. Position stand: The recommended quantity and quality of exercise for developing and maintaining cardiorespiratory and muscular fitness, and flexibility in healthy adults. *Med. Sci Sports Exerc.* 1998;30:975–991.

59. American College of Sports Medicine. Position stand: Appropriate intervention strategies for weight loss and prevention of weight regain for adults. *Med Sci Sports Exerc.* 1994;26:649–660.

60. American College of Sports Medicine. Position stand: Progression models in resistance training in healthy adults. *Med Sci Sports Exerc.* 2002;34:364–381.

61. American Academy of Pediatrics. Policy statement: Strength training by children and adolescents. Available at: http://www.aap.org/policy/pprgtoc.cfm. n.d. Accessed June 17, 2006.

62. National Strength and Conditioning Association. Youth strength training. Available at: http://nsca-lift.org/Publications/posstatements.shtml. n.d. Accessed June 10, 2006.

63. American Diabetes Association. Position statement: Diabetes mellitus and exercise. *Diabetes Care.* 2002;25:S64.

64. American College of Sports Medicine. Position stand: Exercise and type 2 diabetes. *Med Sci Sports Exerc.* 2000;32:1345–1360.

65. American College of Sports Medicine. Position stand: Physical activity and bone health. *Med Sci Sports Exerc.* 2004;36:1985–1996.

66. American College of Sports Medicine. Position stand: Osteoporosis and exercise. *Med Sci Sports Exerc.* 1995;27:i–vii.

67. American College of Sports Medicine. Position stand: Exercise and hypertension. *Med Sci Sports Exerc.* 2004;36:533–553.

68. American College of Obstetricians and Gynecologists. Exercise during pregnancy and the postpartum period. ACOG Committee Opinion No. 267. *Obstet Gynecol.* 2002:99:171–173.

69. American College of Sports Medicine. Position stand: Exercise and physical activity for older adults. *Med Sci Sports Exerc.* 1998;30:992–1008.

70. National Strength and Conditioning Association. Basic guidelines for the resistance training of athletes. Available at: http://nsca-lift.org/Publications/posstatements.shtml. n.d. Accessed June 10, 2006.

71. American College of Sports Medicine. Position stand: The female athlete triad. *Med Sci Sports Exerc.* 2007;39:1867–1882.

72. *ACSM's Guidelines for Exercise Testing and Prescription.* 7th ed. Philadelphia: Lippincott Williams & Wilkins; 2006:29–30.

73. Koeberle BE. *Legal Aspects of Personal Training.* 2nd ed. Canton, Ohio: PRC; 1991.

74. Ohio Board of Dietetics, Bulletin #8, General Non-Medial Nutrition Information. Available at: http://www.dietetics.ohio.gov/bulletins/bulletin8.pdf. n.d. Accessed July 6, 2006: 2.

75. Eickhoff-Shemek J, White C. Internet personal training and/or coaching: What are the legal issues? Part I. *ACSM's Health Fitness J.* 2004;8(3):25–26.

76. Eickhoff-Shemek J, White C. Internet personal training and/or coaching: What are the legal issues? Part II. *ACSM's Health Fitness J.* 2004;8(5):24–25.

77. Eickhoff-Shemek J, White C. Internet personal training and/or coaching: What are the legal issues? Part III. *ACSM's Health Fitness J.* 2005;9(3):29–31.

CHAPTER 8

Instruction and Supervision

LEARNING OBJECTIVES After reading this chapter, health/fitness students and professionals will be able to:

1. Identify the many liability exposures that exist with regard to instruction and supervision.
2. Distinguish specific, transitional, and general supervision and understand how each is applied in a health/fitness facility.
3. Describe the inherent supervisory duties that health/fitness professionals have toward their participants.
4. Describe the various published standards of practice that address instruction and supervision.
5. Develop risk management strategies that will minimize legal liability associated with instruction and supervision.

Providing proper instruction and supervision of programs and services is an important responsibility of all health/fitness professionals. This chapter discusses the liability exposures associated with instruction and supervision by focusing on the many allegations that plaintiffs have made against health/fitness facilities in this area. In addition, published standards of practice and risk management strategies that address instruction/supervision are presented to help guide health/fitness professionals and their risk management advisory committees in the development of their own risk management strategies related to instruction and supervision of their programs and services.

STEP 1 ASSESSMENT OF LEGAL LIABILITY EXPOSURES

Health/fitness personnel and facilities that fail to provide proper instruction and supervision of their programs and services can face serious legal liability problems. Not only can health/fitness professionals be held liable for negligent instruction and/or supervision, but so can their supervisors/managers through the application of a legal doctrine known as *respondeat superior,* as will be discussed in some of the legal cases described in this chapter. This doctrine basically states that employers can be liable for the negligent acts of their employees (and volunteers) while acting within their scope of employment or responsibilities. In other words, "the corporate entity is responsible for the negligent acts of those who represent it in the conduct of activities which it sponsors or facilities and areas which it maintains."[1] Therefore, health/fitness managers and supervisors must not only hire qualified and competent personnel, but also train and supervise them to help ensure they are carrying out their instructional and supervisory responsibilities safely and effectively.

Although there are not many statutory or administrative laws which dictate what health/fitness facilities must provide for proper instruction and supervision, there is ample case law where plaintiffs have sued health/fitness professionals and facilities for the alleged failure to instruct/supervise (omission) or where they have provided alleged improper instruction/supervision (commission). Betty van der Smissen states that the "lack of or inadequate supervision is the most common allegation of negligence."[2] As previously presented in Chapter 3, van der Smissen also states that the duty to supervise occurs by (a) statutory requirement, (b) voluntary assumption of a duty, and (c) the duty inherent in the situation. An example of a statutory requirement would be Wisconsin's state statute[3] that requires fitness centers during all times in which they are open to have at least one employee present on the premises of the fitness center who has completed a courses(s) in basic first aid and CPR taught by an individual, organization, or institution of higher education.

Voluntary supervision occurs when there is generally no duty to provide supervision but because of an action taken by an individual, a duty is created. For example, an employee of a health/fitness facility who is working out during his or her own time does not have a legal duty to correct a participant who is misusing a piece of equipment on how to use it correctly. However, perhaps the employee has a moral duty to do so. If the employee decides to help the participant, he or she has then voluntarily assumed a duty to provide reasonable instruction/supervision. In *Parks v. Gilligan,*[4] discussed in Chapter 3, a participant gratuitously spotted another participant (the plaintiff) who was injured while lifting dumbbells on a bench press. The plaintiff claimed that the volunteer spotter had assumed a duty toward him and failed to carry out that duty. This case resulted in a settlement in which the facility and the volunteer spotter had to pay $15,000 and $5,000, respectively, to the plaintiff.

The third manner in which there is duty to supervise—inherent in the situation—is the focus of this chapter because it involves the "inherent" supervisory duties that health/fitness facilities have toward their participants who are engaged in activities sponsored by them, which for the most part covers "all" programs and services. Therefore, it is not so much whether or not there is duty to supervise, but rather what type of supervision is needed given the situation. Betty van der Smissen classifies supervision as specific, general, and transitional.[5] **Specific supervision** means that the supervisor is "directly" with an individual or small group and most often involves an "instructional" format.[5] In health/fitness facilities, this would typically include personal fitness training, teaching group exercise classes, and providing an initial orientation/instruction to new participants on the proper use of the equipment and facility. From a legal perspective, specific supervision should provide the participant an opportunity to gain knowledge of the activity, an understanding of their own capabilities, and an appreciation of the potential injuries that can occur to the point where the participant can assume the inherent risks of the activity.[5] Once this is achieved, the supervision of the participant can move to transitional and then general categories.

It is also important to realize that specific supervision is not a function of the activity but of the individual participating, meaning the "determinant of likelihood of injury is directly related to the participant's skill capability, physical and mental condition to do the activity, and knowledge/understanding/appreciation of the activity itself."[6] For example, participants who have medical conditions (e.g., high blood pressure, diabetes, pregnancy, etc.) should be provided adequate specific supervision (instruction) that includes knowledge/understanding/appreciation of any specific inherent risks that may exist and any special precautions they should take, given their individual condition.

General supervision involves a supervisor who has the responsibility for overseeing an activity going on in the facility.[5] An example of someone who provides general supervision would be a fitness floor supervisor or anyone else who has responsibilities to supervise facilities such as the locker rooms, saunas, racquetball courts, and child care areas. There are two dimensions of general supervision: individual oriented and group behaviors oriented.[5] An example of individual-oriented supervision would be observing participants to ensure they are using the exercise equipment and facility properly. Group behaviors-oriented supervision involves watching the behaviors of participants (e.g., being sure participants are following the fitness center's policies and procedures) and observing and taking appropriate action if any dangerous conditions occur, such as a piece of equipment that breaks down.

Transitional supervision involves changing from specific to general and back, perhaps several times during any supervisory session.[5] An example of this would be when a staff member has taught a small group of new participants how to use certain exercise equipment during the facility's orientation/instruction program (specific supervision) and then has them exercise on their own while providing general supervision. At times during the general supervision, the staff member may individually and directly help (or reteach) a participant an exercise and then go back to general supervision of all the participants. This also happens when fitness floor supervisors who usually provide general supervision but at times may need to transition to specific supervision (e.g., when they notice a participant misusing the equipment and correction [instruction] is needed).

CASE LAW

Often in negligent claims or lawsuits, plaintiffs allege that the defendant(s) failed to provide proper instruction and supervision—meaning specific supervision (instruction), general, and transitional supervision—as demonstrated in the cases described next. These cases are grouped into the following three categories to help you understand the areas of supervisory duties of health/fitness facilities: (1) general instruction/supervision duties, (2) instruction/supervision duties of group exercise leaders, and (3) instruction/supervision duties of personal trainers.

Case Law: General Instruction/Supervision Duties

Many participants join a health/fitness facility to workout on their own. They do not want to participate in any of the specific programs such as personal fitness training or group exercise. Health/fitness professionals may believe there is no duty to instruct or supervise these individuals. However, there clearly is such a duty, as stated by the appellate court in *Thomas v. Sports City, Inc.*[7] Thomas was injured while using a hack squat machine. After he had completed a set using 180 pounds of free weights that was on the carriage of the machine, Thomas thought he properly engaged the hook to secure the weights. However, he did not secure the hook, and the rack of weights fell, fracturing his ankle and crushing his foot. He claimed that Sport City failed to warn, supervise, and instruct him on the proper use of the hack squat machine. The trial court ruled in favor of the plaintiff, awarding him general damages ($45,000) and special damages ($13,703.35). Comparative fault was assigned as follows: 30% to the plaintiff, 35% to Sport City, and 35% to Capps Welding, the manufacturer of the hack squat machine. (The products liability issue in this case is discussed in Chapter 9.) However, the appellate court reversed the trial court's decision, stating that Sport City was not liable for negligent instruction/supervision and Capps Welding was not liable for a design defect in the machine.

To establish the extent of Sport City's duty to instruct/supervise in this case, the appellate court, citing other court decisions, stated, "members of health clubs are owed a duty of reasonable care to protect them from injury on the premises" and "this duty includes a general responsibility to ensure that their members know how to properly use gym equipment."[8] The appellate court determined that Thomas did know how to use this machine properly and was an experienced, sophisticated user of the machine. Thomas testified that he had been a member of Sport City for several years, worked out at least four times per week, and used the hack squat machine as part of his normal routine. He also testified that he did not need instruction and acknowledged that if he had properly secured the hook, the carriage would not have fallen.

The appellate court concluded that it was not Sport City's failure to warn of dangers or instruct the plaintiff that *caused* his injury. Therefore, there was no negligence on the part of the defendant Sport City. However, the court did state it was uncontested that Sport City had not instructed or supervised the plaintiff on the machine's proper use and that normally this would be a *breach of duty* because the machine could easily cause injury. In other words, health/fitness facilities do have a duty to instruct their participants on the proper use of exercise equipment, warn them of any dangers/risks, and supervise them properly. This is perhaps best accomplished by having all new members/participants attend a facility orientation (discussed later under risk management strategies) that includes instruction on the proper use of the equipment and facility, as well as providing general staff supervision of the fitness floor and other areas within the facility during all operating hours. For example, if a participant is not exercising in a safe manner, it would be the staff supervisor's responsibility to then transition to "specific" supervision (instruction) to help/educate that participant on its proper use. The failure to provide proper supervision of the fitness floor and other areas within a health/fitness facility has been a common allegation made by plaintiffs. See additional cases in Chapters 9 and 10 as well as *Chai v. Sports & Fitness Clubs of America Inc.*[9] in Chapter 5 in which one of the claims was that the defendant failed to monitor the plaintiff properly while he was exercising in the cardiovascular room.

General staff supervision of the facility is not only necessary to help ensure participants are using the equipment and facility properly, but is also important to help enforce the safety policies and procedures established by the facility. For example, if a policy requires participants to replace dumbbells on a rack after use, and a participant is not doing this (e.g., leaving them on the floor or a bench), the staff supervisor should approach and remind the participant of this safety policy.

General supervision of the health/fitness facility must also include observing participants for any inappropriate behavior(s). In a Rhode Island case,[10] a member of a health club was convicted of a second-degree sexual assault after he allegedly sexually assaulted a female patron while both were in the facility's whirlpool. A lifeguard at the facility who observed the defendant's actions testified that when the victim entered the whirlpool she started to observe the defendant. At the criminal trial, one of the questions that the prosecutor asked the lifeguard was "What was the first thing you did when you approached the defendant?"[11] Her answer was that she stated the following to the defendant: "I need to talk to you about what just happened, it can't happen. Those types of things cannot happen here, and I told him that I have seen him bother . . ."[11] She was not able to finish her statement at trial, but it can be inferred perhaps that this lifeguard had previously observed inappropriate behavior by this member toward other members in this facility. The conviction was reversed upon appeal and remanded to the lower court for a new trial because certain testimony of the defendant should not have been allowed as evidence without a cautionary instruction.

Health/fitness professionals (and the organizations they represent) generally are not liable for criminal actions of their participants, but could be potentially liable for negligent supervision when a participant engages in this type of behavior toward another participant. If indeed the lifeguard had observed this type of behavior before the incident in question and did nothing to stop the behavior, and/or management did nothing once informed, the facility could be found negligent and even perhaps grossly negligent. Gross negligence can result when a health/fitness facility has **constructive knowledge** (prior knowledge) of a fact/problem and then does nothing to correct it. Because health/fitness facilities have a duty to provide a reasonably safe environment for their participants, specific policies and procedures must be in place to deal properly with such situations quickly and directly. An example of a negligent supervision case occurred when two children in the shower area of a YMCA were sexually assaulted by an emotionally disturbed teenager. The foster parents of the teen warned the YMCA that he could not be trusted with children. Although the YMCA believed it had properly supervised the boys, the jury did not agree and awarded the plaintiffs $375,000 in damages.[12]

As mentioned earlier and discussed in Chapter 5, employers are generally not liable for criminal actions (e.g., sexual assault) of their employees. These types of actions are not considered within the scope of employment, and therefore imposing vicarious liability on the employer under the doctrine of *respondeat superior* would be quite difficult.[13] However, negligent hiring claims could be made against a health/fitness facility if criminal background checks were not conducted, especially for those employees working with vulnerable populations (e.g., children, older adults, persons with disabilities) as well as those who provide services of a private nature such as massage therapy.[13]

Related to general instruction/supervision duties is the issue of overcrowding in the exercise areas of a health/fitness facility. In *Mannone v. Holiday Health Clubs and Fitness Centers, Inc.,*[14] the plaintiff was injured when his hand was struck by a free weight, causing a subtotal amputation of his left ring fingertip. He claimed that the health club was negligent because it failed to (a) adequately supervise the free-weight room, (b) instruct members on proper use of the free weights, (c) train, qualify, and supervise personnel adequately, and (d) regulate membership numbers to space accommodations. In *Pappalardo v. New York Health & Racquet Club,*[15] the plaintiff fell out of a window after using a leg curl machine. To allow his friend to use the machine, he moved to an area close to the window in an attempt to find room—in what was reported to be a crowded club—to stretch his hamstrings. After noticing his shoe was untied, he squatted down to tie it and bumped against the glass, which shattered, and he fell to the pavement below. The plaintiff alleged a variety of negligence claims against the club and owner of the building including the failure to comply with certain safety codes. "Although the appellate court's decision noted that the club was crowded, nothing further was reported in the decision which would indicate whether or not the issue was raised by the plaintiffs as an allegation of negligence."[15] Health/fitness facilities should make every effort to control for overcrowding in their exercise areas by providing adequate spacing for stretching, walkways (e.g., between machines and windows/walls), and between equipment, as well as regulate the number of members given the size of the facility. In addition, staff members who supervise these areas should be informed on steps/precautions they can take for participants to follow when the facility becomes overcrowded.

Case Law: Instruction/Supervision Duties of Group Exercise Leaders

Group exercise leaders have a duty to instruct and supervise their participants safely. In *Santana v. Women's Workout and Weight Loss Centers, Inc.,*[16] the plaintiff, on her second day in a modified step aerobics class (step aerobics combined with overhead arm strengthening exercises using a Dynaband), fell and fractured her ankle. The injury required surgical intervention involving the insertion of pins in her leg. While performing the combined activities, participants were instructed to look straight ahead at their reflections in a mirror versus looking at their feet. The plaintiff filed a negligence lawsuit against the defendant center, claiming the design of the exercise was unreasonably difficult and dangerous. An expert witness for the plaintiff, Dr. Peter Francis, stated that the combined exercises along with using a mirror for visual orientation created an *inherently dangerous* situation and therefore did not meet the standard of care. In other words, the simultaneous activities "increased" the risks over and above those inherent in a typical step aerobics class, and therefore the instructor was allegedly negligent.

The trial court granted the defendant center's motion for summary judgment stating that the membership agreement that the plaintiff signed, which contained both assumption of risk and waiver statements, barred her suit. Upon appeal, the plaintiff claimed that neither the primary assumption of risk defense nor the waiver defense should apply. The appellate court agreed with the plaintiff, stating that the "defendants generally have a duty to use due care not to increase the risks to a participant over and above those inherent in the sport."[17] It is important to point out that if this injury would have occurred in a typical step aerobics class, the primary assumption of risk defense probably would have protected the defendants from any liability. The plaintiff was not a novice; she had participated in several step aerobics classes at this center before and should have had adequate knowledge/understanding/appreciation of "inherent" risks associated with step aerobics (e.g., that falling and fracturing an ankle could happen).

Regarding the waiver, the plaintiff claimed she was not informed of the waiver (it was hidden on the back side of the agreement) nor was she offered time to read it. When examining the waiver, the appellate court stated there was enough evidence in the circumstances to raise a triable issue of fact as to the validity of the waiver; for example, the plaintiff was unaware of the waiver, there was no advisement near the signature line (on the first page) that a waiver existed on the back side, and the placement and diluted color of the waiver did not make it obvious in the membership agreement. For more on waivers, see Chapter 4.

Remember that the primary assumption of risk defense protects health/fitness professionals and facilities from injuries due to "inherent" risks, not negligence. Interestingly, health/fitness facilities use this defense, claiming that participation in exercise programs is similar to participation in sports. It is common for the primary assumption of risk defense to apply with participation in sports. In its analysis, the *Santana* court stated that sports by their nature (inherently) create extreme risks of injury because they involve (a) competing to score points, racing against time, or accomplishing feats that require strength and speed, and (b) physical contact among individuals/athletes. The court stated that the goal of exercise programs such as step aerobics is to improve health and fitness, and therefore should not be designed to create extreme risks of injury as the directions given by the instructor did in this case.

Although the injury in *Santana* was caused by a fall, injuries involving "naked" resistance tubing have also occurred in group exercise classes.[18] According to a group fitness director at a health club in Utah for more than 10 years, many accidents and injuries have occurred during routine exercise with naked tubing. In one of her classes as the participants were performing a seated row, the tubing broke, snapping back and hitting one of the participants in the eye and resulting in permanent loss of vision in that eye. The club implemented a policy prohibiting the use of the resistance tubing in the frontal plane. Another group fitness director who owned a chain of clubs in Arkansas also reported a similar situation. A participant in a group exercise class was performing a bicep curl with resistance tubing when it broke and hit the participant in the eye. No injury resulted, but the management immediately pulled all naked tubing from the clubs. Fortunately, group exercise programs now have a safer solution to consider in their classes that use resistance tubing. Slastix technology by Stroops has manufactured a nylon cover for the entire length of the latex tubing that prevents the tubing from snapping back if it was to break.[18]

Negligence claims and lawsuits involving the failure to provide proper instruction and/or supervision in group exercise classes have occurred in other cases. For example, in *Contino v. Lucille Roberts Health Spa*,[19] described in Chapter 6, the plaintiff claimed that the aerobics dance class was overcrowded, improperly supervised, and negligently conducted by the defendant's personnel. In a case involving a Pilates instructor,[20] the plaintiff claimed the instructor carelessly, negligently, and recklessly injured her when manipulating the plaintiff's body in two different Pilates exercises. The plaintiff claimed that the actions of the instructor resulted in a serious compression fracture of her thoracic spine, physical and mental pain that will continue, and an adverse effect on her ability to engage in her usual and customary activities. In this case, the plaintiff sought a $100,000 judgment (plus expenses associated with the legal action) against the Pilates instructor and her business.[20]

Case Law: Instruction/Supervision Duties of Personal Fitness Trainers

Certain cases involving instruction/supervision duties of personal fitness trainers were already discussed in Chapter 6, *Rostai v. Neste Enterprises*[21] where the plaintiff claimed that the personal trainer trained him too aggressively in his first workout and did not monitor for signs/symptoms of overexertion; and in Chapter 7, *Makris v. Scandinavian Health Spa, Inc.*[22] where the plaintiff claimed the personal trainer negligently trained, monitored, instructed, supervised, and advised her. Although many negligent claims and lawsuits exist against personal trainers and the organizations they represent, the following two are discussed: *Corrigan v. Musclemakers Inc.*[23] and *Evans v. Pikeway, Inc.*[24]

The plaintiff in *Corrigan* was a 49-year-old woman who was participating in her first personal training session. Toward the end of her session, her personal trainer instructed her to get on a treadmill and set it at 3.5 miles per hour. He provided her with little or no instruction on how to use the treadmill and then left her unattended. After a short while she began to drift back on the belt, and although she attempted to walk faster she was thrown from the treadmill resulting in a fractured ankle. The plaintiff was a novice. She had never participated in a fitness facility of this type, nor had she ever been on a treadmill. She filed a negligence claim against the defendants (the personal trainer and the health club) seeking recovery for her injuries.

The defendants filed a motion for summary judgment claiming the plaintiff voluntarily participated in an athletic activity and therefore assumed the risks. However, the appellate court, quoting another case, stated the "doctrine of primary assumption of risk . . . may be applied in cases where there is typically sporting and recreational events,"[25] but this doctrine does not apply in this case because the fitness activity (exercising on a treadmill) was not an athletic or sporting event. In addition, the plaintiff was a novice who did not fully know, understand, and appreciate the inherent risks associated with using the treadmill—a requirement for the primary assumption of risk to apply. The court concluded that the personal trainer failed to ensure that the plaintiff knew how to use the treadmill, referring to a guideline in the machine's manual that stated knowledge on how to use the treadmill was necessary for safe operation. The court indicated that a jury would need to determine if the plaintiff's injuries were due to the defendant's negligence (breach of duty).

The plaintiff in *Evans* was exercising on a squat machine under the direct supervision of certified personal trainer Janet Kaiser (also the manager of the fitness center) at the time of his injury. He claimed his injury was caused by the negligence of his personal trainer, stating that she "failed to properly and adequately supervise the activities performed by this plaintiff; instructed, permitted and caused the plaintiff to lift a dangerous and hazardous amount of weight; failed to 'spot' this plaintiff when he was lifting the weight bar; failed to ensure that the weight lifted by this plaintiff was appropriate given his experience, ability, weight and size; failed to properly secure the weights to the weight bar lifted by this plaintiff."[26]

The defendant moved for summary judgment requesting the case be dismissed because the assumption of risk and waiver the plaintiff signed prior to participation barred any recovery. The appellate court granted the motion of summary judgment in favor of the defendant because the waiver was valid. Therefore, the case was dismissed protecting the defendant. Because the waiver was valid, the appellate court did not deal with the assumption of risk issue. Waivers that are written and administered properly can protect health/fitness professionals and facilities from their own negligence. See Chapter 4 for more on waivers. Although waivers can be very effective in protecting against negligence, they do nothing to prevent injuries. However, the many other risk management strategies described throughout this text will help prevent injuries from occurring and subsequent litigation.

THE PUBLISHED STANDARDS OF PRACTICE

Of the 10 published standards of practice identified in Chapter 3, nine of them (all except the ACSM/AHA Joint PP-AEDs) have published standards and/or guidelines related to instruction and supervision. The following is a summary of these published statements but should not be considered to be all inclusive.

ACSM/AHA Joint PP, ACSM Guidelines, and ACSM's H/F Standards

The staff qualifications for fitness directors published in the ACSM/AHA Joint PP[27] were presented in Chapter 7. This publication defines an "exercise leader" as someone who "works directly with program participants and provides instruction and leadership in specific modes of exercise" and "helps program participants master behavioral skills needed to adhere to exercise programs."[28] Qualifications for exercise leaders vary depending on the level of the fitness facility (see Table 6.2 in Chapter 6) and are specified as follows:

In level 1, 2, and 3 facilities the exercise leader as a minimum must have a high school diploma or equivalent and entry-level or higher professional certification from a nationally recognized health/fitness organization (comparable to ACSM exercise leader certification). In level 4 facilities, exercise leaders should have education and experience corresponding to that required by ACSM health and fitness instructor certification.[28] (Reprinted with permission. AHA/ACSM scientific statement: Recommendations for cardiovascular screening, staffing, and emergency policies at health/fitness facilities. *Circulation.* 1998;97:2283–2293. © 1998 American Heart Association, Inc.)

The ACSM/AHA Joint PP[27] also indicates that health/fitness facilities need a medical liaison to review medical emergency plans and incident reports as well as to critique emergency drills. In level 4 and 5 facilities, the medical liaison must be a licensed physician, and in level 2 and 3 facilities, he or she can be an emergency medical technician, registered nurse trained in advanced cardiac life support, or a licensed physician (see Table 6-2 in Chapter 6).

Specific staff qualifications (e.g., personal trainers, health/fitness instructors) published in ACSM Guidelines[29] were described in Chapters 6 and 7 with regard to pre-activity health screening and health/fitness assessment and prescription. This publication also provides guidelines with regard to program supervision using a hierarchy—unsupervised, professionally supervised, and clinically supervised. To determine which level of supervision is appropriate, the health status of a participant through risk stratification and functional capacity of the participant must first be obtained, as described in Table 8–1.

TABLE 8-1	General Guidelines for Exercise Program Supervision		
	Level of Supervision		
	Unsupervised	Professional Supervised*	Clinically Supervised†
Health Status	Low risk (from Table 2-4)	Moderate risk (from Table 2-4) Or High risk (from Table 2-4) but with well-controlled, stable CPM disease	High risk (from Table 2-4) with recent onset of CPM that have been cleared by a physician for participation in exercise regimen.
Functional‡ capacity	>7 METs	>7 METs	< 7 METs§

Professionally supervised means supervision by appropriately trained personnel who possess academic training and practical/clinical knowledge, skills, and abilities commensurate with any of the three credentials defined in Appendix F (i.e., ACSM Health/Fitness Instructor, ACSM Exercise Specialist, ACSM RCEP), the ACSM Program Director, or ACSM Health/Fitness Director.

†*Clinically supervised* means supervision by appropriately trained personnel who possess academic training and practical/clinical knowledge, skills, and abilities commensurate with the ACSM Exercise Specialist or ACSM RCEP credentials defined in Appendix F, or the ACSM Program Director.

‡A functional capacity of ≤7 METs is well below the 10th percentile for apparently healthy men, and either at or below the 10th percentile for most apparently healthy women from the Aerobics Center Longitudinal Study (see Table 4-8). *Apparently healthy* individuals within the ACLS cohort would be inclusive of individuals within the ACSM Low and Moderate Risk categories (see Table 2-4).

§For functional capacity of <5 METs, a small staff-to-patient ratio (i.e., one clinical staff member for every five to eight patients) also is recommended.

Abbreviation: CPM, cardiovascular, pulmonary, and/or metabolic disease.

The tables referred to within this table can be found in the following source.

Reprinted with permission from Whaley MH, ed. ACSM's Guidelines for Exercise Testing and Prescription. 7th ed. Philadelphia: Lippincott Williams & Wilkins; 2006.

The ACSM's H/F Standards[30] contain several standards regarding instruction and supervision. Standard #4 states, "All facilities with qualified staff must offer each new member a general orientation to the facility, including identification of resources available for personal assistance with developing a suitable physical activity program and the proper use of any exercise equipment to be used in that program."[31] Standard #8 states, "The fitness and healthcare professionals who have supervisory responsibility for the physical activity programs (supervise and oversee members/users, staff, and/or independent contractors) of the facility must demonstrate the appropriate level of professional education, certification, and/or experience."[32] Standard #17 states, "A facility that offers youth services or programs must provide appropriate supervision."[32] (From American College of Sports Medicine, 2007, *ACSM's Health/Fitness Facility Standards and Guidelines*, 3rd ed., pp. 1–2. © 2007 by American College of Sports Medicine. Reprinted with permission from Human Kinetics, Champaign, IL.) In addition, the ACSM's H/F Standards include several guidelines under Standard #8 (and Standards #9 and #10 listed in Chapter 7) with regard to the recommended levels of education, certification, and experience for positions such as fitness director, group-exercise director, program director, group exercise leader, lifestyle counselor, and personal trainer.

Canadian Standards, NSCA Standards, and MFA Standards

The Canadian Standards[33] addressing fitness-related personnel and their qualifications were listed in Chapter 7. Standard #3 under Fitness Environment states, "The number of participants in an exercise class is based on the square footage that allows each participant unrestricted and safe movement in various types of exercises. Participant numbers may also be defined by building code restrictions and/or fire code regulations."[34]

Under Personnel Qualifications, the NSCA Standards[35] have three guidelines under Personnel Qualifications, which are presented, in part, as follows:

> *Guideline 2.1—The Strength & Conditioning practitioner should acquire a bachelor's or master's degree from a regionally accredited college or university . . . in one or more of the topics comprising the 'Scientific Foundations' domain identified in the Certified Strength & Conditioning Specialist® . . . Examination Content Description . . .*
>
> *Guideline 2.2—The Strength & Conditioning practitioner should achieve and maintain professional certification(s) with continuing education requirements and a code of ethics, such as the CSCS® credential offered through the NSCA CERTIFICATION COMMISSION . . .*
>
> *Guideline 2.3—The productivity of a Strength & Conditioning staff . . . should be enhanced by aligning a performance team comprised of qualified practitioners with interdependent expertise and shared leadership roles.[36]*

Under Program Supervision & Instruction, the NSCA Standards[35] include two standards and one guideline as follows, in part:

> *Standard 3.1—Strength & Conditioning programs must provide adequate and appropriate supervision with well-qualified and trained personnel, especially during peak usage times. In order to ensure maximum health, safety, and instruction, Strength & Conditioning professionals must be present during Strength & Conditioning activities; have a clear view of the entire facility . . . and the athletes in it; be physically close enough to the athletes under their care to be able to see and clearly communicate with them; and have quick access to those in need of spotting or assistance.*
>
> *Standard 3.2—In conjunction with appropriate safety equipment (e.g. power racks), attentive spotting must be provided for athletes performing activities where free weights are supported on the trunk or moved over the head/face . . .*
>
> *Guideline 3.1—Strength & Conditioning activities should be planned—and the requisite number of qualified staff . . . should be available—such that recommended guidelines for minimum average floor space allowance per athlete (100 ft^2), professional-to-athlete ratios (1:10 junior high school, 1:15 high school, 1:20 college), and the number of athletes per barbell or training station (=3) are achieved during peak usage times. Younger participants, novices or special populations engaged in such . . . activities should be provided with greater supervision.[37]*

Under Records & Record Keeping, NSCA Standards[35] Guideline #6.1 states that Strength and Conditioning professionals should develop and maintain various records. Those that relate to instruction and supervision include training logs, progress entries, and/or activity instruction/supervision notes.

Standard #9 from the MFA Standards[38] regarding qualifications for staff members such as fitness directors/supervisors, personal training staff, group fitness instructors, and fitness staff members that provide programming for special populations was presented in Chapter 7. Related to staff training/continuing education and maintaining current certifications, additional MFA Standards state:

> *Standard #10—Facility must provide a variety of training/continuing education opportunities for staff utilizing relationships with and expertise of physicians and other community health care professionals.*
>
> *Standard #11—Staff is required to maintain current certification(s)/license(s) by meeting the continuing education requirements for their specific certifying/licensing bodies.[39]*

The MFA Standards[38] also require that a medical fitness center have medical oversight (Standard #1). The guidelines under this standard are as follows:

1. *The facility should have a Medical Director, a Physician Advisory Committee and/or a Physician Advisor to provide oversight for the center's programming in order to maximize the safety of all participants and ensure medically and scientifically sound programming.*

   a. *The facility leadership and the medical director/advisory committee should meet a minimum of four times per year.*

   b. *The medical director/advisory committee should provide oversight for, but not restricted to:*
      * *Emergency responsibilities/code policy/procedure review*
      * *Facilities' AED program*
      * *Staff emergency response training*
      * *Periodic review of emergency/code response outcomes and identification of opportunities for improvement*
      * *Program content and special populations.*[40]

IHRSA Standards, YMCA Recommendations, and AFAA Standards

There are two IHRSA Standards[41] regarding instruction and supervision. Standard #9 states, "Each person who has supervisory responsibility for a physical activity program or area at the club will have demonstrable professional competence in that physical activity program or area."[42] Supervisory responsibility is defined as "accountability for one or more of the following components: "program scheduling, content and execution of content, program staffing and training, and the space in which the programming takes place" and "demonstrable professional competence suggests a combination of educational and professional experience that would be accepted—by both the industry and public at large."[42]

IHRSA Standard #11 states that "A club that offers youth services or programs will provide appropriate supervision."[43] Under this standard, it states that "Individuals hired to oversee children at the club should be carefully screened, appropriately accredited, thoroughly trained, and closely supervised" and that "Club policy should clearly identify—and place off-limits—any club areas, equipment or activities that might pose a hazard to youngsters."[43]

The YMCA Recommendations[44] for training and qualification of personal trainers and other health/fitness staff members were presented in Chapter 7. In addition, Table 7-1 in Chapter 7 briefly summarized the YMCA Recommendations in the following categories: (a) special populations and/or those with chronic conditions; (b) overweight/obesity, weight loss, diet, eating disorders, and supplements; and (c) youth. Many of the recommendations have instructional and supervisory implications, and it would be necessary to review each in detail to understand these implications.

There are many other YMCA Recommendations that would need to be reviewed in detail that also have instructional/supervisory implications, such as (a) child care issues (e.g., Cytomegalovirus in YMCA Child Care Centers, HIV/AIDS: Participation of Preschool Children with AIDS in YMCA Child Care, Infant and Toddler Sleeping Guidelines for YMCA Child Care Programs); (b) issues involving youth (e.g., Child Abuse Identification and Prevention, Children in Adult Locker Rooms); and (c) specific issues with certain programs/services (e.g., Deer Tick and Lyme Disease Awareness and Education, Exercise and Fluid Replacement, Food Safety and Sanitation, HIV/AIDS: Operating Guidelines for YMCAs; Martial Arts Programs Offered by YMCAs; Massage Therapy in YMCAs; Noise and Music Levels in YMCAs and YMCA programs; Age Guidelines for SCUBA Programs in YMCAs; Guidelines for Skateboard, In-line Skating, Roller Skating and Scooter Safety; and Exposure to Sunlight in YMCA Programs for Children and Adults).

The YMCA Recommendations also provide recommendations regarding a medical advisor or advisory committee: "If a formal medical advisory committee is not practical, an alternate is to have a local practicing physician serve in an advisory capacity on medical and health issues."[45] In addition to a physician(s), members of a medical advisory committee can include nutritionists, exercise physiologists, public health officials, and other experts. Primary functions, in part, are as follows:

- *Review screening and medical requirements for participants*
- *Review and approve medical aspects of all programs*
- *Establish safe operating and adequate emergency response procedures.*[45]

The AFAA Standards[46] in their chapter "Basic Exercise Standards and Guidelines" include many standards and guidelines addressing instruction and supervision issues in group exercise classes. Initially in this chapter, basic principles of exercise training, major components of fitness, health benefits of fitness, and training recommendations are presented. Under professional responsibilities, it is recommended that instructors: (1) have comprehensive liability insurance that includes personal injury liability, general liability, and miscellaneous professional liability insurance (see Chapter 5 for more on liability insurance); (2) complete a training and certification program that includes both theoretical knowledge and practical applications; (3) maintain a current nationally recognized adult-level CPR certification and perhaps also a standard-level first-aid course; (4) be able to recognize an emergency and take appropriate action based on the facility's written emergency response procedures; and (5) check for obvious hazards (e.g., debris, wet floor surfaces, broken exercise equipment) prior to and throughout an exercise class.

Under "Instructional Concerns," the AFAA Standards recommend that group exercise instructors should (1) watch for and take appropriate action if they observe any exercise danger signs in a participant (e.g., nausea, dizziness, tightness in the chest, etc.); (2) modify exercises if a participant exhibits signs/symptoms such as labored breathing, heart rate elevation, and evidence of strain; (3) be aware of certain prescribed and over-the-counter medications that can elicit side effects during exercise; (4) be aware of symptoms of overtraining such as fatigue, anemia, amenorrhea, overuse or stress fractures, etc.; (5) avoid overtraining by varying the type and intensity of the exercises, performing an adequate warm-up and cool-down, etc.; (6) advise participants to hydrate before, during, and after class; (7) recommend proper clothing and footwear; (8) demonstrate instructor etiquette; (9) incorporate factors related to class level, e.g., teach at an intermediate level but explain/demonstrate to the class how to modify to both lower and higher intensities; (10) select appropriate music regarding speed—specific recommendations are provided (bpm) with regard to intensity level; and (11) follow a consistent rhythmic breathing pattern throughout exercise.

Under "Exercise Evaluation," AFAA Standards indicate that group exercise leaders can evaluate an exercise from two perspectives—effectiveness and potential risk of injury—for any participant. Included are the following five questions to determine effectiveness and potential risk:

1. *What is the purpose of this exercise?*
2. *Are you doing that effectively?*
3. *Does the exercise create any safety concerns?*
4. *Can you maintain proper alignment and form for the duration of the exercise?*
5. *For whom is the exercise appropriate?*[47]

Under question 5, a list of 14 exercises are described that AFAA does not recommend in general fitness classes because of their potential increased risks. Also under this section, "Exercise Evaluation," correct body alignment is presented with pictures of the following positions: standing, squats, bent-over, seated, supine, prone, side-lying, kneeling, hands and knees, and while moving.

Under "Group Exercise Format," the AFAA Standards describe the following class components: (a) pre-class announcements, (b) warm-up, (c) cardiorespiratory training, (d) muscular strength and endurance training, (e) flexibility training, and (f) final class segment. For components (b) through (e), the (1) definition, purpose, and duration; (2) common methods; (3) special considerations; and (4) sample exercises are described. The AFAA Standards also include a chapter for the following modes of group exercise, describing specific standards and guidelines for each: aqua fitness, low-impact aerobics, group exercise weighted workouts, cardio-kickboxing, step training, and mat science.

STEP 2 DEVELOPMENT OF RISK MANAGEMENT STRATEGIES

As presented earlier, in ample case law examples plaintiffs have made a variety of negligent claims against health/fitness personnel and facilities involving either the failure to provide instruction and supervision (omission) or improper instruction/supervision (commission). Many professional organizations have also published standards and guidelines with regard to instruction and supervision. Therefore, to apply the law and the published standards of practice, the following risk management strategies are presented that can help minimize injuries and subsequent litigation involving instruction and supervision:

Risk Management Strategy 1: Have only "qualified health/fitness professionals" serve in supervisory roles.

Employees with supervisory responsibilities (e.g., fitness directors/managers, assistant fitness directors, personal training coordinators, and group exercise coordinators) should possess the appropriate credentials as "qualified health/fitness professionals" listed in Chapter 7 as follows:

- Bachelor's degree in exercise science or related field, preferably from an accredited university/college,
- Professional certification commensurate with ACSM's Health/Fitness Instructor (HFI) or NSCA's Certified Strength and Conditioning Specialist (CSCS),
- Current CPR/AED and first-aid certifications, and
- Professional work experience.

In addition, health/fitness professionals that supervise (or teach) certain programs should also possess current certification in that program area (e.g., personal training, group exercise), preferably from a certifying body accredited by the National Commission for Certifying Agencies (NCCA) or some other similar accrediting agency such as those recognized by the United States Department of Education (USDE) or Council for Higher Education Accreditation (CHEA). The NCCA for example, uses a peer review process for certifications offered by various professional organizations to become accredited, meaning the certification meets certain standards established by the NCCA.

Because many health/fitness facilities serve moderate and high-risk populations, these facilities should have at least one (perhaps more) qualified health/fitness professional (e.g., the fitness director and/or a clinical exercise specialist) who has advanced knowledge, skills, and abilities to oversee/direct the programs that serve these populations—for example, a master's degree in exercise science or related area and a certification that correlates to ACSM's Exercise Specialist (ES) or Registered Clinical Exercise Physiologist (RCEP). This will help ensure that these populations receive exercise programs/services that are designed safely and effectively, given their health risks and medical conditions.

Risk Management Strategy 2: Have only qualified group exercise leaders, personal fitness trainers, and fitness floor/facility supervisors provide programs/services to participants.

Employees and independent contractors who serve as personal trainers, group exercise leaders, and fitness floor/facility supervisors should possess the appropriate credentials. As described in Chapter 7, personal trainers who work with low-risk clients should have at a minimum a high school diploma, current personal training certification, current CPR/AED and first-aid certifications, and work experience. Those who work with moderate-risk individuals should possess the same credentials as stated for "qualified health/fitness professionals" and a current personal training certification. Personal trainers who work with high-risk individuals should possess a master's degree in clinical exercise or related field and current certification commensurate with ACSM's Exercise Specialist (ES) or Registered Clinical Exercise Physiologist (RCEP).

Credentials for group exercise leaders, who teach group exercise for general populations, should include a high school diploma, current certification in group exercise, current CPR/AED and first-aid certifications, and work experience. If they teach in specialty areas (e.g., step aerobics, Pilates, aqua fitness, and yoga), they should also possess current certifications in these specific areas. Group exercise leaders who teach classes specially designed for moderate-risk or special populations (older adults, prenatal, postpartum) should possess the credentials described earlier for "qualified health/fitness professionals" and also have experience and certifications in these areas. Those who teach group exercise for high-risk population (e.g., known cardiovascular disease, diabetes, lung disease, etc.) should possess the credentials listed earlier for this category.

Facility and fitness floor supervisors should possess a high school diploma, current certifications in CPR/AED and first aid, current certification in either group exercise or personal training, and work experience. These supervisors, with proper training, could serve in the manager on duty (MOD) role (see Chapter 11)—a designated staff member who is responsible during/after a medical emergency, and so on. However, it would be best to have a "qualified health/fitness professional" to serve in this capacity during all operating hours. Qualified health/fitness professionals should possess the knowledge, skills, and abilities to properly carry out all the responsibilities of the MOD. In addition, while qualified health/fitness professionals are on duty, they are qualified (as described in Chapter 6) to review/interpret pre-activity screening questionnaires for any new members that join, thus providing this process for the new member in a timely fashion.

The issue of a staff member's credentials is likely to be addressed in a negligence claim or lawsuit (e.g., the plaintiff may claim that his or her personal trainer was not qualified to conduct personal training). However, appropriate credentials alone will not serve as an adequate defense for a health/fitness professional. As stated in Chapter 7, the professional standard of care does not vary given the credentials of the professional, but rather it is situationally determined. Betty van der Smissen states, "If one accepts responsibility for giving leadership to an activity or providing a service, one's performance is measured against the standard of care of a qualified professional *for that situation.*"[48] For example, if a personal trainer is training a client who has diabetes and is on medication for hypertension, he or she must know and prescribe exercises that would be appropriate for "that client" and know what exercises not to prescribe (e.g., any contraindications) that could be potentially harmful for "that client." It is more likely that a health/fitness professional who is qualified, that is, possesses the credentials listed earlier to work with high-risk participants, would have the necessary knowledge, skills, and abilities to properly carry out the duty owed toward a participant like this than a health/fitness professional who does not have the appropriate credentials. However, it is not a guarantee that they do.

Therefore, there is a need for training and supervision of all health/fitness professionals, as described under Risk Management Strategy 6, to help ensure the proper duty toward participants is being carried out, given the situation/person(s) served. In addition it is important to realize that some professionals who are highly credentialed (e.g., an academician with a doctorate degree and ACSM ES certification but who has little or no work experience in personal training) may not be adequately qualified to conduct personal training without additional instruction. In other words, it is best to have the health/fitness professional's credentials match up with the job responsibilities or duties. As stated in Chapter 5, health/fitness personnel need to be both "qualified" (possess the proper credentials) and "competent" (know how to carry out the appropriate standard of care properly).

Regarding independent contractors, health/fitness supervisors do not have control over staff members who work in this capacity as described in Chapter 5; for example, supervisors cannot instruct/supervise, conduct performance appraisals, set work schedules, and so on. Any responsibilities that a health/fitness facility wants an independent contractor to have with regard to pre-activity health screening, instruction, supervision, emergency procedures, and so on, should be specified in the contract that all independent contractors sign prior to providing services at the health/fitness facility. It is important that health/fitness managers investigate the qualifications and competence of independent contractors before offering them a contract.

Risk Management Strategy 3: Provide medical oversight if serving moderate- and high-risk populations.

In addition to the need for qualified staff members (described earlier) for health/fitness facilities that serve moderate- and high-risk populations, these facilities also should have medical oversight; that is, a qualified physician or group of physicians and other health/medical experts who serve on a medical advisory committee. This committee has several roles/responsibilities (e.g., see MFA Standards and YMCA Recommendations described previously) and should work regularly with the facility's "qualified health/fitness professionals."

As recommended in Chapter 1 and throughout this book, all health/fitness facilities should have a risk management advisory committee made up of legal, medical, insurance, and exercise science experts. This committee should assist health/fitness professionals in the many decision-making processes necessary in the development of a comprehensive risk management plan. Health/fitness facilities that have a medical advisory committee should make sure this committee works with members of the risk management advisory committee (e.g., the legal and insurance experts) because of the many decisions that these committees make that have both medical and legal implications.

Risk Management Strategy 4: Offer a health/fitness facility orientation for all new participants.

Offering all participants a health/fitness facility orientation is an essential risk management strategy. This orientation is a program that includes instruction and information on (a) proper use of the exercise equipment and facility, (b) awareness of safety policies/procedures and signage, (c) principles of safe/effective exercise, and (d) programs/services offered by the facility that can meet individual needs/interests. This program could be offered in small groups or individually. If offered in small groups, individuals could be put into a couple of different groups such as experienced exercisers (e.g., those who have used exercise equipment before), and beginners (e.g., those who have not used exercise equipment before), and then the orientations could be tailored accordingly. Facilities could also consider offering various levels of facility orientation, perhaps based on an individual's pre-activity health screening results and risk classification of low, moderate, or high. Staff members that meet the credentials listed earlier for fitness floor and facility supervisors (high school diploma, personal training or group exercise leader certification, etc.) could teach the facility orientation program to low-risk participants. "Qualified health/fitness professionals" with the credentials listed previously (bachelor's degree, ACSM HFI certification, etc.) could teach the facility orientation program to moderate-risk participants. If a health/fitness facility serves high-risk participants, they should have health/fitness professionals with the highest credentials (master's degree in clinical exercise, ACSM ES certification, etc.) teach the facility orientation program. However, it would be wise not to label these groups low, moderate and high, but perhaps groups 1, 2, and 3.

The content and extent of the facility orientation program will depend on the participants and their health/fitness levels and degree of experience. For example, for low-risk participants who already have fitness experience, it may be completed in one session. However, for a low-risk participant who is a novice, it may take several sessions or referral to one of the facility's programs for beginners. For participants with health risks or medical conditions, it may also take several sessions, or referral to one of the facility's programs designed especially for them (e.g., senior fitness classes, prenatal exercise classes, personal training sessions with a qualified personal trainer).

As stated earlier under Assessment of Legal Liability Exposures, specific supervision (a facility's orientation program is considered specific supervision because of its instructional nature) should provide the participant an opportunity to gain knowledge of the activity, an understanding of his or her own capabilities, and an appreciation of the potential injuries that can occur, to the point where the participant can assume the inherent risks of the activity.[5] For example, participants who have medical conditions (e.g., high blood pressure, diabetes, pregnancy, etc.) should be provided adequate specific supervision (instruction) that includes knowledge, understanding, and appreciation of any specific inherent risks that may exist and any special precautions they should take, given their individual condition. At what point a participant obtains this necessary knowledge/understanding/appreciation so they can exercise in a general supervision environment is a judgment call for the health/fitness professional teaching the facility orientation program. That is one reason why it is best to have properly credentialed health/fitness professionals serving this function.

At a minimum, all participants should have a facility orientation program that covers proper use of the exercise equipment and facility, the facility's safety policies/procedures, and safe/effective principles of exercise. Proper use of the equipment and the facility should include: (1) instructing participants on the proper position and execution of exercises (flexibility, muscle strength/endurance, and cardiovascular), (2) pointing out to participants any instructional signage that is posted (e.g., pictures of proper stretches, fitness facility safety sign) and instructional placards/warning labels placed on each piece of exercise equipment, and (3) any instructions/signage regarding proper use of facilities such as hot tubs, saunas, swimming pools, and locker/shower areas. The facility's safety policies and procedures should be presented in the form of a handout (or perhaps specified in the membership agreement) and posted within the facility. Staff members who teach the facility orientation program should explain why these policies/procedures are in place and any consequences for participants who do not adhere to them.

Participants must also be educated about the safe and effective principles of exercise. By providing participants some handout materials or a booklet, such as *Physical Fitness: Guidelines for Success*,[49] the teacher can address these basic principles and then the participant can take the handout home to review it in more detail. *Physical Fitness: Guidelines for Success*, is a 32-page booklet which covers the following topics:

- Top-25 reasons to exercise
- Fitness components
- Principles of exercise
- Pre-activity screening
- Aerobic principles
- Weight training principles
- Flexibility principles
- Potential risks associated with exercise
- Motivational tips to maintain your exercise program
- Sample workouts

In addition to minimizing medical emergencies and possible subsequent litigation, a facility orientation can help reduce a variety of other problems. Often problems and/or participant complaints occur because the participants have not been made aware of the policies/procedures established by the facility and the importance of following them. Although not recommended, health/fitness facilities that want to allow participants the option to refuse participation in the facility orientation program should have them read and sign a refusal form (see Figure 8-1).

Risk Management Strategy 5: Have staff supervision during all operational hours.

All health/fitness facilities should be supervised by a qualified staff member(s) during all operational hours. At a minimum, this should be a person who meets the qualifications of the fitness floor/facility supervisor listed earlier. Preferably, this person should meet the credentials for a "qualified health/fitness professional" as described previously. Some facilities that are large or have facilities such as racquetball/basketball courts, saunas/hot tubs, locker/shower areas, and so on, may need more than one facility supervisor during all operational hours.

All health/fitness facilities should have a fitness floor supervisor in the fitness area(s) at all times where the exercise equipment is located. There should be regular, periodic supervision of all other areas within the facility. How often staff members should check these other areas is a judgment call, but during peak times the frequency of supervision should increase. Health/fitness facilities should consider the published standards of practice that have specified guidelines in this regard. With their risk management advisory committees, they should develop supervision guidelines that would be appropriate, given the facility's programs, populations served, and needs. Although facility/fitness floor supervisors should have a job description that describes their job responsibilities, here is a list of some of the responsibilities of a typical fitness floor supervisor:

- Serves as the manager on duty (MOD) who has oversight in case of a medical emergency or any other emergency (see Chapter 11).
- Provides specific, general, and transitional supervision to participants so they are exercising safely and following the facility's policies and procedures; provides spotting when needed.
- Takes appropriate action if a problem occurs (e.g., a piece of equipment breaks, a risk or hazard of some type develops, a behavior problem with a participant occurs, a participant misuses the equipment or facility, the facility becomes overcrowded).
- Documents and reports to management any situations that arise (such as those stated directly earlier). Note: Some facilities may want to develop a special form that is completed for documentation purposes. Documentation can serve as evidence that the proper standard of care was carried out.
- Ensures that equipment and facility signage is properly in place at all times.

Refusal to Participate in the Health/Fitness Facility Orientation

To help ensure safe participation in health/fitness activities, several major professional fitness organizations have published standards and/or guidelines that require or recommend that health/fitness facilities provide all new members an orientation to the facility that includes proper use of the exercise equipment. Therefore, to comply with these national standards and guidelines, _____ (name of health/fitness facility) ("Facility") has established a policy that requires all participants to participate in the Facility's Orientation. However, though not recommended, participants may refuse to participate in this process by reading and signing the following:

I _____ (name of participant) understand that Facility requires all participants to complete a Facility Orientation that includes instruction/information regarding: (a) proper use of the exercise equipment and facility; (b) awareness of safety policies and procedures; (c) principles of safe/effective exercise such as warm-up, progression, and monitoring of sign/symptoms of overexertion; and (d) programs/services offered by the Facility to meet individual needs and interests.

However, I have chosen not to participate in the Facility Orientation.

Risks associated with refusal to participate in the Facility Orientation

I understand and appreciate that there exists the possibility of adverse effects occurring during exercise testing and exercise. The purpose of my participation in a facility orientation is to familiarize myself with the facility and its equipment, the proper use of the facility and that equipment, the proper methods of my participation in the activities carried on within the facility, and the rules and regulation for use of the facility and the equipment, amenities, and activities carried out in the facility. If I do not participate in the orientation, I acknowledge and agree that I may not fully understand and appreciate how equipment and amenities in the facility are to be operated and used and accordance with applicable rules and regulations, and that the risks of harm to me and others may be increased. I have been informed that the risks of activity, though remote, include abnormal blood pressure, fainting, disorders of heart rhythm, stroke, and very rare instances of heart attack or even death. In addition, I understand that I may experience musculoskeletal conditions or injuries such as fractured bones, muscle strains, muscle sprains, muscular fatigue, contusions, muscle soreness, joint injuries, torn muscles, heat-related illnesses, and back injuries. I understand that other risks not listed here, both minor and major, can also occur. By my refusal to participate in the facility/equipment orientation the chances of the occurrence of one or more of these or other risks may be increased. Moreover, I recognize that I may hurt myself or others by not fully understanding how to use the equipment or amenities in the facility, or how to use the facility itself or during my participation in activities in the facility due to my failure to participate in the orientation or ability to identify the rules and regulations applicable thereto. I understand that the benefits of participating in the Facility Orientation are to enhance my safety and to possibly minimize some of the risks stated above. I assert that my participation is voluntary and that I knowingly assume all such risks.

Waiver/Release

My signature below indicates that I have been fully informed of, understand, and appreciate the benefits of participating in the Facility Orientation, as well as the potential risks of not participating in the Facility Orientation. In addition, my signature also indicates that I have executed a release and waiver document with the Facility which, among other things, contractually binds me and my estate not to bring any type of legal claim and/or lawsuit against the Facility and/or its staff members for among other things, the failure of the Facility and/or its staff to conduct a Facility Orientation. I also understand that this release/waiver gives up and relinquishes my right to institute a claim or lawsuit against the Facility and/or its staff members for a number of other acts and/or omissions related to the ordinary negligence of those released. I hereby reaffirm my understanding and agreement to that release and waiver documents and to this statement.

_____   _____
Signature of Participant   **Date**

_____   _____
Signature of Staff Member   Date

FIGURE 8-1 Refusal to Participate in the Health/Fitness Facility Orientation

Risk Management Strategy 6: Establish training programs for all health/fitness staff members.

Training programs (initial and ongoing) for all health/fitness professionals should be established. The manager or owner has the ultimate responsibility for risk management for the health/fitness facility. When he or she hires supervisors—professional staff members who have oversight of the programs/services as well as supervisory responsibilities—training must be provided for them on their respective instruction and supervisory responsibilities. In turn, these supervisors need to train their subordinates on their respective instruction and supervision responsibilities.

Generally, health/fitness supervisors, along with their manager/owner and the facility's risk management advisory committee, develop the risk management strategies (e.g., policies and procedures that need to be carried out) and then train their subordinates so they know how to carry out the policies and procedures. An example in the area of instruction and supervision would be for the group exercise coordinator to provide an initial training program for all new group exercise leaders so they become familiar with proper instruction/supervision techniques and the philosophy/policies related to the facility's group exercise program.

Realize that just because a health/fitness professional has certain credentials, it does not automatically mean the person can perform the job effectively. Initial training is likely needed for all health/fitness professionals. Once initial training has occurred, ongoing in-service training (or other types of training such as community workshops, conferences, online learning) should be provided throughout the year. An example of an effective initial and ongoing training program for group exercise leaders has been published[50,51] and serves as a good model for training other health/fitness professionals. Part I of this two-part article described the necessary planning steps and content of a successful "initial" training program that focuses on safe and effective teaching. Part II addresses the importance of "ongoing" training to help ensure that group exercise leaders are carrying out the facility's safety policies and procedures properly, as well as always learning new and advanced teaching strategies. For more on staff training, see Chapter 12.

Risk Management Strategy 7: Conduct evaluations of job performance on all health/fitness staff members.

Evaluation of job performance is a critical risk management function. The job performance of all health/fitness professionals should be evaluated by their superiors. Evaluation entails regular observation and feedback, but it should also include a formal annual performance appraisal. For example, how would a group exercise coordinator know if the group exercise leaders are teaching safely and effectively if their job performance has not been evaluated? An article describing the procedures on how to conduct job performance appraisals of group exercise leaders (GELs) has been published[52] with application to the comprehensive performance appraisal tool for GELs found in Figure 8-2. This tool was developed using principles of performance appraisal theory[53] and was validated by group exercise coordinators who participated in a study.[52] In the *Santana* case, described earlier, it is not known if a job performance of the step aerobics instructor was ever evaluated, but it is probably unlikely. If an experienced, qualified group exercise coordinator had observed this instructor's performance, it is likely he or she would have informed the exercise leader not to teach the combined exercises anymore. If the instructor then no longer taught these exercises, perhaps the injury would not have happened, which demonstrates how effective an important risk management strategy like conducting a job performance appraisal can be.

PERFORMANCE APPRAISAL TOOL: GROUP EXERCISE LEADER (GEL)

Name of GEL _____ Name of Supervisor_____
Date of Class Observation _____ Name of Class _____
Number of participants attending _____ Date/Time of Class _____
Reason for Appraisal: _____ Introductory _____ Follow-Up _____ Regular Interval

Rate the performance as I, M, E, or NA as follows:

I - Improvement is needed; performance standard is not met
M – Meets performance standard
E – Exceeds performance standard
NA – Not Applicable

Note: **Explanation** sections are available to describe any particular rating.

SECTION 1: IN-CLASS EVALUATION

	I	M	E	NA
Behavior-Based Performance				
Criterion #1 – Pre-class Conduct				
1. Arrives prior to class time	__	__	__	__
2. Sets up equipment	__	__	__	__
3. Greets participants as they arrive	__	__	__	__

Explanation: _____

	I	M	E	NA
Criterion #2 – Beginning of Class Conduct				
1. Starts class on time	__	__	__	__
2. Introduces self and class format	__	__	__	__
3. Welcomes everyone	__	__	__	__
4. Makes announcements, e.g., anything related to today's class	__	__	__	__
5. Encourages participants to exercise at own level	__	__	__	__

Explanation: _____

	I	M	E	NA
Criterion #3 – Safe Instruction				
Warm-Up				
1. Teaches warm-up which is specifically appropriate for the class	__	__	__	__
2. Incorporates appropriate duration of warm-up	__	__	__	__
Stimulus				
3. Teaches appropriate intensity given fitness levels of participants	__	__	__	__
4. Incorporates proper progression of intensity	__	__	__	__
5. Incorporates proper progression of complexity	__	__	__	__
6. Monitors intensity by having participants take their heart rates	__	__	__	__
7. Monitors intensity by having participants rate via RPE	__	__	__	__
8. Observes each participant for signs of overexertion	__	__	__	__
9. Takes proper action if a participant appears to be overexerted	__	__	__	__
10. Incorporates appropriate duration of stimulus	__	__	__	__
11. Gradually decreases the intensity of exercises prior to cool-down	__	__	__	__
Cool-Down				
12. Incorporates appropriate stretching in the cool-down	__	__	__	__
13. Incorporates appropriate duration of cool-down	__	__	__	__

Safe Instruction throughout Class	I	M	E	NA
14. Teaches and demonstrates proper form and execution of exercises	__	__	__	__
15. Corrects improper form/execution of exercises	__	__	__	__
16. Demonstrates modifications given various levels of fitness	__	__	__	__
17. Teaches exercises in an appropriate sequence and progression	__	__	__	__
18. Avoids contraindicated exercises	__	__	__	__
19. Avoids patterns/combinations that can contribute to balance/coordination problems	__	__	__	__
20. Incorporates appropriate number of sets/reps when teaching muscle strength/endurance exercises	__	__	__	__
21. Incorporates exercises that utilize a variety of muscle groups	__	__	__	__
22. Incorporates exercises that provide muscle balance	__	__	__	__
23. Incorporates exercises to address muscles that are commonly tight and/or weak	__	__	__	__
24. Incorporates safe transitions, e.g., standing to non-standing	__	__	__	__

Explanation: _____
_____
_____

FIGURE 8-2 Performance Appraisal Tool: Group Exercise Leader (GEL)

Criterion #4 – Effective Teaching Methods

	I	M	E	NA
1. Uses simple, command or cue words	—	—	—	—
2. Incorporates proper timing of command or cue words	—	—	—	—
3. Provides verbal encouragement/positive feedback	—	—	—	—
4. Utilizes appropriate voice quality including projections, volume, and enunciation	—	—	—	—
5. Utilizes appropriate nonverbal communication	—	—	—	—
6. Moves around the room while teaching	—	—	—	—
7. Uses appropriate music volume	—	—	—	—
8. Uses appropriate music tempo	—	—	—	—
9. Selects appropriate music	—	—	—	—
10. Teaches to the beat of the music; demonstrates proper rhythm	—	—	—	—
11. Utilizes room space effectively	—	—	—	—
12. Teaches exercise concepts/principles	—	—	—	—

Explanation: _____
_____

Criterion #5 – Class Management

1. Comes to class prepared	—	—	—	—
2. Demonstrates control and command of the class	—	—	—	—
3. Uses class time effectively	—	—	—	—

Explanation: _____

Criterion #6 – Professionalism

1. Dresses appropriately	—	—	—	—
2. Demonstrates professional conduct and attitude	—	—	—	—
3. Supports policies and procedures of the facility	—	—	—	—
4. Handles equipment properly	—	—	—	—

Explanation: _____

Criterion #7 – Interaction with Participants

1. Uses an appropriate approach when correcting form/execution	—	—	—	—
2. Shows maturity when dealing with difficult participants	—	—	—	—
3. Encourages a noncompetitive atmosphere	—	—	—	—
4. Establishes a positive rapport	—	—	—	—
5. Incorporates humor appropriately	—	—	—	—
6. Demonstrates enthusiasm	—	—	—	—
7. Creates an enjoyable class	—	—	—	—
8. Welcomes late comers and encourages them to warm-up	—	—	—	—

Explanation: _____

Criterion #8 – End of Class Conduct

1. Ends class on time	—	—	—	—
2. Thanks participants	—	—	—	—
3. Gives positive feedback	—	—	—	—
4. Makes announcements, e.g., promotes other classes/upcoming events	—	—	—	—
5. Available to address participant questions/comments	—	—	—	—

Explanation: _____

Criterion #9 – Post-class Conduct

1. Puts away equipment	—	—	—	—
2. Leaves classroom on time	—	—	—	—
3. Follows procedures, e.g., turning off lights, locking door, etc.	—	—	—	—

Explanation: _____

SECTION 2: OUT-OF-CLASS EVALUATION

Behavior-Based Performance

	I	M	E	NA
Criterion #1 – Behavior outside the Classroom				
1. Demonstrates dependability regarding teaching responsibilities	—	—	—	—
2. Makes prior arrangements for class when absent	—	—	—	—

FIGURE 8-2 *(Continued)*

	I	M	E	NA
3. Attends required in-service trainings regarding emergency plan	___	___	___	___
4. Attends required in-service trainings and meetings	___	___	___	___
5. Maintains current CPR/AED certification	___	___	___	___
6. Maintains current First-Aid certification	___	___	___	___
7. Maintains current GEL certification	___	___	___	___
8. Available to substitute classes for other instructors	___	___	___	___
9. Responds to phone/email messages in a timely manner	___	___	___	___

Explanation: _____

Trait-Based Performance
Criterion #1 – Communication Traits

	I	M	E	NA
1. Demonstrates appropriate interpersonal communication	___	___	___	___
2. Responds to constructive criticism appropriately	___	___	___	___

Explanation: _____

Criterion #2 – Professional/Personal Traits

	I	M	E	NA
1. Demonstrates a positive attitude	___	___	___	___
2. Demonstrates an unbiased attitude	___	___	___	___
3. Exhibits creativity	___	___	___	___
4. Shows a desire to learn	___	___	___	___
5. Takes responsibility for actions	___	___	___	___
6. Demonstrates self-motivation	___	___	___	___

Explanation: _____

Results-Based Performance
Criterion #1 – Accomplishments Related to Participants

	I	M	E	NA
1. Obtained high attendance adherence in classes taught	___	___	___	___
2. Obtained positive participant evaluations	___	___	___	___

Explanation: _____

Criterion #2 – Accomplishments Related to Program/Facility

	Yes	No	In Progress
1. Created a new program or class	___	___	___
2. Improved an operational procedure(s)	___	___	___
3. Developed skills to teach another class or perform another job	___	___	___

Explanation: _____

Criterion #3 – Professional Accomplishments

	Yes	No	In Progress
1. Obtained additional degree or certification	___	___	___
2. Obtained an award or recognition	___	___	___
3. Attended conferences/workshops for continuing education	___	___	___

Explanation: _____

SECTION 3: PERFORMANCE APPRAISAL FEEDBACK

Discussion/Feedback Date _____ (Discussed self-performance appraisal, supervisor performance appraisal and developed an action plan).

Action Plan: (Steps to address performance standards rated "I" with a projected timeframe)

General/Positive Feedback:

GEL Signature _____   Date: _____

Supervisor Signature _____   Date: _____

Copy of written Performance Appraisal Tool given to GEL and original placed in GEL Personnel File on _____ (date).

FIGURE 8-2 (Continued)

Risk Management Strategy 8: Establish the maximum number of participants in group exercise classes.

A policy on the maximum number of participants in group exercise classes should be established. Group exercise leaders at all times should be able to adequately observe all class participants for proper position/execution of the exercises as well as signs/symptoms of overexertion. Again, this is a judgment call; no definitive numbers can be recommended. However, the following factors should be considered when establishing this policy for each type of group exercise class: space available in the classroom, level of expertise and experience of the instructor, type of participants (e.g., novices, general population, special populations, low-high risk, children, etc.), type of group exercise class, and building/fire codes.

Risk Management Strategy 9: Provide proper instruction and supervision for all youth programs and services.

Youth programs (e.g., physical activities such sports, aquatics, and dance) and services (e.g., child care) should be properly taught and supervised by adults to provide a safe environment and experience. However, never assume that because someone is an adult, the person is qualified to instruct/supervise kids. Although some specific qualifications may be necessary, it is critical for the health/fitness facility to provide training for adult instructors and supervisors whether they are employees or volunteers. This training should cover not only how to instruct and supervise kids, but should also address the policies and procedures of the facility (e.g., pre-activity health screening, forms such as agreements to participate and waivers, and the facility's emergency action plan).

All children should be taught how to participate in activities safely and why that is important. A minor, along with his/her parent/guardian, should sign an agreement to participate that explains the expectations and the rules/policies they should follow, along with a listing of the inherent risks associated with participation in any specific activity (see Chapter 4). These documents should be written so they are appropriate to the age of the participant.

Health/fitness facilities that provide child care services also have numerous supervision responsibilities. Child care in health/fitness facilities can be basic babysitting services or full day care services. Babysitting is probably more common. Full day care services are subject to state and local laws. When developing the supervision risk management strategies for babysitting and/or full day care services, health/fitness facilities need to consider any applicable state/local laws in addition to published standards of practice such as the YMCA Recommendations[44] that provide guidelines on a variety of child care supervision issues.

In addition, as already discussed under Assessment of Legal Liability Exposures, criminal background checks should be conducted on staff members/volunteers who will be working with youth or other vulnerable populations (e.g., older adults, persons with disabilities) as well as those who provide services of a private nature such as massage therapy. Continual supervision of these staff members/volunteers is also important. These risk management steps may be helpful to refute claims or lawsuits involving negligent hiring and/or negligent supervision.

Risk Management Strategy 10: Establish procedures for proper documentation related to instruction and supervision.

Procedures for proper documentation/record keeping involving instruction and supervision should be in place. Examples include (a) dates of the facility orientations (and names of individuals who participated); (b) situations that arise during general supervision of the facility such as when a piece of equipment breaks, a risk or hazard of some type develops, a behavior problem with a participant occurs, a participant misuses the exercise equipment/facility, or the facility becomes overcrowded; (c) exercise prescription/instruction/supervision notes of personal trainers and GELs; (d) dates of staff training programs and names of staff members who attended; and (e) performance appraisals of staff members.

PUT INTO PRACTICE CHECKLIST 8-1

Rate your phase of development for each of following risk management strategies related to instruction and supervision:

	Developed	Partially Developed	Not Developed
1. Having only "qualified health/fitness professionals" serve in supervisory roles.			
2. Having only qualified group exercise leaders, personal fitness trainers, and fitness floor/facility supervisors provide programs/ services to participants.			
3. Providing medical oversight if serving moderate- and high-risk populations.			
4. Offering a health/fitness facility orientation for all new participants.			
5. Having staff supervision during all operational hours.			
6. Establishing training programs for all health/fitness staff members.			
7. Conducting evaluations of job performance on all health/fitness staff members.			
8. Establishing the maximum number of participants in group exercise classes.			
9. Providing proper instruction and supervision for all youth programs and services.			
10. Establishing procedures for proper documentation related to instruction and supervision.			

SUMMARY

Health/fitness professionals must recognize the numerous liability exposures that exist with regard to instruction and supervision. As presented in this chapter, the lack of adequate instruction and supervision is a common allegation of negligence. This is perhaps consistent with the results from the study (described in Chapter 1) conducted by an insurance company over a 12-year period that analyzed the number of claims and costs in the health clubs they insured. "Member malfunction" was the most common claim (see Table 1-2 in Chapter 1). This category of claims where members hurt themselves while working out (e.g., straining a muscle, dropping a weight on their foot, and smashing fingers on selectorized machines) can many times be related to lack of proper instruction and supervision. In addition, this study included a substantial number of professional liability claims that directly reflected incidents involving improper instruction by health/fitness facility personnel.

Because almost all programs and services that health/fitness facilities provide for their participants require some level of instruction and/or supervision, it is essential that this area of liability be addressed in the risk management plan. Health/fitness professionals and their risk management advisory committees need to review legal cases in which the issue of inadequate instruction/supervision has been raised, as well as the many published standards of practice in this area. The development of risk management strategies in this area may take more effort than in other areas presented in this book. However, this effort will pay off with fewer injuries because of inadequate instruction/supervision and subsequent litigation, as well as in high-quality programs/services that will help increase participant satisfaction and retention.

RISK MANAGEMENT ASSIGNMENTS

1. Prepare a PowerPoint presentation describing the three types of supervision (specific, transitional, and general) that could be used in a staff training program.

_____

_____

_____

_____

2. Develop a "supervision" plan for all programs and services within your health/fitness facility.

_____

_____

_____

_____

3. Develop a job description for the fitness floor supervisor, specifically describing his or her many instruction/supervision duties.

_____

_____

_____

_____

4. Develop a detailed outline describing the content for the facility orientation program for all new participants.

_____

_____

_____

_____

5. Adapt/revise the GEL performance appraisal tool in Figure 8-2 to develop a performance appraisal tool that could be used to evaluate the job performance of personal trainers.

_____

_____

_____

_____

6. Make a list of the types of signs (and their content) that should be posted within the facility that address instruction and supervision.

_____

_____

_____

_____

7. Develop a policy regarding the necessary staff qualifications needed for each educational program provided in your facility.

_____

_____

_____

_____

KEY TERMS

Constructive knowledge   Specific supervision   Transitional supervision
General supervision

REFERENCES

1. van der Smissen B. *Legal Liability and Risk Management for Public and Private Entities.* Vol 1. Cincinnati, Ohio: Anderson; 1990:83.
2. van der Smissen B. *Legal Liability and Risk Management for Public and Private Entities.* Vol 2. Cincinnati, Ohio: Anderson; 1990:163.
3. Wis. Stat. Ann. §100.178 (West), 1987.
4. Suit against volunteer spotter settled. *Exercise Standards and Malpractice Reporter.* 1998;12:41.
5. van der Smissen B. *Legal Liability and Risk Management for Public and Private Entities.* Vol 2. Cincinnati, Ohio: Anderson; 1990.
6. van der Smissen B. *Legal Liability and Risk Management for Public and Private Entities.* Vol 2. Cincinnati, Ohio: Anderson; 1990:170.
7. *Thomas v. Sport City, Inc.,* 738 S0.2d 1153 (La. 2 Cir., 1999).
8. *Thomas v. Sport City, Inc.,* 738 S0.2d 1153 (La. 2 Cir., 1999): 1157.
9. *Chai v. Sports & Fitness Clubs of America, Inc.* Analyzed in: Failure to defibrillate results in new litigation. *Exercise Standards and Malpractice Reporter.* 1999;13:55–56.
10. Herbert D. Patron of health club convicted of sexual assault—but conviction reversed on appeal. *Exercise Science and Malpractice Reporter.* 2002;16:49, 52.
11. Herbert D. Patron of health club convicted of sexual assault—but conviction reversed on appeal. *Exercise Science and Malpractice Reporter.* 2002;16:49, 52.
12. McKibben G. YMCA must pay in rape suit. *Denver Post.* April 16, 1997:A-01.
13. Moorman A, Eickhoff-Shemek J. Risk management strategies for avoiding and responding to sexual assault complaints. *ACSM's Health & Fitness J.* 2007;11(3):35–37.
14. *Mannone v. Holiday Health Clubs and Fitness Centers, Inc.* Analyzed in: New exercise related case claims that alleged overcrowding and lack of instruction/supervision lead to his injuries. *Exercise Science and Malpractice Reporter.* 1993;7(1):15.
15. *Pappalardo v. New York Health & Racquet Club.* Analyzed in: Herbert D. Alleged overcrowding of health club facility—correlation to injury? *Exercise Science and Malpractice Reporter.* 2001;15(3):38.
16. *Santana v. Women's Workout and Weight Loss Centers, Inc.* (2001 Cal. App. LEXIS 1186)
17. *Santana v. Women's Workout and Weight Loss Centers, Inc.* (2001 Cal. App. LEXIS 1186): 26.

18. Naked tubing costing companies big money due to liability issues—a safer solution is now available. *Exercise Science and Malpractice Reporter.* 2006;20:61.

19. *Contino v. Lucille Roberts Health Spa,* 509 N.Y.S 2d 369 (N.Y. App. Div. 2d 1986).

20. Herbert DL. New case filed against Pilates instructor. *Exercise Science and Malpractice Reporter.* 2003;17:65, 68–71.

21. *Rostai v. Neste Enterprises,* 41 Cal. Reptr.3rd 411 (Cal. Ct. App., 4th Dist. 2006).

22. *Makris v. Scandinavian Health Spa, Inc.,* Ohio App. LEXIS 4416 (Ohio Ct. App., 1999).

23. *Corrigan v. Musclemakers, Inc.,* 686 N.Y.S2d 143 (1999 N.Y. App. Div. LEXIS 1954).

24. *Evans v. Pikeway, Inc.,* 2004 N.Y. Slip Op. 24556 (2004 WL 3196946).

25. *Corrigan v. Musclemakers, Inc.,* 686 N.Y.S2d 143 (1999 N.Y.App. Div. LEXIS 1954): 145.

26. *Evans v. Pikeway, Inc.,* 2004 N.Y. Slip Op. 24556 (2004 WL 3196946), 862.

27. American College of Sports Medicine and American Heart Association Joint Position Statement. Recommendations for cardiovascular screening, staffing, and emergency policies at health/fitness facilities. *Med Sci Sports Exerc.* 1998;30:1009–1018.

28. American College of Sports Medicine and American Heart Association Joint Position Statement. Recommendations for cardiovascular screening, staffing, and emergency policies at health/fitness facilities. *Med Sci Sports Exerc.* 1998;30:1009–1018, 1016.

29. Whaley MH, ed. *ACSM's Guidelines for Exercise Testing and Prescription.* 7th ed. Philadelphia: Lippincott Williams & Wilkins; 2006.

30. Tharrett SJ, McInnis, KJ, Peterson, JA, eds. *ACSM's Health/Fitness Facility Standards and Guidelines.* 3rd ed. Champaign, Ill: Human Kinetics; 2007.

31. Tharrett SJ, McInnis, KJ, Peterson, JA, eds. *ACSM's Health/Fitness Facility Standards and Guidelines.* 3rd ed. Champaign, Ill: Human Kinetics; 2007:1.

32. Tharrett SJ, McInnis, KJ, Peterson, JA, eds. *ACSM's Health/Fitness Facility Standards and Guidelines.* 3rd ed. Champaign, Ill: Human Kinetics; 2007:2.

33. *Canadian Fitness Safety Standards & Recommended Guidelines.* 3rd ed. 2004. Available at: http://www/oases.on.ca/safety/safetyStdsCurrent.htm. Ontario, Canada: Ontario Association of Sport and Exercise Sciences (OASES). Accessed September 2, 2007.

34. *Canadian Fitness Safety Standards & Recommended Guidelines.* 3rd ed. 2004. Available at: http://www/oases.on.ca/safety/safetyStdsCurrent.htm. Ontario, Canada: Ontario Association of Sport and Exercise Sciences (OASES). Accessed September 2, 2007:2.

35. *NSCA Strength & Conditioning Professional Standards & Guidelines.* May 2001. Available at: http://www.nscalift.org/Publications/standards.shtml. Colorado Springs: National Strength and Conditioning Association (NSCA). Accessed September 2, 2007.

36. *NSCA Strength & Conditioning Professional Standards & Guidelines.* May 2001. Available at: http://www.nscalift.org/Publications/standards.shtml. Colorado Springs: National Strength and Conditioning Association (NSCA). Accessed September 2, 2007:13.

37. *NSCA Strength & Conditioning Professional Standards & Guidelines.* May 2001. Available at: http://www.nscalift.org/Publications/standards.shtml. Colorado Springs: National Strength and Conditioning Association (NSCA). Accessed September 2, 2007:13–14.

38. *The Medical Fitness Model: Facility Standards and Guidelines.* Richmond, Va: Medical Fitness Association (MFA); May 2006.

39. *The Medical Fitness Model: Facility Standards and Guidelines.* Richmond, Va: Medical Fitness Association (MFA); May 2006:11–12.

40. *The Medical Fitness Model: Facility Standards and Guidelines.* Richmond, Va: Medical Fitness Association (MFA); May 2006:7–8.

41. IHRSA Club Membership Standards. In: *IHRSA's Guide to Club Membership & Conduct.* 3rd ed. Boston: International Health, Racquet & Sportsclub Association (IHRSA); 2005.

42. IHRSA Club Membership Standards. In: *IHRSA's Guide to Club Membership & Conduct.* 3rd ed. Boston: International Health, Racquet & Sportsclub Association (IHRSA); 2005:4.

43. IHRSA Club Membership Standards. In: *IHRSA's Guide to Club Membership & Conduct.* 3rd ed. Boston: International Health, Racquet & Sportsclub Association (IHRSA); 2005:5.

44. *Medical Advisory Committee Recommendations: A Resource Guide for YMCAs.* Chicago: YMCA of the USA; February 2007.

45. *Medical Advisory Committee Recommendations: A Resource Guide for YMCAs.* Chicago: YMCA of the USA; February 2007:84.

46. *Exercise Standards & Guidelines Reference Manual.* 4th ed. Sherman Oaks, Calif: Aerobics and Fitness Association of America (AFAA); 2005.

47. *Exercise Standards & Guidelines Reference Manual.* 4th ed. Sherman Oaks, Calif: Aerobics and Fitness Association of America (AFAA); 2005:10–11.

48. van der Smissen, B. Elements of negligence, In: Cotten DJ, Wolohan JT, eds. *Law for Recreation and Sport Managers.* 3rd ed. Dubuque, Iowa: Kendall/Hunt; 2003:60–61.

49. Eickhoff-Shemek J, Berg K. *Physical Fitness: Guidelines for Success;* 2003. Available by contacting lead author at eickhoff@tempest.coedu.usf.edu.

50. Brathwaite AC, Davidson D, Eickhoff-Shemek, JM. Recruiting, training, and retaining qualified group exercise leaders: Part I. *ACSM's Health Fitness J.* 2006;10(2):14–18.

51. Davidson D, Brathwaite AC, Eickhoff-Shemek, JM. Recruiting, training, and retaining qualified group exercise leaders: Part II. *ACSM's Health Fitness J.* 2006;10(3):22–26.

52. Eickhoff-Shemek JM, Selde S. Evaluating group exercise leader performance: An easy and helpful tool. *ACSM's Health Fitness J.* 2006;10(1):20–23.

53. Mathis RL, Jackson JH. *Human Resource Management.* 10th ed. Mason, Ohio: Thomson South-Western; 2003.

CHAPTER 9

Exercise Equipment

LEARNING OBJECTIVES After reading this chapter, health/fitness students and professionals will be able to:

1. Recognize the different liability exposures that are potentially incurred by those who are merely making space available for physical activity as opposed to those who provide a fully equipped and staffed health/fitness facility.

2. Appreciate the breadth of risk exposures associated with a virtual myriad of exercise and fitness devices.

3. Understand the need to select, install, and maintain equipment, as well as the need to properly remove from use equipment in need of repair/replacement and repair/replace such exercise equipment in health/fitness facilities.

4. Learn and understand the need to provide proper instruction and supervision to fitness clients in the use of exercise equipment.

5. Describe the various published standards of practice that address exercise equipment issues.

6. Develop various risk management strategies to reduce the chance of fitness client injuries associated with the use of exercise equipment.

Injuries arising from participant use of exercise equipment in health/fitness facilities are a frequent source of negligence claims and lawsuits against health/fitness personnel and the facilities within which programs and services are provided to those participants. As presented in Chapter 1, liability claims associated with equipment malfunction (e.g., failure to maintain the equipment properly) and member malfunction (e.g., failure to instruct/supervise participants properly on the correct use of equipment) are quite common. See Table 1-2 in Chapter 1. In addition to these types of negligent acts/omissions claims made against a health/fitness facility and its personnel, injuries resulting from using exercise equipment can also be related to the negligent conduct of the participant (e.g., misuse of the equipment) and defects in the equipment for which the manufacturer may be liable (**product liability**) (see Figure 9-1). This chapter describes many legal cases involving exercise equipment injuries as well as various standards of practice published

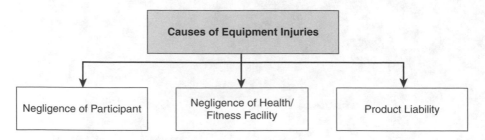

FIGURE 9-1 Causes of Equipment Injuries

by professional and independent organizations relevant to exercise equipment. Specific risk management strategies are also presented that will help minimize exercise equipment injuries and resultant claims and lawsuits.

STEP 1 ASSESSMENT OF LEGAL LIABILITY EXPOSURES

Negligence claims and lawsuits against health/fitness facilities and their personnel arise out of a number of acts/omissions associated with the selection, assembly, installation, and maintenance of such equipment, together with those claims that arise out of participant instruction and/or supervision in the use of equipment. These claims include allegations related to the following:

- The purchase of substandard, improperly designed, or defective equipment.
- The improper assembly/installation of equipment.
- The failure to maintain equipment properly or to follow manufacturers' or industry promulgated maintenance schedules for equipment.
- The failure to remove equipment from service when it is in need of maintenance, repair, or replacement and to repair or replace such equipment.
- The failure to keep fitness equipment clean, sanitary, and in proper working order.
- The failure to provide appropriate and proper instruction in the use of exercise equipment.
- The failure to appropriately supervise equipment use by fitness clients.
- The failure to provide access to equipment to those who are disabled as required by law.

The legal risks associated with providing mere space as opposed to equipment and services are different and increase decidedly as equipment and services are added to the mix. In the 1986 case of *Dillon v. Keatington Racquetball Club*,[1] the court held that absent special circumstances, one who merely rents space for a particular activity owes no duty toward users to supervise the space's use. Despite the ruling in the case, however,

> [O]nce a facility does more than merely rent space, it is likely that it will be required to exercise due care to protect users from unreasonable risk of harm or to insure compliance with safety related game rules. This does not mean that the facility is required to act as an insurer against all risks; but rather, that the facility and its personnel act in accordance with principles of due care toward its patrons when they are engaged in leading, instructing or supervising those participants. Negligence in performing these activities can well result in liability.[2]

As stated earlier, the manufacturer (and sometimes the distributor/seller as well) can be held liable for equipment injuries because of defects in the exercise equipment. A defect is anything making a product *unreasonably dangerous*.[3] The Restatement of the Law (Third) of Torts defines three types of defects: **manufacturing defect, design defect,** and **marketing defect** as described in Figure 9-2.[4]

Categories of Product Defects

Manufacturing Defect: A product contains a manufacturing defect when the product departs from its intended design even though all possible care was exercised in the preparation and marketing of the product.

Design Defect: A product is defective in design when the foreseeable risks of harm posed by the product could have been reduced by the adoption of a reasonable alternative design by the seller or a predecessor in the commercial chain of distribution and the omission of the alternative design renders the product not reasonably safe.

Marketing Defect: A product is defective because of inadequate instructions or warnings when the foreseeable risks of harm posed by the product could have been reduced by the provision of reasonable instructions or warnings by the seller or a predecessor in the commercial chain of distribution and the omission of the instructions or warnings renders the product not reasonably safe.

FIGURE 9-2 Categories of a Product Defect (*Restatement of the Law (Third) of Torts: Products Liability. Tentative Draft No.* 1 § 2. Categories of product defects. April 12, 1994, 9–10. Copyright [1994] by the American Law Institute. Reprinted with permission. All rights reserved[4].)

CASE LAW: EQUIPMENT SPACING, PLACEMENT, AND INSTALLATION

Improper spacing, placement, and installation of exercise equipment can increase the risks of untoward events and then result in related claims and suits. For example, in a report of a case from the state of New York, *Pappalardo v. New York Health & Racquet Club,*[5] the facts would indicate that the plaintiff fell out of a second-story window while using a leg curl machine. He fell when he dismounted the machine so a friend could use the device. The machine was in a row somewhere between 18 inches to 3 feet from a window. The plaintiff contended that the space between the windows and the machines was not sufficient. The actual fall occurred when the plaintiff squatted down to tie his shoe and came into contact with the window, which shattered, and then he fell. Although summary judgment was granted by the trial court, the appellate court returned the case to the lower court for determination of safety code issues.

Such issues have also been raised in other cases. For example, in *Mannone v. Holiday Health Clubs and Fitness Centers,*[6] a complaint was filed in which the plaintiff alleged that the overcrowding of facilities, inadequate instruction in the use of equipment, and the lack of appropriate supervision resulted in his hand being struck by a free weight, this in turn causing a "subtotal amputation of his left ring fingertip." The amended complaint included the following specific allegations:

- Failure to supervise adequately the use of the free weights in the free-weight room;
- Failure to instruct the members on safe use of the free weights in the free-weight room;
- Failure to provide a safe place for members to use the reclining chair for use with the free weights in the free-weight room;
- Failure to provide adequate warnings;
- Failure to regulate adequately and limit member access to a safe number of members in the free-weight room for the limited space available;
- Failure to train, qualify and supervise personnel adequately; and
- Failure to regulate membership numbers to space accommodation.[6]

Also remember that the second edition of *ACSM's Health/Fitness Facility Standards and Guidelines*[7] provided some information about placement and space issues for exercise devices and machinery, as well as equipment and instructor/supervisor-to-patron ratios. Specific advice, equipment placement and layout recommendations, diagrams, and spacing considerations are often provided for fitness facilities by equipment manufacturers and some facility designers, such as architects/engineers. The third edition of *ACSM's Health/Fitness Facility Standards and Guidelines* moved away from providing specific information on these issues.[8]

Aside from overcrowding issues, equipment installation and placement issues can also create particular risks and concomitant claims and suits. For example, in the Ohio case of *Darling v. Fairfield Medical Center,*[9] the plaintiff contended that she lost her balance and fell from a treadmill without side rails when she briefly closed her eyes. Although the trial court granted summary judgment to the defendants, the appellate court reversed on the basis of an expert affidavit.

The affidavit of William Herbert, Ph.D., an expert in exercise physiology, stated that:

> *7. As well, the Sports Clinic failed to set up the treadmill in compliance with the mandates set forth in the manufacturer's operation manual and also failed to provide Mrs. Darling with the cautions and warnings contained in that manual. For instance . . . the Clinic failed to set the treadmills up with appropriate clearance and floor space between other equipment and the walls, as required by the manufacturer's manual and this was unreasonable.*

***

> *11. The fact that Mrs. Darling momentarily closed her eyes prior to the fall does not change my opinion or the obligations of the Sports Clinic. Mrs. Darling had a medical history that made her obviously susceptible to instability. In fact, every person using a treadmill at the Sports Clinic was susceptible to instability by virtue of the injury or illness that brought them there. The Clinic's patients were not young, healthy members of a private health club. These patients, including Mrs. Darling, had the potential to become unstable and lose their balance for countless reasons ranging from becoming fatigued, dizzy or having a knee buckle to tripping over a shoestring left untied. The Clinic knew or should have known this and had an obligation to provide side safety rails for its treadmills to prevent significant injury to a patient, like Linda Darling, who loses her balance.*[10]

Although this case involved a clinical type facility as opposed to a typical health/fitness facility, it does adequately demonstrate the relevant issues related to equipment installation and placement. As noted in one article commenting on this case,

> *Among other things, the decision in this case readily points out the importance of facilities' compliance with manufacturer's instructions as to set-up, use, instructions, and warnings. Instructions and warnings which are delineated within manufacturer's materials but which are not communicated to users do little to achieve compliance with the requested provision of important information to those who utilize such equipment.*[11]

In another case against a fitness center that was also described in Chapter 3, *Xu v. Gay,*[12] the facts were stated by the court as follows:

> *In February 1999, Ning Yan went to defendant's fitness center to use a one-week complimentary pass. Yan visited the fitness center on February 16 and 18, 1999. Each time he visited he was required . . . to sign-in and did so. At the top of the sign-in sheet was a paragraph that purportedly constituted a release of liability.*

On February 18, 1999, while using one of the treadmills, Yan fell and hit his head. The head injury Yan sustained was severe, and he died on March 12, 1999. The parties dispute the circumstances of Yan's fall. Plaintiff contends that Yan stumbled while jogging and that the belt of the treadmill threw Yan back into the wall or the window ledge, which were only $2^{1}/_{2}$ feet behind him. Defendant asserts that Yan was ill and fell down, hitting his head on the floor. No one actually saw Yan hit the wall, floor, or window ledge.[13]

Based on these facts:

[P]laintiff filed this suit alleging ordinary negligence by defendant, loss of consortium, and wrongful death. Defendant filed a motion for summary disposition under MCR 2.116(C)(7), arguing that the release at the top of the sign-in sheet that Yan signed precluded any claims of ordinary negligence against defendant. Following a hearing on May 10, 2000, the trial court agreed with defendant, and on May 19, 2000, the Court granted defendant's motion regarding the claim of ordinary negligence, but also granted plaintiff leave to file his second amended complaint, which was actually filed on April 5, 2000, without the court's permission, and alleged a claim of gross negligence against defendant.[13]

In response to these claims, the defendant:

[R]enewed her motion for summary disposition to dismiss plaintiff's claims of gross negligence and wrongful death. . . . On September 12, 2001, following a hearing, the trial court concluded that reasonable minds could not differ and there was insufficient evidence to support a claim of gross negligence. Therefore, because the wrongful-death claim was derivative, both claims failed. On September 24, 2001, the trial court entered an order granting defendant summary disposition on plaintiff's remaining claims.[14]

The plaintiff appealed. In support of her claim of gross negligence, the plaintiff:

[O]ffered the testimony of Dr. Marc Rabinoff, an expert in recreational safety. Rabinoff testified with respect to the industry's standard of care regarding the safety distance behind treadmills, which should be a minimum of five feet. Rabinoff admitted that these are only recommended standards and are not mandatory. Rabinoff also stated that a similar accident was sure to happen again if the treadmill was not moved farther from the wall. However, we note that there was no evidence establishing that Yan actually hit his head on the wall, as opposed to the floor.

Defendant admitted that she knew a treadmill user could stumble while on the moving belt. However, defendant denied knowing that such a loss of balance could cause the user to be propelled backwards off the treadmill. Rabinoff testified that defendant's statement was "the dumbest statement I have ever heard from anyone I think in thirty years who had anything to do with the fitness field about a treadmill." Further, Rabinoff found defendant's lack of knowledge regarding safety standards for a fitness club to be incredulous, stating that defendant was "the worst, poorly educated owner/operator of a health club I have ever seen in twenty-five years." The evidence also indicated that the treadmills were placed in their current positions by the fitness club's previous owner. Defendant bought the club approximately one year before the accident, and did not move the treadmills.

Plaintiff also asserted that the manufacturer recommended that the treadmill be . . . placed at least five to six feet from a wall. However, plaintiff offered no admissible evidence to establish this point. . . . In fact, the evidence showed that the manufacturer of this treadmill had no setback recommendation in its operator's manual for the model of treadmill involved in this case.

Essentially, plaintiff argues that there were industry standards, that defendant should have known about these standards, and that defendant's ignorance of and failure to implement these standards constituted gross negligence. However, this establishes a case of ordinary negligence, not gross negligence. Evidence of ordinary negligence does not create a question of fact regarding gross negligence. . . . Viewing the evidence in the light most favorable to plaintiff, we find that reasonable minds could not differ; defendant's mere ignorance does not constitute conduct so reckless as to demonstrate a substantial lack of concern for whether an injury resulted to Yan. Jennings, supra; Vermilya, supra. Therefore, we hold that the trial court did not err in granting summary disposition in favor of defendant on plaintiff's gross-negligence claim.[15]

Although the case was reversed on the grounds that the sign-in sheet the plaintiff had signed did not bar the action, the case again readily points out the equipment placement issues that can arise in equipment claims and litigation.

Each of these categories of potential risk associated with exercise equipment create avenues of injury exposure for clients and legal exposure to claims and lawsuits for personnel and facilities. The diversity of available exercise devices and the number of different equipment manufacturers of such equipment require a certain kind of expertise for those who identify and select equipment for use in heath/fitness facilities. Equipment that turns out to be improperly designed, substandard, or inherently defective is often the focus of relevant claims of negligence lodged against equipment manufacturers rather than those who simply secure and install equipment for use in their facilities. However, health/fitness facilities are often joined in lawsuits that arise out of alleged design or manufacturing defects. Such suits are commonly referred to as *product liability claims* and in the fitness field typically also include other relevant allegations to the effect that facilities did not properly instruct or supervise users in the operation of such equipment. For example, in the case of *Thomas v. Sport City, Inc.,*[16] also described in Chapter 8, a health club patron who was injured at the defendant's facility while using a hack squat machine filed suit against the health club and the device manufacturer. The appellate court ruled that neither the club nor the manufacturer were liable. In regard to the claim against the club dealing with improper instructions, the appellate court ruled:

Under the particular facts and circumstances of this case, we find that Sport City's failure to warn or instruct plaintiff in the proper use of the hack squat machine was not a cause of plaintiff's accident and injury. It was known or understood by plaintiff, a sophisticated user of the exercise machine, that the hook had to be completely over the peg to lock the carriage and prevent it from falling. Therefore, instruction or warning would have served no purpose. The trial court clearly erred in finding Sport City at fault.[17]

As described in Chapter 8, Thomas failed to engage the hook to secure the weights properly, which caused the weights to fall and crush his foot. This case is a good example in which the injury was the plaintiff's fault (i.e., Thomas's own carelessness caused his injury).

In the product liability claim against Capps Welding, manufacturer of the hack squat machine, Thomas claimed there was a design defect in the machine. To determine if there was a design defect, the appellate court required Thomas to prove there was an alternate design that would meet the purpose of the hack squat machine—a machine that would allow for a full squat—and be capable of preventing his injury. Expert witnesses testified that the design of the hack squat machine was similar in design to other manufacturers' hack squat machines. Therefore, Thomas was not able to establish an alternate design, and the court concluded that the Capps Welding hack squat machine did not have a design defect.

Similar claims have been set forth in a number of other cases and in a number of jurisdictions. Such lawsuits have also included allegations that equipment was improperly installed. In the case of *Homer v. Bally Total Fitness Corporation*,[18] a health club member was injured when she was using an arm curl machine. She alleged that the injury occurred because of the negligence of the defendant in its installation of the exercise machine. Although the plaintiff alleged that the defendant facility ignored its duty "to stabilize the arm curl machine," the court determined that her execution of a membership contract containing a waiver and release provision barred the action.

Although it is unclear if the club followed the manufacturer's instructions in the installation of the device in question, another case, *Craig v. Lake Shore Athletic Club, Inc.*,[19] involved a similar device. The untoward event in this case occurred as the device in question, a dip station, was being used as intended. The plaintiff alleged that the "defendant facility was negligent and grossly negligent because it did not bolt the device to the floor, using predrilled holes in accordance with the manufacturer's instructions."[20] He did not prevail on these claims however, because of his execution of a pre-participation waiver and release like the one signed in the *Homer* case.

Although standards of practice published by professional organizations (described later) vary with regard to equipment installation, manufacturers providing instructions mandating that equipment be bolted to the floor would seem to provide a rather clear standard for facilities to follow. Another similar case, *Ayre v. Santa Clarita Athletic Club*,[21] was reported in 2005. Like the preceding cases it also involved a piece of equipment that fell over because it was allegedly not fastened to the floor. The action, however, was barred because of an executed pre-participation release.

CASE LAW: EQUIPMENT INSPECTION, MAINTENANCE, AND REPAIR

Alleged failures to inspect, maintain, and repair exercise devices can also lead to claims and litigation. In the state of Washington case of *Marshall v. Bally's Pacwest, Inc.*,[22] a health club member was injured when she was allegedly thrown from a treadmill. She subsequently filed suit against the defendant club, the manufacturer of the device, and a treadmill repairer. The plaintiff alleged that she was exercising on the treadmill at the defendant health club's facility when the machine abruptly stopped. She claimed that when she then pressed the start button, the machine started at 6.2 mph rather that the usual 2.5 mph, causing her to be thrown from the machine and injured. She contended "that because of the sudden and unexpected start, she was violently thrown from the treadmill, causing severe injuries when her head struck the Plexiglas wall behind the machine."[23] However, she also testified in her pretrial deposition that "(1) she did not recall how abruptly the treadmill reached full speed; (2) she did not recall being 'thrown' from the treadmill; and (3) she did not recall hitting the glass behind the wall."[23] Because of the incident, she filed suit and alleged "(1) Bally's negligently failed to maintain safe premises; (2) Life Fitness negligently designed and manufactured the treadmill; and (3) Washington Athletic negligently failed to repair and maintain the treadmill."[24]

Some four years after the injury, the plaintiff's attorney requested an inspection of the treadmill in question. By that time, the treadmill had been sent back to the manufacturer for replacement. It had been installed by the Defendant Washington Athletic, which, according to the court's statement of facts, had "assembled the treadmill along with other identical treadmills at Bally's. After installing the machines, Washington Athletic ran the treadmills to ensure they were operating correctly. All treadmills operated properly."[24]

According to the reported case facts, before the machine was sent back to the manufacturer for replacement, "the treadmill was used continuously and routinely cleaned and maintained. On November 18, 1993, Washington Athletic installed new central processing units (CPUs) in all Life Stride 9500 model treadmills, including the subject treadmill. No request was made to retain or preserve the CPU removed from the machine. The treadmill was operational until its frame broke on April 22, 1997, nearly four years after Marshall's accident. At the request of Life Fitness, Bally's returned the machine to Life Fitness in Chicago for replacement."[24]

Based on the previous facts, the defendants moved for summary judgment, contending there was insufficient evidence of proximate cause, one of the elements necessary for a successful negligence action. The defendant health club also moved for judgment in its favor because of the plaintiff's execution of a waiver/release document in her membership contract. The trial court granted those motions and the plaintiff appealed. Although the appellate court concluded that issues related to proximate cause were not generally subject to summary adjudication, they contended that the plaintiff, "in short . . . provides no evidence that she was thrown from the machine . . . or how she was injured. Given this failure to produce evidence explaining how the accident occurred, proximate cause cannot be established. [footnote omitted] Because Marshall did not produce evidence of proximate cause, she failed to produce evidence sufficient to withstand summary judgment."[25] As a consequence of this reasoning, the appellate court affirmed the trial court's decision.

In a somewhat older case, *Alack v. Vic Tanny International of Missouri, Inc.*,[26] the plaintiff health club member was engaged in a specific cardiovascular workout routine known as a "Super Circuit." While engaged in this routine using ten different weight machines and then running a lap between each exercise, he was injured on an upright row machine. He "suffered injuries to his mouth and lips, including several loose and broken teeth" when "the machine's handle disengaged from the weight cable and smashed into . . . [his] mouth and jaw."[27] The injured club member ultimately brought suit after two surgeries and incurring $17,000 in medical expenses. He contended that the club negligently maintained the equipment that caused his injuries. Despite the plaintiff's execution of a membership agreement that contained an explicit waiver of liability, the trial court ruled the clause did not bar the suit. As a consequence, the trial court permitted the case to go to a jury for determination, which returned a $17,000 verdict. On final appeal to the Missouri Supreme Court that verdict was upheld.

In the case of *Calarco v. YMCA of Greater Metropolitan Chicago*,[28] the plaintiff brought suit against the defendant YMCA alleging negligence when she was injured while using a weight machine. The facts of that case were reported as follows:

> *Plaintiff alleged that she was injured when weights on a "Universal Centurion 1020 Variable" gym machine fell on her hand in the weight room at the Buehler YMCA, one of the facilities operated by the YMCA, and sought recovery for her injury. Plaintiff appeals from the granting of the YMCA's motion for summary judgment based on an exculpatory clause included on the YMCA's application for membership and signed by plaintiff. . . . Plaintiff's complaint alleged that plaintiff was injured when metal weights fell on her hand causing broken bones and injuring her permanently. She alleged that the YMCA was negligent in failing to adequately inspect and maintain the "Universal Centurion 1020 Variable" gym machine, in failing to repair the machine, and in failing to warn or notify plaintiff that the machine was in a state of disrepair and unsuitable for use. Plaintiff later added Universal Gym Equipment, Inc., manufacturer of the machine, as a defendant, alleging negligence in the design and construction of the weight machine.*[29]

The trial court granted the defendant YMCA's motion for summary judgment on the basis of the plaintiff's execution of a membership waiver. However, the appellate court reversed that ruling and held that the exculpatory clause "was not sufficiently clear, explicit and unequivocal to show an intent to protect [the] facility from liability arising from use of its equipment under [the] circumstances presented."[30] The plaintiff in this case, at least implicitly, alleged that the device in question, because of its "state of disrepair" was "unsuitable for use" and should have been removed from service.

In the case of *Peso v. American Leisure Facilities Management Corp.*,[31] the plaintiff, who was injured while using a treadmill at the defendant club, brought suit alleging that her injuries were the result of a fall because of the presence of a "sticky substance" on the belt of the treadmill. In another case based on a somewhat similar claim dealing with an alleged failure to keep equipment clean, *Hoffman v. New Life Fitness Centers, Inc.,*[32] a health club patron brought suit against the defendant facility claiming that she contracted the herpes simplex type II virus while using a tanning bed at the defendant's facility. She recovered a default judgment on the claim but because of a procedural issue, the default judgment in her favor was overturned on appeal. As a consequence, the litigation was returned to the trial court for determination.

CASE LAW: HOME, DONATED, AND USED EQUIPMENT

There are also clear drawbacks in using exercise equipment designed for home use in health/fitness facilities because equipment generally used in such facilities is typically more durable than that designed/manufactured for home use. As a consequence, equipment designed for home use should probably not be used in facilities where it would be potentially subject to much greater use by a multitude of individuals working out in such facilities. Applicable risks may therefore immensely increase. Moreover, used equipment should only be put into commercial use after it has been inspected, refurbished as necessary, and tested before further use. To demonstrate what can occur, consider the case of *Zacharias v. City of Bloomington*.[33] In the case, a spring-driven rower exercise machine was donated to a community recreation center operated by the defendant. The court described the machine as follows:

> *The rower consisted of two pedals with attached stirrups connected to a spring, which in turn was connected to a handle. To use the rower, a person placed her feet on the pedals beneath the stirrups and pulled up on the handle with her hands, causing the spring to extend. The rower could be used from a sitting, standing, or prone position.*[34]

When the machine was donated it came in a brown paper bag along with an instruction sheet. Because neither the city nor the community center wanted to keep the rower, it was offered to the center's senior exercise class. The plaintiff and another member of the class were in the exercise area when the device arrived. The center's coordinator asked the plaintiff if she wanted to try it. The plaintiff was not shown the instruction sheet or provided with any instruction. According to the court's description of what happened, the plaintiff at that point:

> *[T]ried the rower. She testified that she placed her feet on the pedals and under the stirrups and pushed her feet in as tightly as she could; she pulled the rower's handle up to her chest level and then a little higher; and as she went to pull the handle even higher, she heard a loud snap, and the rower struck her in the right eye. Zacharias did not know what caused the accident, and no one witnessed the accident. As a result of the accident, Zacharias lost the sight in her right eye.*
>
> *Zacharias testified that she understood how a spring works, specifically, that the more one pulls, the more tension is created. Zacharias also testified that she understood the importance of placing one's feet securely on the pedals because, otherwise, one's feet could slip off of the rower.*[34]

Suit was subsequently filed and summary judgment was granted to the defendant based on governmental immunity grounds.

A similar case, dealing with other equipment purchased at a garage sale, was determined in the Illinois case of *Catberro v. Naperville School District No. 203*.[35] The case was also decided on governmental immunity grounds. One commentator advised:

> *While the case previously dealt with state immunity law issues, professionals in sport, recreation and fitness should always insure that equipment used in activity is appropriate and safe for use. Equipment purchased in a used or second hand condition must be very carefully inspected prior to putting such*

equipment into service. Equipment which is not appropriate for use in a commercial setting, moreover, should not be used in such settings. Inattention to these details as well as others may well lead to needless injuries, claims and suits.[36]

CASE LAW: EQUIPMENT INSTRUCTION, SUPERVISION, AND WARNINGS

Failure to provide appropriate and proper instruction in the use of exercise equipment or in the supervision of that use has led to a number of litigations. An example of these cases should be of particular benefit to those seeking to learn about the applicable risks and then to develop a plan to reduce the related legal risks in this area of concern. Many of these cases deal with a number of intertwined issues impacting not only the topics of instruction and supervision in the use of equipment, but also equipment design and manufacturing concerns, equipment placement and maintenance issues, emergency response topics, waiver and release matters, and a whole host of other subjects.

Perhaps one of the most basic issues in this area can be best exemplified by an examination of the litigation in *Sicard v. University of Dayton.*[37] In this case, a student at the defendant university was injured when a school-employed spotter and two volunteer spotters allegedly failed to contain 365 pounds of weights the student was using during a bench press. The student, a scholarship basketball player, was required to engage in this weight training as part of his basketball training. The student's pectoral muscle was ruptured when the weights struck him during a repetition.

The student subsequently filed suit against the employee "who was hired by the University to assist in its weight lifting program for student athletes" and the University of Dayton. In his suit, the student claimed that the employee engaged in reckless and wanton misconduct by his acts/omission and that he and the university, his employer, were thus responsible for the injuries which the student athlete suffered.

In response to these allegations, the defendants moved for the entry of summary judgment in their favor, contending the evidence could not constitute reckless or wanton misconduct. The trial court granted this motion finding there was not genuine issue of material fact for jury determination. The student appealed, contending that the trial court erroneously granted judgment to the defendants because there were disputed materials facts at issue. In analyzing the activity engaged in by the student, the appellate court noted:

Weight lifting is not a contact sport; weight lifters compete against the limits of their own strength and skill, not against each other. They obtain the assistance of spotters to help them lift a substantial weight and to avoid an injury that failure to perform the lift successfully may entail. Spotters are considered participants in the lifting activity, according to . . . [the student athlete], who testified that "they should follow the lift so [sic] almost like reenacting it from where they are standing."[38]

In this regard, the court also noted,

Participation in the sport of weight lifting manifests a willingness to submit to injuries from stress and strain entailed in lifting very heavy objects. Participation in weight lifting does not manifest a willingness to submit to injury from falling weights. The rules of weight lifting allow for the assistance of spotters to avoid such injuries, not merely to secure the better performance of a lift as a test of the weight lifter's strength and skill. A spotter who intentionally fails to provide the assistance necessary to avoid injuries from falling weights may be found to have engaged in reckless act or omission if he knew or should know that the failure creates an unreasonable risk of physical harm to the weight lifter.[39]

The appellate court ruled there were issues of disputed fact and that a jury could conclude the defendant employee acted recklessly in his alleged failure to spot the athlete, thereby exposing the student to serious injury. Therefore, the court ruled that summary judgment had been improperly granted and reversed the trial court's ruling. The case was remanded to the lower court for full trial. Although the preceding case was against a university's strength and conditioning program as opposed to a typical health/fitness facility, it readily points out the potential supervision issues that can arise related to similar activities. Such issues can even arise when volunteers offer to assist equipment users (*Parks v. Gilligan*[40]). Not all such claims can be successfully prosecuted, however (see *Arnold Schaeffer v. Harborfield Central School District*[41]).

In a case that was also discussed in Chapters 4 and 5, *Mathis v. New York Health Club, Inc.*,[42] the plaintiff suffered injuries while being supervised by a personal fitness trainer as the client used a weight machine. Despite the client's expressed concerns, the trainer had him using up to 270 pounds on the machine. With the trainer's supervision he did various repetitions and was ultimately injured. He subsequently brought suit and contended that the trainer and the facility were negligent in the trainer's instruction and supervision of the client in his use of the equipment. The defendants moved for summary judgment, but the court denied their request even though the court noted the plaintiff was not a novice to the weight machine activity under examination. In response to the issue of whether or not the plaintiff assumed the risks of the activity, the court noted that the client "cannot be said to have assumed risks in excess of those usually encountered in the activity, particularly unreasonably increased risks attributable to lapses in judgment by a trainer."[43]

In another case, *Corrigan v. Musclemakers, Inc.*,[44] involving a health/fitness facility member's use of a treadmill, the member on her first visit to the facility met with a personal trainer who placed her on a treadmill. The machine was set at 3.5 miles per hour and the trainer allegedly without instruction to her about adjusting the speed, stopping the machine, or the operation of the controls, left her unattended. She ultimately was thrown from the machine and injured. Although the defendants attempted to assert, in a summary judgment motion filed in response to the member's suit, that the member assumed the risks of her participation, the court denied the motion and determined that the case should be decided by a jury.

At least one court has determined that "members of health clubs are owed a duty of reasonable care to protect them from injury while on the premises . . . [This duty] necessarily includes a general responsibility to ensure that their members know how to properly use gym equipment."[45] Although a number of other cases have also been filed dealing with instruction and supervision issues, this case, *Thomas v. Sport City, Inc.*,[45] because of its clarity and specific application to the health/fitness field, is of significant importance.

The lack of exercise equipment warnings or the provision of warnings that are alleged to be inadequate has also been the subject of claim and litigation. For example, in the case of *Parish v. Icon Health & Fitness, Inc.*,[46] a plaintiff brought a product liability action against a trampoline manufacturer after he was injured on the device and became a quadriplegic. The suit was predicated on defective design and negligent failure to warn. The defendant's motion for summary judgment was granted by the trial court. The Iowa Supreme Court affirmed this ruling on appeal. The negligent warning claim involved in the case—a type of claim that could also be asserted against health/fitness facilities in an appropriate case—was based on a claim that the "trampoline did not incorporate adequate warnings and that a genuine issue of fact was generated on that issue."[47] The plaintiff contended the motion should not have been determined on summary judgment.

The Iowa Supreme Court analyzed this claim and determined under the Restatement (Third) of Torts that a product could be defective in design due to "inadequate instructions or warnings." See Figure 9-2 for this Restatement's definitions of design defect and marketing defect. In this case, however, the court found that the trampoline and its attachments provided minimum warnings permanently placed on this device advising the user as follows:

WARNING

Do not land on head or neck.

Paralysis or death can result, even if you land in the middle of the trampoline mat (bed).

To reduce the chance of landing on your head or neck, do not do somersaults (flips).

Only one person at a time on trampoline.

Multiple jumpers increase the chances of loss of control, collision, and falling off.

This can result in broken head, neck, back, or leg.

This trampoline is not recommended for children under 6 years of age.[48]

Based on these warnings, the court concluded,

These warnings also include nationally recognized warning symbols cautioning against those activities. During manufacture . . . one warning [is placed] on each of the eight legs of the trampoline, and the design is such that the only way to assemble the trampoline is to have these warnings facing out so they are visible to the user. . . . two printed (nonpictorial) warnings . . . are sewn onto the trampoline bed itself. It also provides a warning placard for the owner to affix to the trampoline that contains both the pictorial warning and the language regarding safe use of the trampoline, and it provides an owner's manual that contains the warnings as found on the trampoline as well as additional warnings regarding supervision and education. It is undisputed that these warnings exceed the warnings required by the American Society for Testing and Material (ASTM).[48]

On its evaluation of the warnings issue, the court reviewed comments in the Restatement and noted,

The Restatement recognizes that users must pay some attention for their own safety:

Society does not benefit from products that are excessively safe—for example, automobiles designed with maximum speeds of 20 miles per hour—any more than it benefits from products that are too risky. Society benefits most when the right, or optimal, amount of product safety is achieved. From a fairness perspective, requiring individual users and consumers to bear appropriate responsibility for proper product use prevents careless users and consumers from being subsidized by more careful users and consumers, when the former are paid damages out of funds to which the latter are forced to contribute through higher product prices [emphasis in opinion].[48]

Based on all of the preceding, the court concluded,

In this case, it is undisputed that the three warnings affixed to the pad of the trampoline and the placards that came with both the trampoline and the fun ring warned against the specific conduct in which the plaintiff was engaged at the time of his injury, i.e., attempting somersaults or flips. We conclude that a reasonable fact finder could not conclude that the defendant's warnings were inadequate, and we affirm the district court's summary judgment on that claim.[49]

THE PUBLISHED STANDARDS OF PRACTICE

This section describes the standards of practice published by professional organizations related to exercise equipment. In addition, standards of practice published by independent agencies or companies such as the American Society of Testing and Materials (ASTM) and manufacturers of exercise equipment are presented.

The Published Standards of Practice: Professional Organizations

The ACSM's H/F Standards[50] contain a few guidelines regarding exercise equipment and Standard #21 as follows: "All cautionary, danger, and warning signage must have the required signal icon, signal word, signal color, and layout, as specified by the American National Standards Institute (ANSI) and reflected in the American Society of Testing and Materials (ASTM) standards for fitness equipment and fitness facility safety signage and labels."[51] (From American College of Sports Medicine, 2007, *ACSM's Health/Fitness Facility Standards and Guidelines,* 3rd ed., pp. 1–2. (©) 2007 by American College of Sports Medicine. Reprinted with permission from Human Kinetics, Champaign, IL.)

The ACSM Guidelines[52] provide some recommendations associated with the calibration of exercise testing equipment, and the ACSM/AHA Joint PP[53] recommends that the variety and quantity of exercise equipment should meet the needs of individuals and be well maintained.

The NSCA Standards[54] provide, in part, the following standards under Facility & Equipment Set-up, Inspection, Maintenance, Repair & Signage:

#4.1—Exercise devices, machine and equipment—including free weights—must be assembled, set up and placed in activity areas in full accordance with manufacturer's instructions, tolerances and recommendations; and with accompanying safety signage, instruction placards, notices and warnings posted or placed according to the ASTM standards . . . so as to be noticed by users prior to use.

#4.2—Prior to being put into service, exercise devices, machines or free weights must be thoroughly inspected and tested by Strength & Conditioning professionals to ensure that they are working and performing properly.

#4.3—Exercise machines, equipment and free weights must be inspected and maintained at intervals specified by manufacturers.

#4.4—Exercise devices, machines, equipment and free weights which are in need of repair, as determined by regular inspections or as reported by users, must be immediately removed from service and locked "out of use" until serviced and repaired; and be reinspected and tested to ensure that they are working and performing properly before being returned to service. If such devices are involved in incidents of injury, legal advisors or risk managers must be consulted for advice prior to service/repair or destruction.[55]

In addition, under Records & Record Keeping, Guideline #6.1 states that "Strength & Conditioning professionals should develop and maintain various records including: manufacturer provided user's manuals, warranties and operating guides; equipment selection, purchase, installation, set-up, inspection, maintenance and repair records."[56]

IHRSA Standard #12 states that "The club will be kept clean and the equipment will be maintained in working order." The interpretation provided states that "The club should ensure cleanliness in all areas through regularly scheduled cleanings with appropriate substances. Any equipment known to be malfunctioning should be repaired or replaced within a reasonable period of time. Signs should be posted on or near any equipment that, due to its malfunctioning, poses a risk of injury to club patrons."[57]

Under Fitness Environment, Canadian Standard #1 states, "All fitness related environments and equipment shall be clean, well maintained, and free from hazards" and Standard #4 states that "All fitness testing equipment shall be checked, cleaned and calibrated as required."[58]

The AFAA Standards[59] include a chapter entitled "Standards and Guidelines for Group Exercise Weighted Workouts." The chapter includes safety information related to the use of weights (e.g., handheld weights, ankle weights) in group exercise classes, such as precautions, when to use weights, when not to use weights, types of low weights, how much weight, when to increase weight, and exercise danger signs when using low weights and other general precautions.

The YMCA Recommendations[60] include information on passive exercise equipment and trampolines. The YMCA of the USA discourages the use of passive exercise equipment except for rehabilitation of certain medical conditions and strongly recommends that YMCAs should not use trampolines for recreational purposes. If trampolines are used, several precautions are recommended, such as checking liability insurance polices to ensure trampolines are covered, posting manufacturer warning labels and rule charts, and using them only under the supervision of qualified instructors.

The Published Standards of Practice: Independent Organizations

The American Society for Testing and Materials (ASTM) has published standards for fitness equipment and facilities. These standards, which are voluntary, can be accessed via the Internet at www.astm.org. Although many of these standards are directed at manufacturers of equipment, one ASTM standard—F1749[61]—addresses warning labels and fitness facility safety signage, and another ASTM standard—F2115[62]—includes, among many other specifications, spacing recommendations for treadmills. To quote one knowledgeable commentator, the ASTM Standard F 1749:

> [S]ets forth guidelines for the design and placement of warning labels and signage on fitness products and in fitness facilities. Following the ANSI Z 535 guidelines, the standard first instructs as to the proper hazard classification, signal word choice [DANGER, WARNING or CAUTION] and background color. With these basics established, the standard then defines how a hazard information or general warning label for fitness products is to be designed. If a company is in compliance with this standard then it will be affixing a general warning label on its products.
>
> The next portion of the standard addresses the design of labels to be affixed at specific hazard locations. These are called site specific labels. These labels often make use of pictorials to convey the hazard in the immediate location. As with the general warning label, specific colors and shapes need to be used and these are dependent on the severity of the hazard being addressed.
>
> The individual safety standards for fitness equipment [bikes, treadmills, weight machines, etc.] each have a warnings section that outlines the minimum information that needs to be present in the general warning label and specific references as to the locations on the products where site specific labels should be used.
>
> The remaining section of the warnings and signage standard introduces to the industry the Facility Safety Sign. The purpose of this sign is to reiterate and draw a person's attention to the potential hazards present in all fitness products. As the name implies, this sign is to be installed in a prominent location in the fitness facility where it will be encountered and read by the club's members. To be in compliance with ASTM F1749 a manufacturer must provide one of these signs with each equipment order and the facility operator must follow the posting instructions provided with the sign . . .
>
> If you attend any of the industry trade shows you will now observe that the products are, for the most part, in compliance with this standard. The manufacturers are using more warnings and the look and placement of these labels is becoming more uniform. This was the primary goal of this standard.[63]

See Figure 9-3 for the necessary specifications for a warning label as described in ASTM F1749 and page 1–3 in Appendix 9 for an example of an actual warning label provided for the Cybex Eagle Chest Press. Also, see Figure 9-4 for the Facility Safety Sign specifications as provided in ASTM F1749. This same ASTM Standard[61]

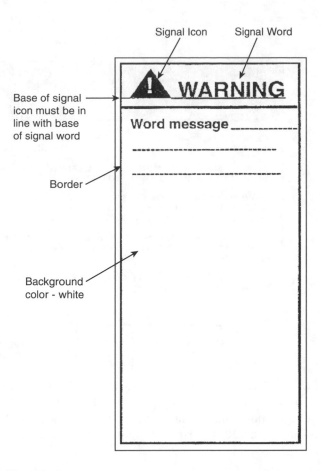

FIGURE 9-3 Vertical General Warning Label Layout (Reprinted, with permission, from ASTM F1749–96 Standard Specification for Fitness Equipment and Fitness Facility Safety Signage and Labels, copyright ASTM International, 100 Barr Harbor Drive, West Conshohocken, PA 19428.)

provides classifications (noted by signal words—danger, warning, and caution) for product safety signs and labels based on the relative seriousness of the potential hazards as follows:

4.1.1 Danger—Indicates an imminently hazardous situation which, if not avoided, will result in death or serious injury. This signal word is to be limited to the most extreme situations.

4.1.2 Warning—Indicates a potentially hazardous situation which, if not avoided, could result in death or serious injury.

4.1.3 Caution—Indicates a potentially hazardous situation which, if not avoided, may result in minor or moderate injury. It may also be used to alert to unsafe practices.[64] (Reprinted, with permission, from ASTM F1749–96 Standard Specification for Fitness Equipment and Fitness Facility Safety Signage and Labels, copyright ASTM International, 100 Barr Harbor Drive, West Conshohocken, PA 19428.)

In addition to a variety of specifications for motorized treadmills, ASTM Standard F2115[62] provides recommended minimum clearance dimensions that are "required around each treadmill for access to, passage around, and emergency dismount."[65] These are "0.5 m (19.7 in.) on each side of the treadmill and 1 m (39 in.) behind the treadmill."[65]

Manufacturers of exercise equipment also publish an owner's manual for each piece of exercise equipment. These manuals contain important information for health/fitness

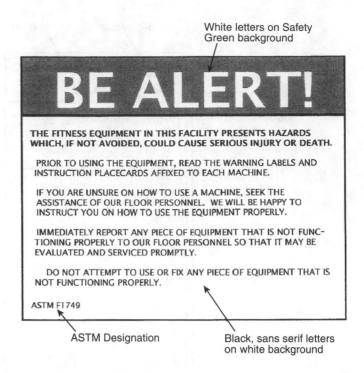

White letters on Safety Green background

BE ALERT!

THE FITNESS EQUIPMENT IN THIS FACILITY PRESENTS HAZARDS WHICH, IF NOT AVOIDED, COULD CAUSE SERIOUS INJURY OR DEATH.

PRIOR TO USING THE EQUIPMENT, READ THE WARNING LABELS AND INSTRUCTION PLACECARDS AFFIXED TO EACH MACHINE.

IF YOU ARE UNSURE ON HOW TO USE A MACHINE, SEEK THE ASSISTANCE OF OUR FLOOR PERSONNEL. WE WILL BE HAPPY TO INSTRUCT YOU ON HOW TO USE THE EQUIPMENT PROPERLY.

IMMEDIATELY REPORT ANY PIECE OF EQUIPMENT THAT IS NOT FUNC-TIONING PROPERLY TO OUR FLOOR PERSONNEL SO THAT IT MAY BE EVALUATED AND SERVICED PROMPTLY.

DO NOT ATTEMPT TO USE OR FIX ANY PIECE OF EQUIPMENT THAT IS NOT FUNCTIONING PROPERLY.

ASTM F1749

ASTM Designation

Black, sans serif letters on white background

FIGURE 9–4   Example of Facility Safety Sign to Be Posted in the Equipment Room (Reprinted, with permission, from ASTM F1749–96 Standard Specification for Fitness Equipment and Fitness Facility Safety Signage and Labels, copyright ASTM International, 100 Barr Harbor Drive, West Conshohocken, PA 19428.)

facilities (e.g., procedures for user safety precautions and preventive maintenance). See Appendix 9 for excerpts (Chapter 1 on Safety and Chapter 5 on Maintenance) from the Owner's Manual for the Cybex Eagle Chest Press. This owner's manual has incorporated the specifications of ASTM Standard F1749. See also Appendix 10 (p. 1–3) where Cybex (manufacturer of the 750T Treadmill) specifies 79 inches of clearance behind the treadmill, almost double the ASTM Standard F2115 specification.

STEP 2   DEVELOPMENT OF RISK MANAGEMENT STRATEGIES

As presented earlier in the case law examples, plaintiffs have made negligence claims against the health/fitness personnel and facilities that have involved a variety of exercise equipment issues. Professional and independent organizations also have published standards of practice that address procedures that health/fitness facilities can follow to help minimize exercise equipment injuries. To implement the law and the published standards of practice, health/fitness facilities can practice a variety of risk management strategies and techniques in their efforts to reduce the risks applicable to the assertion of claims and suits related to exercise equipment. These might be summarized as follows:

Risk Management Strategy 1: Use care in the selection of exercise equipment.

Professional judgment needs to be exercised in the selection of equipment. Commercial-grade equipment from reputable manufacturers is surely superior to equipment designed for home use or made by nonmainstream manufacturers. Reasonable care should be exercised in the selection of equipment for installation and use in health/fitness facilities. Used equipment needs to be carefully inspected and approved for use prior to installation by qualified individuals from a reputable exercise equipment maintenance company.

Risk Management Strategy 2: Assemble, install, inspect, and test exercise equipment properly before use.

Equipment needs to be assembled and installed in full accordance with manufacturer and industry standards. Such equipment should be bolted or otherwise secured to floor surfaces if designed to be installed in such a manner and/or where equipment is top heavy or unstable. Special attention should be given to spacing dimensions as indicated by the manufacturer and other industry standards. Equipment needs to be inspected and tested before it is released for use.

Risk Management Strategy 3: Post exercise equipment signage.

Manufacturer and/or industry instructional and warning signs need to be prominently posted for participants to see while they are preparing to use and using the equipment. For example, warning labels that meet the ASTM specification should be posted on each piece of exercise equipment. See Figure 9-3 and Appendix 9 (p. 1–3). Instructional placards (available from the manufacturer) should also be placed on or near each piece of equipment. In addition, the ASTM Facility Safety Sign (see Figure 9-4) needs to be prominently displayed in each exercise equipment area.

Risk Management Strategy 4: Provide appropriate instruction and supervision for exercise equipment use.

Participants need to be instructed properly in exercise equipment use, supervised in the use of the equipment, preferably during their initial use of the equipment, and reinstructed and supervised as often as necessary thereafter. For example, as discussed in Chapter 8, health/fitness facilities should provide a facility orientation for all participants prior to their use of exercise equipment and have qualified staff supervision of the exercise equipment area(s) during all operational hours.

Health/fitness professionals who provide individual instruction (e.g., personal fitness trainers) need to understand the importance of teaching their clients how to use the exercise equipment properly and then supervise them to be sure they are using the equipment correctly. In addition, personal trainers need to know how to apply principles of safe exercise (e.g., warm-up, progression, cooldown, monitoring signs/symptoms of overexertion, etc.) when training clients and how to design safe programs to meet client's individual needs. As mentioned in Chapter 8, personal fitness trainers not only should be qualified but also be competent. There are many case law examples described in this book where it appears from the facts that the personal fitness trainers were not competent.

Group exercise leaders that use exercise equipment in their classes (hand weights, resistance tubing, stability balls, etc.) should incorporate the proper and safe use of this type of equipment while teaching. For example, as mentioned in Chapter 8, Slastix technology by Sroops has manufactured a cover for resistance tubing that prevents it from snapping back. In addition, as stated earlier, The AFAA has published several standards and guidelines for group exercise weighted workouts that should be followed.

"Instruction" guidelines published in the owner's manuals of exercise equipment may be introduced in a court of law as admissible evidence in determining the standard of care. For example, in *Corrigan v. Musclemakers, Inc.*,[44] which was also described in Chapter 8, the plaintiff was not instructed by her personal trainer on how to use the treadmill. The court referred to a guideline in the owner's manual of the treadmill, which stated that knowledge on how to use the treadmill was necessary for safe use. Also, see Appendix 9 (p. 1–2) where it states, "Make sure that all users are properly trained on how to use the equipment."

Risk Management Strategy 5: Inspect and maintain exercise equipment and remove from use if in need of repair.

Equipment has to be inspected and maintained in full accordance with manufacturer/industry requirements and schedules. Although health/fitness facilities may contract with service providers who periodically conduct inspections and maintenance on the exercise equipment, designated, qualified health/fitness staff members should also be involved in the regular maintenance of the exercise equipment. For example, see Appendix 9 for "daily" and "weekly" procedures that should be implemented for one piece of equipment, the Cybex Eagle Chest Press.

Regarding service providers, they must be qualified or "authorized" to provide inspection and maintenance services. Cybex International offers a three-day training program designed for service providers. At the end of the training a certification exam is given, and those who pass the exam become "authorized service providers." Cybex International also encourages health/fitness staff members who have responsibility for their facility's exercise equipment to attend these trainings so they learn how to troubleshoot when a potential problem occurs with their own facility's exercise equipment. These staff members receive a "certificate of completion" for attending the training program (Personal Communication, Doug Ackerman, Cybex International, December 10, 2007).

Equipment in need of repair must be removed from service until it is fixed. As one of the NSCA Standards states, "Exercise devices, machines, equipment and free weights which are in need of repair, as determined by regular inspections or as reported by users, must be immediately removed from service and locked 'out of use' until serviced and repaired; and be re-inspected and tested to ensure that they are working and performing properly before being returned to service. If such devices are involved in incidents of injury, legal advisors or risk managers must be consulted for advice prior to service/repair or destruction."[55]

Risk Management Strategy 6: Keep exercise equipment clean and disinfected.

Equipment needs to be kept clean by facility personnel and members and disinfected in accordance with manufacturer/industry requirements. As an example, see Appendix 9 for specific cleaning procedures for the Cybex Eagle Chest Press.

Risk Management Strategy 7: Comply with exercise equipment recall/repair/warranty notices.

Equipment subject to manufacturer or other forms of repair notices, warnings, or recalls needs to be handled in accordance with these recalls.

Risk Management Strategy 8: Maintain exercise equipment records.

Appropriate equipment records as to selection, installation, maintenance, repair, and usage should be maintained for a period of time commensurate with the applicable life of the machine in question, as well as the period defined by state and/or federal law as to when a claim or suit might be instituted against a facility and its personnel related to that equipment under the statute of limitations.

For example, NSCA Guideline #6.1, under Records & Record Keeping, states that "Strength & Conditioning professionals should develop and maintain various records including: manufacturer provided user's manuals, warranties and operating guides; equipment selection, purchase, installation, set-up, inspection, maintenance and repair records."[56] Maintaining these records may serve as a good defense for health/fitness facilities because it can help demonstrate that the proper standard of care (duty) was carried out.

✓ PUT INTO PRACTICE CHECKLIST 9-1

Rate your phase of development for each of the following risk management strategies related to exercise equipment:

	Developed	Partially Developed	Not Developed
1. Using care in the selection of exercise equipment.			
2. Assembling, installing, inspecting, and testing exercise equipment properly prior to use.			
3. Posting exercise equipment signage.			
4. Providing appropriate instruction and supervision for exercise equipment use.			
5. Inspecting and maintaining exercise equipment and removing from use if in need of repair.			
6. Keeping exercise equipment clean and disinfected.			
7. Complying with exercise equipment recall/repair/warranty notices.			
8. Maintaining exercise equipment records.			

SUMMARY

Diverse exercise equipment is widely used in essentially all health/fitness facilities. Exercise equipment must be identified and purchased for use in such facilities with an understanding that it needs to be assembled, installed, maintained, and repaired in accordance with manufacturer requirements and recommendations, as well as industry standards and guidelines. Such equipment needs to be serviced, cleaned, and maintained regularly. Records about the equipment should be maintained in accordance with an overall risk management plan. Facility users should be introduced properly to such equipment, instructed in the use of that equipment, and supervised in their activities with that equipment.

Risks and concerns associated with exercise equipment might be summarized as follows:

- Equipment should be selected, purchased, assembled, installed, and maintained in accordance with manufacturer/industry recommendations and standards.
- Equipment designed for home use should probably not be used in commercial settings.
- Written records regarding equipment use/assembly and maintenance need to be maintained and preserved.
- Replacement parts put on exercise machines should be provided from the manufacturer or be commensurate with the original parts.
- Equipment associated with an injury should be immediately removed for service and inspected. Pictures should be taken and equipment and parts that are removed or replaced should be preserved for later examination and testing if necessary (and to avoid potential compromise of evidence claims).
- Incident reports should be completed—providing information as to *what* happened, *when* it happened, *where* it happened, *why* it happened, and *who* was involved and witnessed the event. No attribution of fault should be directed at the facility or to facility personnel when these reports are completed. The reports should be directed to the facility's legal counsel and marked "privileged."[66]

RISK MANAGEMENT ASSIGNMENTS

1. Develop a list of the equipment most frequently made available and used in health/fitness facilities. Indicate how each piece of equipment is typically used in such facilities.

   _____

   _____

   _____

   _____

2. Design a draft installation diagram for the placement of the equipment identified in assignment 1 in a typical health/fitness facility. Using published standards of practice, consider how that equipment should be installed and how each piece should be placed in reference to other equipment, walkways, walls, facility boundaries, access points, and so on.

   _____

   _____

   _____

   _____

3. Consider what facility signage should be used for various items of equipment and how and in what manner that signage should be placed in a facility.

   _____

   _____

   _____

   _____

4. For one piece of equipment usually found in a facility and identified in assignment 1, develop an outline including appropriate instruction for the proper use of that piece of equipment as well as possible warnings applicable to that piece of equipment.

   _____

   _____

   _____

   _____

5. Using the specifications from the owner's manual, propose an equipment maintenance record form and determine how a facility should maintain those records.

   _____

   _____

   _____

   _____

KEY TERMS

Design defect   Marketing defect   Product liability
Manufacturing defect

REFERENCES

1. *Dillon v. Keatington Racquetball Club,* 151 Mich. App. 138 (Mich. App., 1986).
2. Herbert DL. Provide services or just facilities? The legal concerns are different. *Fitness Manage.* 1988:45:45.
3. Keeton WP, Dobbs DB, Keeton RE, Owen DO. *Prosser and Keeton on Torts.* 5th ed. St. Paul, Minn: West; 1984.
4. *Restatement of the Law (Third) of Torts: Products Liability.* Tentative Draft No. 1. § 2. Categories of product defects. Philadelphia: American Law Institute; April 12, 1994: 9–10.
5. *Pappalardo v. New York Health & Racquet Club.* Analyzed in: Herbert DL. Alleged overcrowding of health club facility—Correlation to injury? *Exercise Standards and Malpractice Reporter.* 2001;15(3):38.
6. *Mannone v. Holiday Health Clubs and Fitness Centers.* Analyzed in: New exercise related case claims that alleged overcrowding and lack of instruction/supervision lead to his injuries. *Exercise Science and Malpractice Reporter.* 1993;7(1):15.
7. Tharrett SJ, Peterson JA, eds. *ACSM's Health/Fitness Facility Standards and Guidelines.* 2nd ed. Champaign, Ill: Human Kinetics; 1997.
8. Tharrett SJ, McInnis KJ., Peterson JA, eds. *ACSM's Health/Fitness Facility Standards and Guidelines.* 3rd ed. Champaign, Ill: Human Kinetics; 2007.
9. *Darling v. Fairfield Medical Center,* 142 Ohio App.3d 682 (Ohio Ct. App., 2001).
10. *Darling v. Fairfield Medical Center,* 142 Ohio App.3d 682 (Ohio Ct. App., 2001):687.
11. Herbert DL. Treadmill lawsuit to proceed to trial: The case of *Darling v. Fairfield Medical Center. Exercise Standards and Malpractice Reporter.* 2001;15(6):94–95, 94–95.
12. *Xu v. Gay,* 257 Mich.App. 263 (Mich. App., 2003).
13. *Xu v. Gay,* 257 Mich.App. 263 (Mich. App., 2003):265.
14. *Xu v. Gay,* 257 Mich.App. 263 (Mich. App., 2003):266.
15. *Xu v. Gay,* 257 Mich.App. 263 (Mich. App., 2003):270–271.
16. *Thomas v. Sport City, Inc.,* 738 S0.2d 1153 (La 2 Cir., 1999).
17. *Thomas v. Sport City, Inc.,* 738 S0.2d 1153 (La 2 Cir., 1999):1158.
18. *Homer v. Bally Total Fitness Corporation,* 2001 WL 1528517 (Cal. App. 2 Dist., 2001).
19. *Craig v. Lake Shore Athletic Club, Inc.,* 1997 WL 305228 (Wash. App. Div., 1997).
20. Herbert DL. Must exercise devices be bolted to the floor? *Exercise Standards and Malpractice Reporter.* 2002;16(2):17,20–21, 21.
21. *Ayre v. Santa Clarita Athletic Club,* 2005 WL 1683596 (Los Angeles County Superior Court, 2005).
22. *Marshall v. Bally's Pacwest, Inc.,* 94 Wash. App. 372 (Wash. Ct. App., 1999).
23. *Marshall v. Bally's Pacwest, Inc.,* 94 Wash. App. 372 (Wash. Ct. App., 1999):375.
24. *Marshall v. Bally's Pacwest, Inc.,* 94 Wash. App. 372 (Wash. Ct. App., 1999):376.
25. *Marshall v. Bally's Pacwest, Inc.,* 94 Wash. App. 372 (Wash. Ct. App., 1999):380.
26. *Alack v. Vic Tanny International of Missouri, Inc.,* 923 S.W.2d 330 (Mo., 1996).
27. *Alack v. Vic Tanny International of Missouri, Inc.,* 923 S.W.2d 330 (Mo., 1996):332.
28. *Calarco v. YMCA of Greater Metropolitan Chicago,* 149 Ill. App.3d 1037 (Ill. App. Ct., 1986).
29. *Calarco v. YMCA of Greater Metropolitan Chicago,* 149 Ill. App.3d 1037 (Ill. App. Ct., 1986):1038–1039.
30. *Calarco v. YMCA of Greater Metropolitan Chicago,* 149 Ill. App.3d 1037 (Ill. App. Ct., 1986):1044.
31. *Peso v. American Leisure Facilities Management Corp.,* 277 A.D.2d 48 (N.Y.A.D., 2000).
32. *Hoffman v. New Life Fitness Centers, Inc.,* 116 Ohio App.3d 737 (Ohio Ct. App., 1996).
33. *Zacharias v. City of Bloomington,* 1998 WL 846506 (Minn. Ct. App., 1998).
34. *Zacharias v. City of Bloomington,* 1998 WL 846506 (Minn. Ct. App., 1998):1.
35. *Catberro v. Naperville School District No. 203,* 739 N.E.2d 115 (Ill. App. Ct., 2000).
36. Herbert DL. Equipment allegedly purchased at garage sale results in injury and suit. *Exercise Standards and Malpractice Reporter.* 2001;15(1):13, 13.
37. *Sicard v. University of Dayton,* 104 Ohio App.3d 27 (Ohio Ct. App., 1995).
38. *Sicard v. University of Dayton,* 104 Ohio App.3d 27 (Ohio Ct. App., 1995):31–32.
39. *Sicard v. University of Dayton,* 104 Ohio App.3d 27 (Ohio Ct. App., 1995):32.

40. *Parks v. Gilligan*. Analyzed in: Volunteer spotter may be liable for weight lifter's injury. *Exercise Standards and Malpractice Reporter*. 1998;12(2):24.

41. *Arnold Schaeffer v. Harborfield Central School District*. Analyzed in: Fried DH. Student injured while participating in weight training program—Defense verdict. *Exercise Standards and Malpractice Reporter*. 1999;13(1):9.

42. *Mathis v. New York Health Club, Inc.*, 690 N.Y.S. 2d 433 (N.Y. App. Div., 1999).

43. *Mathis v. New York Health Club, Inc.*, 690 N.Y.S. 2d 433 (N.Y. App. Div., 1999) (affirmed on appeal, 732 N.Y.S.2d 341):346.

44. *Corrigan v. Musclemakers, Inc.*, 686 N.Y.S. 2d 143 (N.Y. App. Div., 1999).

45. *Thomas v. Sport City, Inc.*, 738 S0.2d 1153 (La 2 Cir., 1999):1157.

46. *Parish v. Icon Health & Fitness, Inc.*, 719 N.W. 2d 540 (Iowa, 2006).

47. *Parish v. Icon Health & Fitness, Inc.*, 719 N.W. 2d 540 (Iowa, 2006):545.

48. *Parish v. Icon Health & Fitness, Inc.*, 719 N.W. 2d 540 (Iowa, 2006):546.

49. *Parish v. Icon Health & Fitness, Inc.*, 719 N.W. 2d 540 (Iowa, 2006):546–547.

50. Tharrett SJ, McInnis KJ, Peterson JA, eds. *ACSM's Health/Fitness Facility Standards and Guidelines*. 3rd ed. Champaign, Ill: Human Kinetics; 2007.

51. Tharrett SJ, McInnis KJ, Peterson JA, eds. *ACSM's Health/Fitness Facility Standards and Guidelines*. 3rd ed. Champaign, Ill: Human Kinetics; 2007:2.

52. Whaley MH, ed. *ACSM's Guidelines for Exercise Testing and Prescription*. 7th ed. Philadelphia: Lippincott Williams & Wilkins; 2006.

53. American College of Sports Medicine and American Heart Association Joint Position Statement. Recommendations for cardiovascular screening, staffing, and emergency policies at health/fitness facilities. *Med Sci Sports Exerc*. 1998;30:1009–1018.

54. *NSCA Strength & Conditioning Professional Standards & Guidelines*. May 2001. Available at: http://www.nscalift.org/Publications/standards.shtml. Colorado Springs: National Strength and Conditioning Association (NSCA). Accessed September 2, 2007.

55. *NSCA Strength & Conditioning Professional Standards & Guidelines*. May 2001. Available at: http://www.nscalift.org/Publications/standards.shtml. Colorado Springs: National Strength and Conditioning Association (NSCA). Accessed September 2, 2007:14.

56. *NSCA Strength & Conditioning Professional Standards & Guidelines*. May 2001. Available at: http://www.nscalift.org/Publications/standards.shtml. Colorado Springs: National Strength and Conditioning Association (NSCA). Accessed September 2, 2007:15.

57. IHRSA Club Membership Standards. In: *IHRSA's Guide to Club Membership & Conduct*. 3rd ed. Boston: International Health, Racquet & Sportsclub Association (IHRSA); 2005:5.

58. *Canadian Fitness Safety Standards & Recommended Guidelines*. 3rd ed. 2004. Available at: http://www.oases.on.ca/safety/safetyStdsCurrent.htm. Ontario, Canada: Ontario Association of Sport and Exercise Sciences (OASES). Accessed September 2, 2007:2.

59. *Exercise Standards & Guidelines Reference Manual*. 4th ed. Sherman Oaks, Calif: Aerobics and Fitness Association of America (AFAA); 2005.

60. *Medical Advisory Committee Recommendations: A Resource Guide for YMCAs*. Chicago: YMCA of the USA; 2007.

61. American Society for Testing and Materials. *Standard Specification for Fitness Equipment and Fitness Safety Signage and Labels. F 1749*. West Conshohocken, Pa: American Society for Testing and Materials (ASTM) International; 1996.

62. American Society for Testing and Materials. *Standard Specification for Motorized Treadmills. F 2115*. West Conshohocken, Pa: American Society for Testing and Materials (ASTM) International; 2001.

63. Voris HC. Fitness equipment safety standards: Part II—Warning labels and signage. *Exercise Standards and Malpractice Reporter*. 2001;15(4):49, 52–53, 52–53.

64. American Society for Testing and Materials. *Standard Specification for Fitness Equipment and Fitness Safety Signage and Labels. F 1749*. West Conshohocken, Pa: American Society for Testing and Materials (ASTM) International; 1996:2.

65. American Society for Testing and Materials. *Standard Specification for Motorized Treadmills. F 2115*. West Conshohocken, Pa: American Society for Testing and Materials (ASTM) International; 2001:5.

66. Case against hotel for exercise machine related injury to proceed to trial. *Exercise Standards and Malpractice Reporter*. 2000;14(1):8–9, 9.

APPENDIX 9

The following information has been reprinted from the Owner's Manual of the Cybex Eagle Chest Press:

1. Chapter 1 – Safety (Pages 1-1 – 1-4)
2. Chapter 5 – Maintenance (Pages 5-1 – 5-8)

Cybex Eagle Chest Press Owner's Manual

1 - Safety

(Safety)

Read the Owner's Manual carefully before assembling, servicing or using the equipment.

It is the responsibility of the facility owner and/or owner of the equipment to instruct users on proper operation of the equipment and review all labels.

! WARNING: Serious injury could occur if these safety precautions are not observed:

USER SAFETY PRECAUTIONS

- Obtain a medical exam prior to beginning an exercise program.

- Read and understand warning labels and user manual prior to exercising. Obtain instruction prior to use.

- Keep body and clothing free from and clear of all moving parts.

- Inspect machine prior to use. **DO NOT** use if it appears damaged or inoperable.

- **DO NOT** attempt to fix a broken or jammed machine. Notify floor staff.

- Use the machine only for the intended use. **DO NOT** modify the machine.

- Be sure that the weight pin is completely inserted. Use only the pin provided by the manufacturer. If unsure seek assistance.

- Never pin the weights in an elevated position. **DO NOT** use the machine if found in this condition. See assistance from floor staff.

- Children must not be allowed near these machines. Teenagers must be supervised.

- **DO NOT** use if guards are missing or damaged.

- **DO NOT** use dumbbells or other incremental weights, except those provided by the manufacturer.

- Inspect all cables and belts and connections prior to use. **DO NOT** use if any components are worn, frayed or damaged.

- **DO NOT** remove any labeling from equipment. Replace any damaged labels.

- Stop exercising if you feel faint, dizzy or experience pain at any time while exercising and consult your physician.

Cybex Eagle Chest Press Owner's Manual

Facility Safety Precautions

- Read the Owner's Manual carefully before assembling, servicing or using the equipment.

- Securely anchor each machine to the floor using the anchor holes provided in each machine.

> **NOTE:** *Cybex is not responsible for the actual anchoring of equipment. Consult with a professional contractor.*
>
> **NOTE:** *Use fasteners having a minimum of 500 lbs. tensile capacity (3/8" grade 2 bolts or better).*
>
> **NOTE:** *If legs/frame does not contact surface, DO NOT pull down with anchors. Shim any leg or frame not in contact with surface using flat washers.*

- Make sure that each machine is set up and operated on a solid level surface. **Do not install equipment on an uneven surface.**

- Make sure that all users are properly trained on how to use the equipment.

- Make sure there is enough room for safe access and operation of the equipment.

- Perform regular maintenance checks on the equipment. Also pay close attention to all areas most susceptible to wear, including (but not limited to) cables, pulleys, belts and grips.

- Immediately replace worn or damaged components. If unable to immediately replace worn or damaged components then remove from service until the repair is made.

- Use only Cybex supplied components to maintain/repair the equipment.

- Keep a repair log of all maintenance activities.

- Inspect all cables and belts and connections prior to use. **DO NOT** use if any components are worn, frayed or damaged.

NOTE: *It is the sole responsibility of the user/owner or facility operator to ensure that regular maintenance is performed.*

Warning/Caution Decals

Warning decals indicate a potentially hazardous situation, which, if not avoided, could result in death or serious injury.

Caution decals indicate a potentially hazardous situation, which, if not avoided, could result in minor or moderate injury.

The warning and caution decals are shown on the following page. The diagrams following the decals show where each decal is located.

Cybex Eagle Chest Press Owner's Manual

⚠ WARNING

A

SERIOUS INJURY COULD OCCUR IF THESE PRECAUTIONS ARE NOT OBSERVED

1. Obtain a medical exam prior to beginning an exercise program.

2. Read and understand warning labels and user manual prior to exercising. Obtain instruction prior to use.

3. Keep body and clothing free from and clear of all moving parts.

4. Inspect machine prior to use. DO NOT use if it appears damaged or inoperable.

5. DO NOT attempt to fix a broken or jammed machine. Notify floor staff.

6. Use the machine only for the intended use. DO NOT modify the machine.

7. Be sure that the weight pin is completely inserted. Use only the pin provided by the manufacturer. If unsure seek assistance.

8. Never pin the weights in an elevated position. DO NOT use the machine if found in this condition. Seek assistance from floor staff.

9. Children must not be allowed near this machine. Teenagers must be supervised.

10. DO NOT use if guards are missing or damaged.

11. DO NOT use dumbbells or other incremental weights, except those provided by the manufacturer.

12. Inspect all cables and belts and connections prior to use. DO NOT use if any components are worn, frayed, or damaged.

13. DO NOT REMOVE THIS LABEL. REPLACE IF DAMAGED.

4605-381-4 A

B

⚠ CAUTION

Personal injury may occur.

Keep away from moving parts to avoid injury.

4000Y316-4

C

⚠ CAUTION

Seat may fall if improperly engaged.

Verify seat is secure before exercising to avoid injury.

4520-362-4

Safety
Page 1-3

Cybex Eagle Chest Press Owner's Manual

Chest Press - 11000

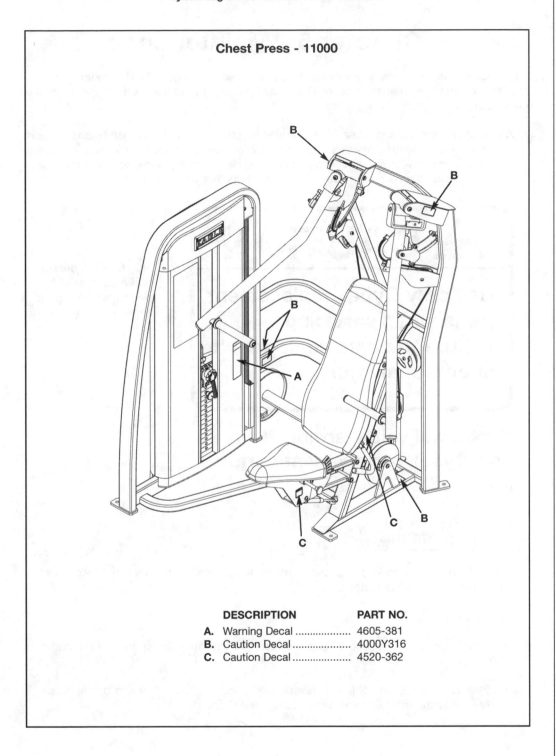

DESCRIPTION	PART NO.
A. Warning Decal	4605-381
B. Caution Decal	4000Y316
C. Caution Decal	4520-362

Cybex Eagle Chest Press Owner's Manual

Chapter 5 - Maintenance

All preventive maintenance activities must be performed on a regular basis. Performing routine preventive maintenance actions can aid in providing safe, trouble-free operation of all Cybex Strength Systems equipment.

NOTE: Cybex is not responsible for performing regular inspection and maintenance actions for your machines. Instruct all personnel in equipment inspection and maintenance actions and also in accident reporting/recording. Cybex phone representatives are available to answer any questions or concerns that you may have.

⚠ CAUTION

Use only Cybex replacement parts when servicing. Failure to do so could result in personal injury.

NOTE: All inspections and repairs must be performed by trained service personnel only.

Cybex will void warranty if non-Cybex replacement parts are used.

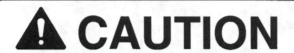

Daily Procedures

1. **Upholstery -** Wipe down all upholstery as per the recommendations listed below for light soiling and more difficult stains.

   Light Soiling

   • A solution of 10% household liquid dish soap with warm water applied with a soft damp cloth.

   • If necessary, a solution of liquid cleanser and water applied with a soft bristle brush. Wipe away the residue with a water dampened cloth.

Cybex Eagle Owner's Manual

More Difficult Stains

• Dampen a soft white cloth with a solution of 10% household bleach (sodium hypochlorite), 90% water. Rub gently. Rinse with a water dampened cloth to remove bleach concentration.

• The same procedure can be used with full strength household bleach, if necessary.

• Allow bleach to puddle on the affected area or apply with a soaked cloth for approximately 30 minutes. Rinse with a water dampened cloth to remove any remaining bleach concentration.

Alternative Method for Difficult Stains

• Dampen a soft white cloth with rubbing alcohol and rub gently. Rinse with a water

dampened cloth to remove any remaining rubbing alcohol concentration.

NOTE: *To restore luster, a light coat of spray furniture wax can be used. Apply for 30 seconds and follow with a light buffing using a clean white cloth.*

Please Review Carefully

When using strong cleaning agents such as rubbing alcohol or bleach, it is advisable to first test in an inconspicuous area. Other cleaning agents may contain harsh or unknown solvents and are subject to formula changes by the product manufacturer without notice. Should you desire to use other cleaning agents, carefully try them in an inconspicuous area to determine potential damage to the material. Never use harsh solvents or cleaners which are intended for industrial applications. To clean stained or soiled areas, a soft white cloth is recommended. Avoid use of paper towels.

Cleaning products may be harmful/irritating to your skin, eyes, etc. Use protective gloves and eye protection. Do not inhale or swallow any cleaning product. Protect surrounding area/clothing from exposure. Use in a well ventilated area. Follow all product manufacturer's warnings. CYBEX and its vendors cannot be held responsible for damage or injuries resulting from the use or misuse of cleaning products.

2. **Frames -** Wipe down all frames using a mild solution of warm water and car wash soap. Be sure to dry thoroughly. ***AVOID*** acid or chlorine based cleaners and also cleaners containing abrasives as these could scratch or damage the equipment.

3. **Chrome -** Clean chrome tubes, first using chrome polish and then using a car wax seal. Neutral cleaners with a pH between 5.5 and 8.5 are recommended. Be sure to dry thoroughly. ***AVOID*** acid or chlorine based cleaners and also cleaners containing abrasives as these could scratch or damage the equipment.

Cybex Eagle Chest Press Owner's Manual

4. Guidelines for cleaning front panel:

- Use clean soft cloths or sponges for application of cleaners and again for washing and rinsing.

- Follow up the application with warm water rinse.

- Don't use abrasives or high alkaline cleaners.

- Don't leave cleaners on for long periods, wash immediately.

- Don't apply cleaners in direct sunlight or at elevated temperatures.

- Don't use scrapers, squeegees or razors.

- Don't clean with gasoline.

Compatible Cleaners and Detergents:

- Formula 409

- Top Job

- Joy

- Palmolive

- Windex with Ammonia D

To Minimize Fine or Hairline Scratches:

Mild automotive polish applied and removed with a soft, clean cloth will help fill scratches.

Suggested Polishes:

- Johnson Paste Wax

- Mirror Glaze #10 Plastic Polish (by Mirror Bright Polish Co.)

- Novus Plastics Polish #1, #2 (by Novus Inc.)

Cybex Eagle Chest Press Owner's Manual

Weekly Procedures

1. Check all nuts and bolts for looseness. Tighten as required.

2. Inspect all belts (entire length) for any ***non-uniformity and wear.***

Immediately replace belt if any of the following conditions are present:

	3D View	3D or Side View
• **Peeling of the belt's skin.**		
• **Wave in the belt.**		
• **Belt is necked down (narrow section).**	Replace belt if any section is over 1/32" (.03") narrower than rest of the belt.	Examine edge of belt (both sides). Replace belt if any section is narrower than the rest.
• **Cracks or splits.**		
• **One or more strands of kevlar hanging out.** *NOTE: Also replace belt if there is a significant amount of frayed kevlar.*		

Cybex Eagle Chest Press Owner's Manual

3. Some machines use cables in addition to belts. Inspect all cables for wear or damage and proper tension. When inspecting cables, run your fingers on the cable, paying particular attention to bends in the cable and attachment points.

Replace all worn cables immediately. The following conditions may indicate a worn cable:

- A tear or crack in the cable sheath that exposes the cable. See Figure 1

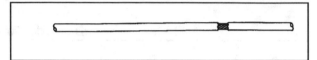

Figure 1

- A kink in the cable. See Figure 2.

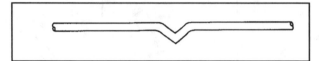

Figure 2

- A curled sheath. See Figure 3.

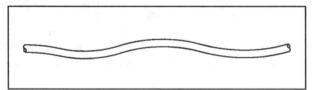

Figure 3

- "Necking", a stretched cable sheath. See Figure 4.

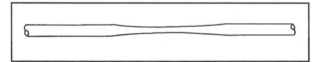

Figure 4

Cybex Eagle Owner's Manual

4. Inspect bars and handles for wear, paying particular attention to tab area connecting points.

   Replace all worn handles immediately.

5. Inspect snap links for proper latching (indicates wear).

   Replace all worn snap links immediately.

6. Inspect for loose or worn grips.

   Replace all loose or worn grips immediately.

7. Inspect all labeling for readability. This includes instructional placards, warning and caution decals.

   Replace all worn labeling immediately.

8. Inspect all weight stacks for proper alignment and operation.

   Correct all improper alignment and operation issues immediately.

9. Wipe *Weight Stack Guide Rods* clean over entire length. Lubricate with a light coat of medium weight automotive engine oil.

Yearly Procedures

1. Replace all belts and cables at least annually.

Cybex Eagle Chest Press Owner's Manual

Environment

Static Electricity - Depending upon where you live, you may experience dry air, causing a common experience of static electricity. This may be especially true in the winter time. You may notice a static build-up just by walking across a carpet and then touching a metal object. The same can hold true while working out on your unit. You may experience a shock due to the build-up of static electricity on your body and the discharge path of the unit. If you experience this type of situation, you may want to increase the humidity to a comfortable level through the use of a humidifier.

Humidity - The unit is designed to function normally in an environment with a relative humidity range of 30% to 75%.

NOTE: *Do not install or use the unit in an area of high humidity, such as in the vicinity of a steam room, sauna, indoor pool or outdoors. Exposure to extensive water vapor, chlorine and/or bromine could adversely affect the electronics as well as other parts of the machine.*

Temperature - The unit is designed to function normally in an environment with an ambient temperature range of 50°F (10°C) to 104°F (40°C) degrees.

Storage

Humidity - The unit can be shipped and stored in an environment with a relative humidity range of 10% to 90%.

NOTE: *Do not store the unit in an area of high humidity, such as in the vicinity of a steam room, sauna, indoor pool or outdoors. Exposure to extensive water vapor, chlorine and/or bromine could adversely affect the electronics as well as other parts of the machine.*

Temperature - The unit can be shipped and stored in an environment with an ambient temperature range of 32°F (0°C) and 140°F (60°C) degrees.

Cybex Eagle Chest Press Owner's Manual

CHAPTER 10

Facility Risks

LEARNING OBJECTIVES After reading this chapter, health/fitness students and professionals will be able to:

1. Identify the relevant risks associated with the physical plant of health/fitness facilities and those other areas where activities are conducted, as well as those areas "off premises" where some activities are carried out.

2. Understand the applicable duties owed to participants of health/fitness facilities based on their status as business invitees.

3. Appreciate the need to comply with applicable laws such as the ADA so as to accommodate those with special needs under the law.

4. Learn the applicable published standards of practice associated with the development and maintenance of physical plant facilities for health/fitness activities.

5. Develop risk management strategies to eliminate or reduce some of the applicable risks that arise in health/fitness facilities.

This chapter outlines the law, describes various standards of practice published by professional organizations, and offers risk management strategies to reduce health/fitness facility risks. This chapter focuses on facility risks that are common to most health/fitness facilities but does not include all facility risks. For example, risks related to swimming pools are not included. However, health/fitness facilities that have swimming pools need to comply with any states laws that may be applicable and should also adhere to safety standards and guidelines published by organizations including but not limited to the American Red Cross, YMCA, National Swimming Pool Foundation, National Spa & Pool Institute, U.S. Water Fitness Association, Aquatic Exercise Association, Canadian Lifesaving Society, National Safety Council, and pool manufacturers.

In the area of facility risks, health/fitness students and professionals are encouraged to refer to one of the most authoritative and comprehensive books in the field: *Facility Design and Management for Health, Fitness, Physical Activity, Recreation and Sports Facility Development.*[1] It was developed by the Council on Facilities and Equipment

(CFE) of the American Association for Active Lifestyles and Fitness—an Association of the American Alliance for Health, Physical Education, Recreation, and Dance (AAHPERD). This book provides numerous guidelines for facility design and operation. It is in its 11th edition and was written by numerous experts in the field. This book contains chapters on topics such as: (a) the ADA and architectural barriers, (b) indoor surfaces, (c) electrical and mechanical considerations, (d) signage, (e) aquatic facilities, (f) strength and cardiovascular training areas, (g) indoor and outdoor courts, (h) saunas/Jacuzzis, and much more.

STEP 1 ASSESSMENT OF LEGAL LIABILITY EXPOSURES

Before describing the law and the published standards of practice related to facility risks, it is important to review the law with regard to invitees, which was presented previously in Chapter 3. Individuals using health/fitness facilities will more likely than not be classified in reference to those facilities, as "business invitees." **Business invitees** are those persons who are expressly or implicitly invited on defined premises for a purpose that will be of benefit to the inviter—the premise occupier. Such individuals are to be distinguished from a **trespasser** or mere **licensee** to whom a lesser degree of care is required by business owners. The duty owed to business invitees is among the highest required by law and requires facilities to do the following:

- Make their premises free from reasonably discernable defects, or
- Warn such persons of any known defects or those unknown defects that could be discovered on the application of reasonable care.

This defined duty of care can also be extended to areas that may not be part of the normally defined physical plant of most facilities and into areas where members and guests may be invited—even under circumstances where those areas are not under the control or within the maintenance responsibility of facility management.

In a 1971 Oregon Supreme Court decision, *Bertrand v. Palm Springs and European Health Spa, Inc.,*[2] the plaintiff health spa member was injured when she slipped and fell in the defendant's locker room on a wet floor. She thereafter filed suit, which was determined by a jury in favor of the plaintiff. The defendant spa appealed to Oregon's highest state court, which ruled that the plaintiff was a business invitee to whom the defendant owed "the duty to keep the premises in a reasonably safe condition for . . . [the member's] protection."[3] Although the court noted that the defendant "may not have known of the particular puddle in this locker room [that the plaintiff stepped in] . . . it did know that water was not uncommon in this area and that the [floor] tile was hazardous when it had water on it."[4] A similar result was rendered in another slip and fall case from Pennsylvania.[5] This result was reached even though a release had been executed by the member (but did not specifically release the facility from "negligence").

In the health/fitness setting, various specific duties owed by facilities to their members have been litigated dealing not only with slip and fall cases but also with whirlpools,[6] hot tubs,[7] saunas, steam rooms,[8] tanning beds,[9] and swimming pools.[10] Although many such cases also involve the enforceability of prospectively executed releases/waivers, the exact scope of duty owed in particular cases, the issue of whether or not published standards should be used to assist in duty determinations, and a host of other issues, the status of a plaintiff as a business invitee—on the premises for the defendant's benefit—is almost always an initial important issue put forth for court determination.

THE LAW

This section addresses Title III of the Americans with Disabilities Act (ADA)—a federal statutory law that was previously described in Chapter 6. In addition, several case law examples are described relevant to facility risks associated within the premises (inside and outside) as well as off-premise activities.

The ADA

Often individuals believe that Title III of the ADA only addresses those matters dealing with the restitution of architectural barriers such as those providing for the installation of ramps, elevators, rest rooms with grab bars, and so on. However, Title III also addresses the provision of access to programs and services offered by health/fitness facilities that are the focus of the cases that follow. As a brief review, Herbert and Herbert,[11] state that the ADA (Public Law 101–336):

> [P]rohibits discrimination by places of public accommodation against those with disabilities. Places of public accommodation include, among others, professional offices of healthcare providers or service establishments, places of recreation, gymnasiums, health spas and other places of exercise or recreation. The provisions of the law cover activities conducted by and at health and fitness facilities. The law essentially prohibits discrimination on the basis of disability and the full and equal enjoyment of the goods, services, facilities, privileges, advantages or accommodations of any place of public accommodation by any person who owns, leases (or leases to) or operates a place of public accommodation (see Section 302). The utilization of safety screening criteria by health and fitness facilities is probably permissible under the Act (and mandated by the accepted standard of care) provided such criteria are based upon actual risks and not upon stereotypes or generalizations. This conclusion is further reinforced when taking into consideration the stated legislative history comparisons to the Federal Rehabilitation Act and judicial interpretations of that Act, which have allowed the use of such screening criteria. Health and fitness facilities with admission/participation policies that would exclude or limit certain individuals from program activities would be well advised to review the requirements of the law with their legal counsel. While certain other requirements are also necessary under the law, including architectural changes where they are readily achievable, the provisions dealing with access and participation would seem to be of particular interest to most facilities. There are also similar legislation in existence at the state and local levels providing similar protections.[12]

Claims litigated against health/fitness facilities and personnel based on alleged failures to allow access to or use of facilities or equipment have been lodged principally based on alleged violations of the Americans with Disabilities Act (ADA). One such suit, *Montalvo v. Radcliffe*,[13] worked its way through the court system all the way to the U.S. Supreme Court, which, however, denied the petition for writ of certiorari.[14] In this case, according to a reported analysis of this ruling,

> [A] mother enrolled her 12-year-old son into a traditional, Japanese, combat-oriented martial arts school owned and operated by the defendants. The classes involved substantial body contact which often resulted in bloody injuries. At the time the mother enrolled her son, she filled out a membership application and agreement in which she represented and warranted that her son was "in good health and suffer[ed] from no illness or condition . . . which would possibly be infectious to others."[15] The form also provided that 'no member . . . [could] use the facility with any open cuts, abrasions, open sores, infections [or other] maladies with the potential of harm to others."[15] At the time that the mother filled out these papers her son in fact had AIDS. She apparently chose not to disclose this fact because she felt that if the defendants knew of her son's condition, they would not allow him to participate with his friends in the instruction.[16]
>
> The defendants received an anonymous telephone call that dealt with the child's infectious condition. As a result the defendants made inquiries to the mother which ultimately led to a disclosure that the child had AIDS. Based upon the mother's admission as to the child's true condition, the defendants refused to allow the boy to commence karate classes "because of the risk of

transmitting HIV to other students through frequent bloody injuries and physical contact."[15] *The defendants did however offer to provide the child with private karate lessons. The mother rejected that alternative and filed suit under the Americans with Disabilities Act (ADA) and analogous state statutes. The plaintiff sought an injunction requiring the defendants to admit the son into the classes and for damages, costs and attorneys fees.*

After a trial to the Court, the Court ruled in favor of the defendants and held "placing plaintiff directly into the martial arts classes . . . would present a direct threat to the health and safety of the instruction personnel and the students in violation of [the ADA] . . ." and that the defendants' "offer to provide plaintiff with private lessons in lieu of class instruction "was a reasonable accommodation"[17] *under the ADA. The court rejected the state law charges on essentially the same basis.*

In response to the court's ruling, the plaintiffs appealed. On appeal, the appellate court affirmed the trial court's ruling and noted that there were instances when there was a need to protect the public health which would outweigh the rights of disabled individuals. The appeals court also noted that when an individual posses a "direct threat" which cannot be readily accommodated, that the requirements of the Act will not be violated by exclusion from participation. Thus that court upheld the lower court's ruling.[18]

Facilities should note that this ruling placed significant emphasis on the combative nature of this activity and even noted that it was different from "the more prevalent family-oriented fitness programs offered by most martial arts schools."[19] *As a consequence, the decision, while of significance, may be limited to combat style programs and not all karate, boxing or even wrestling programs.*[20] (Note: Portions of the previous case (Montalvo) were reprinted with permission from D. Herbert.[18])

In another case, *Kuketz v. Petronelli*,[21] the Massachusetts Supreme Court ruled that: "a fitness club's refusal to permit a wheelchair racquetball player to compete in a club league under the condition that the wheelchair player receive two bounces and his able-bodied (referred to by the parties as 'footed' player) opponents receive one bounce" was "not an act of discrimination on the basis of physical disability in violation of Federal and State antidiscrimination laws."[22]

The facts indicated the following:

Stephen B. Kuketz, a paraplegic since 1991, was by 1995 a nationally ranked wheelchair racquetball player. In the fall of 1994, Kuketz joined the Brockton Athletic Club (club), a fitness club then owned and operated by MDC Fitness Corporation (MDC). . . . The club sponsored a racquetball league in which men and women competed in divisions organized by gender and ability. The men's "A" league was the most competitive division. In January 1995, Kuketz paid a nominal league fee and requested placement on the men's "A" league roster. . . . Because of his disability, Kuketz is not competitive at any level of racquetball unless permitted to return the ball after its second bounce. He presumed that in the club's league play he would be granted this accommodation, while his footed opponents would be required to return the ball after no more than one bounce. . . .

The official rules of racquetball (rules), which govern league play, provide that the "objective" of the game is "to win each rally" and that a player loses a rally when he is "unable to hit the ball before it touches the floor twice." . . . The rules further provide for a modification to the "standard rules" for wheelchair competition, and establish five different levels or "divisions" for such competition. . . . Wheelchair players competing within these divisions must return the ball before the third bounce (i.e., "[t]he ball may hit the floor twice before being returned"), except in the "Multi-Bounce Division," where the "ball may bounce as many times as the receiver wants though the player may swing only once to return the ball to the front wall." . . . *These modified rules also provide that a player "can neither intentionally jump out of his chair to hit a ball nor stand up in his chair to serve the ball."* . . . *The rules have no provision governing competitive play between a wheelchair player and a footed player.[23]*

In February 1995, the general manager of the club, Roslyn Petronelli, after consulting with other players in the league, informed Kuketz that he would not be allowed to play in the men's "A" league. . . . Petronelli cited safety concerns as the primary reason . . . and offered Kuketz two alternative options: he could play in a lower-level league under the one-bounce rule or he could play in a wheelchair league that she would assist him in organizing. . . . Kuketz declined both offers.

Kuketz subsequently filed a complaint with the Massachusetts Commission Against Discrimination (commission) against the club, charging that it violated Title III of the Americans with Disabilities Act of 1990 (ADA), 42 U.S.C. §§ 12101 et seq. (2000); G. L. c. 151B, § 5; and G. L. c. 272, § 98, by refusing to allow him to participate in the men's "A" league. . . . In defense of their actions, the club contended that Kuketz was denied the accommodation he requested for safety reasons and because to grant it would fundamentally change the nature of the game.

Before the commission completed its investigation, the club ceased operations. Kuketz then moved to amend his complaint by substituting MDC and Charles M. Mirrione, MDC's president, as respondents, and by adding Petronelli as a respondent. . . . Prior to a ruling by the commission on that motion, Kuketz removed his charges from the commission pursuant to G. L. c. 151B, § 9, and filed a complaint in the Superior Court.[24]

Based on these facts and on cross motions for summary judgment, a Superior Court judge granted judgment for the defendants on all of Kuketz's claims. Specifically, the judge ruled that the defendants were not required under Title III of the ADA to permit Kuketz two bounces in league-sponsored racquetball games against footed players because such a modification would "fundamentally alter the nature of the racquetball competition," . . . and that Kuketz's state law disability claim failed because the interpretation of G. L. c. 272, § 98, proceeds "hand in hand" with the interpretation of the ADA. Kuketz appealed, asserting that the judge erred in finding that his requested modification constituted a fundamental alteration of the game of racquetball, and that the absence of an individualized assessment of his abilities and the reasonableness of the requested modification precluded summary judgment for the defendants.[25]

In analyzing the facts and law the Supreme Judicial Court of Massachusetts analyzed relevant state and federal law and determined as follows:

The ADA was enacted in 1990 for the express purpose of providing "a clear and comprehensive national mandate for the elimination of discrimination against individuals with disabilities." 42 U.S.C. § 12101(b)(1). Title III of the ADA confers rights to disabled patrons of places of public accommodation, "thus enabling individuals with disabilities to participate more fully in the mainstream of society with improved access to hotels, convention centers, entertainment and sporting events, and commercial establishments." 1 H.H. Perritt, Jr., Americans with Disabilities Act Handbook § 6.01, at 389 (2003). Section 12182 of Title III of the ADA sets out the general rule:

"No individual shall be discriminated against on the basis of disability in the full and equal enjoyment of the goods, services, facilities, privileges, advantages, or accommodations of any place of public accommodation by any person who owns, leases (or leases to), or operates a place of public accommodation."[26]

The statute then defines discrimination to include:

[A] failure to make reasonable modifications in policies, practices, or procedures, when such modifications are necessary to afford such goods, services, facilities, privileges, advantages, or accommodations to individuals with disabilities, unless the entity can demonstrate that making such modifications would fundamentally alter the nature of such goods, services, facilities, privileges, advantages, or accommodations. Id. at § 12182(b)(2)(A)(ii).

It is undisputed that Kuketz is an individual with a disability as defined in the ADA. . . . There is also no dispute that the club was a place of public accommodation covered under Title III of the ADA. . . . The issue we must decide is whether the club unlawfully discriminated against Kuketz when it refused to modify its policies and practice to allow Kuketz to play in the men's 'A' league. . . . There is significant dispute, however, as to the reasonableness of the modifications sought in light of the safety concerns raised by the defendants. There is also disagreement on whether the modifications would fundamentally alter the nature of the game. Because we conclude that affording Kuketz two bounces against footed players in league play would fundamentally alter the nature of the competition, we need not otherwise address the reasonableness of Kuketz's requested modifications.[27]

In determining the relevant legal issues, this Massachusetts Court looked to a previous decision of the U.S. Supreme Court for guidance and stated that the fundamental alteration inquiry:

[W]as the central issue before the United States Supreme Court in Martin. Casey Martin, a professional golfer afflicted with a degenerative circulatory disorder that made walking an eighteen-hole golf course a physical impossibility, requested permission to use a golf cart during the final stage of a professional tour qualifying tournament . . . [T]he sponsor of the tournament refused to waive its walking rule. At trial and subsequently on appeal, the PGA TOUR argued that walking constituted a substantive rule of golf and that waiving this rule in any circumstances would fundamentally alter the nature of the competition. . . . The Supreme Court disagreed, deciding, inter alia, that permitting Martin to use a golf cart would not work a fundamental alteration of the game of golf.[28]

According to the Court,

[A] modification of [the PGA TOUR's] golf tournaments might constitute a fundamental alteration in two different ways. It might alter such an essential aspect of the game of golf that it would be unacceptable even if it affected all competitors equally; changing the diameter of the hole from three to six inches might be such a modification. Alternatively, a less significant change that has only a peripheral impact on the game itself might nevertheless give a disabled player, in addition to access to the competition as required by Title III, an advantage over others and, for that reason, fundamentally alter the character of the competition. . . . The Court concluded that the PGA TOUR's walking rule, which was "based on an optional condition buried in an appendix to the Rules of Golf," was neither an essential element of the game, nor "an indispensable feature of tournament golf." . . . ("essence of the game has been shot-making"). The Court also rejected the PGA TOUR's contention that Martin would gain unfair advantage over his competitors if permitted to use a golf cart.[28]

In applying this law to the facts just outlined, the Massachusetts court determined that summary judgment had been properly granted. The court noted, "Fitness and athletic clubs open to the public may choose to 'level the playing field' in any number of ways, and such practices are not to be discouraged, but the law does not require modifications that change the fundamental rules of the sport."[29] (Note: Portions of this case

[*Kutetz*] were reprinted with permission from Herbert D. Club decision to bar wheelchair-bound racquetball player from competition results in suit. *The Sports, Parks, and Recreation Law Reporter.* 2005;19(1):6–8.)

Inside Premises: Floor Surfaces

Efforts should be made to provide a proper floor surface for all activity programs so as to avoid what is commonly called "slip-and-fall" incidents. Slippery, oily, over-waxed, wet, or dusty floors can cause serious falls or collisions and related injuries and lawsuits.[5,30,31] Liability can attach from such injuries and falls, particularly where the injured party can establish knowledge of the dangerous condition and a failure to correct despite actual or implied knowledge of the condition by the facility. Such conditions should not go uncorrected. A system of periodic checks should be instituted to discover and remedy these so that the duty owed to the participant can be completed and established if necessary in a legal setting. Consequently, records of facility checks should be maintained, including items pertinent to the safety and condition of floor surfaces.

Floor surfaces that are defectively constructed, inadequately maintained, or deteriorated as a result of severe weather, overuse, or other conditions can also result in participant injuries and lawsuits. Generally, the same basic rules apply as with slippery floors; however, some states impose liability only where the defect causing the fall and injury exceeded certain established, set parameters (e.g., floor surface irregularities greater than 1 inch). In these states, defects under the set measurement would not result in any liability. In majority of states, such defects are almost always jury questions and not subject to hard and fast measurement rules. As with slippery floors, periodic and documented checks or similar inspections should be made of the program floor area for defects in construction, contour, composition, and the like, to discover cracks, depressions, uneven areas, weakened materials, crumbling concrete, or similar deteriorating defects. Such defects obviously should be corrected as soon as possible after discovery; moreover, inaction after discovery could even provide more evidence of knowing maintenance of an unsafe condition and, in essence, provide the injured party with a better legal case.

A failure to correct dangerous conditions that result in subsequent injuries may even result in claims of willful or wanton negligence.[32] Upon discovery, the simple solution should be to correct the condition, inform participants of the temporary hazard, or modify program activities to avoid exposure until correction is made. In addition, published standards of practice should be implemented. See Published Standards of Practice later.

With some specialized activities (e.g., dance exercise and aerobics), the use of specialized floor surfaces must be considered. It appears quite clear that harder floor surfaces such as concrete or tile/linoleum over concrete are inappropriate and in fact contribute to a variety of injuries and activities.[33] Even padded and carpeted surfaces appear to be incapable of reducing the correlations between injuries and floor surfaces. Specialized floor surfaces clearly appear to be required and are probably indicated to meet the appropriate standard of care for dance exercise and other aerobic exercise activities and routines, the tempo of which is set to music.[33] Recommended footwear for certain activities may also have legal implications.[34]

Other cases have also dealt with floor issues. For example, in the case of *Goynias v. Spa Health Clubs, Inc.,*[35] the plaintiff health club patron was injured at the defendant's facility when he fell on a slippery and wet floor after he left the men's shower area and returned to the locker room. In response to his suit, the defendant moved for summary judgment and denied any negligence. The trial court granted that request. The plaintiff appealed. On appeal, the plaintiff contended that the defendant's motion should not have been granted. The North Carolina appellate court affirmed the trial court's ruling. In doing so, that court acknowledged that:

A property owner is required to exercise reasonable care to provide for the safety of all lawful visitors on his property . . . whether the care provided is reasonable must be judged against the conduct of a reasonably prudent person under the circumstances. . . . [This duty] includes the duty to exercise ordinary care to keep the premises in a reasonably safe condition and to warn the invitee of hidden perils or unsafe conditions that can be ascertained by reasonable inspection and supervision.[36]

The appellate court in this case also ruled that for a plaintiff to demonstrate negligence, the plaintiff must prove that the defendant "either: (1) negligently created the condition causing injury, or (2) negligently failed to correct the condition after actual or constructive notice of its existence."[37] In addressing these issues, the court examined the facts and determined:

In the case before us, plaintiff has failed to show that defendant negligently created the situation which caused plaintiff's injury. Plaintiff's own expert testified in his deposition that the tile floor was textured and possessed a .64 coefficient of friction, significantly higher than the .04 standard for a bathtub or shower floor. Plaintiff's expert testified the floor was sloped; however, the expert performed no tests which would indicate what that slope was or if it was significant enough to be the cause of the accident. Plaintiff's expert testified the lighting in the room was such that a person could not see a puddle which had formed; however, the expert examined the area two and a half years after the accident, and offered no evidence or factual basis as to what the lighting conditions were at the time of the accident. Plaintiff's expert offered that the slip resistance of the floor was determined with clean water, and that resistance could be lessened by the presence of soap or other oils. However, neither plaintiff nor plaintiff's expert offered any evidence of the presence of soap or oils in the water on the date of the accident. "Negligence is not presumed from the mere fact of injury. Plaintiff is required to offer legal evidence tending to establish beyond mere speculation or conjecture every essential element of negligence, and upon failure to do so, nonsuit is proper."[37]

The record shows defendant installed a tile floor which was textured in order to create a slip-resistant floor with a much greater slip resistance than is required. Defendant placed several non-skid mats in the area where plaintiff fell, and defendant installed a floor with a slope to facilitate the drainage of water. There is no evidence the slope caused plaintiff to fall or was constructed at an angle that would be considered too steep.

[I]n this case, plaintiff has failed to offer any evidence which would tend to prove defendant was aware dangerous puddles had formed or were forming on the floor. Plaintiff testified he did not notice any puddles immediately before or immediately after he slipped. He did not notice any standing water until he returned a few minutes later to the place where he fell, accompanied by an employee of the health club. Furthermore, a proprietor has no duty to warn an invitee of an obvious danger or of a condition of which the invitee has equal or superior knowledge. Reasonable persons are assumed, absent a diversion or distraction, to be vigilant in the avoidance of injury in the face of a known or obvious danger. . . .

While we acknowledge plaintiff did not slip in a bathtub, we still deem the area where he slipped to be an area where one might be expected to exercise extra caution. The chances of water, and even soapy water, on the floor of an area where people walk out of a shower across to a locker room appear to be high. Plaintiff admitted he saw the black nonskid mats on the floor and that he knew the purpose of the mats was to help in preventing falls. He also admitted that the nonskid mats indicated to him that the floors could be slippery.

Defendant was required to keep its premises in a reasonably safe condition. The record shows defendant placed mats on the floor and provided a drain with a slope. Also, the texture of the floor exceeded the required slip resistant standard for bathroom flooring. There is no evidence defendant was actually or constructively aware of an unobvious dangerous condition which it failed to correct. Therefore, plaintiff failed to show defendant breached its duty to plaintiff.[38]

As a consequence of the case just described, it is important to understand that the particular facts and circumstances of individual cases may well dictate the outcome of a court's ruling based on a judicial determination of those facts as well as prior similar court rulings.

Inside Premises: Other Potential Facility Risks

The principal risk exposures for health/fitness facilities include floor surfaces, water-based amenities, heat, humidity and air pollutants, maintenance issues, and facility access. A look at each of these matters should be of benefit.

Some program activities might require special services and precautions. For example, certain flexibility and muscular toning exercise might require floor mats of a particular minimum thickness or resilience, so that friction burns of the skin or possible trauma to soft tissue and bone may be avoided. Failure to provide such mats, or insistence on exercise without such equipment, could clearly result in litigation.

Other serious problems can occur in special exercise testing and training facilities. Design of the physical plant and instructions to participants about facility use and monitoring practices by staff will affect the likelihood of mishaps and consequently, the likelihood of litigation.[39-41] For instance, when activity areas require electrical power, the facilities must be properly equipped with grounded electrical outlets and, in areas where wet or perspiring participants will come in contact with electrically powered devices, such devices must be equipped with ground-fault circuit interrupters that automatically shut down power in the event that deteriorated insulation or another incident allow potentially dangerous current leakage to ground wires (e.g., treadmills, ECG systems, whirlpools, saunas, etc.). Likewise, exclusive use of electrically powered equipment fitted with heavily insulated and grounded power cords and larger plugs must also be standard for all programs.

Many other examples of risk could be cited in relation to program facilities, including those associated with locker rooms, shower areas, steam rooms, saunas, hot tubs, and swimming pools.[42] Inappropriate and harmful conditions in health/fitness facilities may increase the risk of lacerations related to sharp objects that protrude into participant pathways or access ways. Injury can occur when (a) water temperature control devices do not function properly, (b) instructions on proper use are not clearly written nor appropriately posted, or (c) safe egress is not possible (e.g., sauna doorways). Substantial claims have already been brought forth regarding these conditions. For example, in the case of *Leenen v. Ruttgers Ocean Beach Lodge Ltd.*,[43] the plaintiff, a pregnant (19 weeks of gestation) guest at the defendant resort entered a resort-owned hot tub that she alleged reached a temperature as high as 110°F. Although she indicated that she left the tub when it seemed too hot, she contended her unborn child was affected detrimentally. The child was later born with cerebral palsy, which she contended was related to the hot tub exposure. After the third or fourth day of trial, the case was settled for $560,000.[44] Similar cases have also been filed related to similar issues.[45,46] Cases related to alleged supervision deficiencies concerning whirlpool use have also arisen.[47] Individuals with cardiac or circulatory problems, and those who have other adverse health conditions, should seek expert advice and clearance prior to using hot tubs, saunas, steam rooms, or similar devices.

Physiologically stressful levels of heat, humidity, and air pollutants coupled with poor air circulation or other conditions represent additional risks for exercisers that can contribute to exercise injury or death and must be addressed.[48] Claimed failures of participants or program staff to consider such factors properly may contribute to serious injuries or death.[49]

In general, facilities should be properly designed, equipped, and maintained in all program areas if liability is to be controlled at manageable levels. All areas should be regularly checked and kept free of defects and nuisances to minimize the chances of participant injury, illness, or death. Some items present in certain health/fitness facilities may also pose risk of claims and suit. For example, the provision of tanning beds may expose facilities to the claim of some patrons because of the long-term use of such beds if they cause certain diseases. In other situations, the transmission of disease processes from surfaces of such beds to others may also result in suit.[50]

Appropriately designed and correctly worded warnings contained in properly posted signage can greatly assist facilities in meeting their obligations in this regard. Several published standards of practice provide standards and guidelines regarding facility signage. See published standards of practice later.

Published standards of practice also address controlling facility access. Because health/fitness facilities have an obligation to provide a reasonably safe environment for their participants, it will be important to have a system that will help safeguard entrance into the facility so only authorized individuals have access. Health/fitness facilities and professionals should know they may be liable for certain kinds of criminal activity that takes place on their premises even though they may not, as a somewhat general rule, be liable if a third party not under their control criminally attacks a business invitee on their premises with whom it has no special relationship. Theft of property of a facility member in this regard may well be actionable against the facility.[51]

Outside Premises: Ground Surfaces

Accumulations of ice and snow can also result in dangerous conditions to participants entering and exiting program locations, or perhaps to those individuals exercising in such conditions at the recommendation or prescription of program professionals. Most states, particularly those in which cold and snow are an annual occurrence, have developed rules, or, as lawyers call them, "precedents" making the prosecution of fall cases in ice and snow almost impossible to maintain successfully. Courts usually reason that in such climates everyone knows and appreciates the slippery conditions of ice and snow accumulation and must consequently take certain precautions to protect themselves. Different rules can apply, however, if the ice and snow buildups are not natural but reflect artificial accumulations, or if snow is allowed to accumulate without adequate maintenance, or if such accumulations conceal hidden defects. In such cases, proper maintenance is again the best prevention against liability to the program and its personnel.

Off Premises: Outdoor and Offsite Activities

An exercise session carried out in ice and snow conditions, which results in a participant injury, could well result in litigation of a slightly different character from the normal slip-and-fall situation. For example, if exercise sessions were needlessly conducted under such conditions, a strong case might be developed against the program and its personnel for negligence and perhaps intentional misconduct in the event of participant injury. However, defenses such as contributory negligence and assumption of risk may be available to program operators.

Such defenses will not greatly assist under some circumstances where the participant is merely carrying out the instructions of the exercise staff. Obviously, therefore, common sense should always be part of planning and consideration before prescription of activity. When conditions dictate delivery of activity or substitution of indoor exercise for outdoor functions, leaders should respond accordingly.[52] Prescription of activity to be carried out off premises and without supervision should contain some

---

**EXERCISER'S ALERT
WEATHER AND ENVIRONMENTAL
CONSIDERATIONS**

In carrying out your exercise activities, you should always be alert to environmental conditions and changing weather. Exercise in high temperatures (above 80° Fahrenheit) or at high humidity should be undertaken only in moderation. Prolonged activity in sustained heat, humidity, and/or sun should be avoided. If you choose to exercise in periods of high heat, humidity, and temperature, such activity should be undertaken before 11:00 a.m. or after 3:00 p.m. Fluid should be taken liberally during exercise, particularly at high temperatures and before thirst is indicated.

Exercising during severe weather, snow, sleet, severe rain, hail, high winds, storms, or similar conditions should also be avoided.

Activity at high altitudes should be undertaken gradually and a step at a time. Fluid intake should be increased during high altitude exercise. Such exercise should be progressively undertaken, beginning slowly and increasing over several days until normal activity can be undertaken.

FIGURE 10-1   Exerciser's Alert: Weather and Environmental Conditions

instruction or warning as to severe or adverse weather conditions.[53] Alert messages like those in Figure 10-1 may be in order. Consideration must be given to various climatic conditions in which contemplated activity will be carried out.[54] Possible deficiencies in the consideration of such environmental factors may lead to untoward events[48,55] and even successful claim and suit.[56] One 1993 race event that led to the heat stroke of a 12-year-old Arizona girl resulted in a $4.5 million settlement.[57] The race in this case was carried out on a bright sunny day in Arizona, with the temperature about 110°F and humidity at 20%. The girl, who had recently returned to Arizona after having spent most of her summer in Minnesota, did not practice at least 10 days before the competition as required by the applicable interscholastic rules. Although she won her race, she collapsed, became disoriented, incoherent, and suffered a severe seizure and irreversible brain damage. Such events may be avoidable with proper planning and some event scheduling flexibility. Again, an environmental alert like that in Figure 10-1 should be considered.

Aside from weather and other environmental factors that must be taken into account when prescribing off-premises activity, other concerns must also be addressed. If exercise is prescribed along set trails or areas, consideration must be given to pedestrian and vehicular traffic patterns along such trails, composition and consistency of the terrain, availability of lighting for the surface (for early morning and late evening use), and even the proximity of the trail to public telephones that will accommodate no-cost activation of an emergency medical response system. Such factors are of particular importance to some groups (e.g., cardiac, preventive, and rehabilitative patients).[53,58]

Prescription of activity to be carried out at set locations or particular sites should be preceded by inspection prior to commencement of activity, and at specified intervals, inasmuch as the same rules that apply to business invitees may also be applicable to established off-premises activities to be carried out at preset locations. The establishment of such areas should be subject to pre-use planning activity and consultation with a variety of professionals, including police, fire, emergency response groups, and telephone utility companies, as well as park and other governmental officials if applicable. *Personal trainers who provide service to clients in the clients' own homes or offices need to consider all of these issues in advance of service delivery.* Not only must these areas be appropriate for the services being offered, but considerations related to space, floor surfaces, transportation, lighting, and even emergency response must all be reviewed.

The establishment of activity areas within high-crime districts or where trails are poorly illuminated or marked might well be deemed to be causative of injury in the event of an untoward event occurring within such areas.[59] Although the general rule may well be stated to the effect that a facility owes no duty to protect a plaintiff from criminal attack by a third party,[60] there are exceptions. At least one court (*Simpson v. Big Bear Stores Co.*) has defined this duty as follows: "a business owner has a duty to warn or protect its business invitees from criminal acts of third parties when the business owner knows or should know that there is a substantial risk of harm to its invitees on the premises in the possession and control of the business owner. The duty does not extend to premises not in the possession and control of the business owner."[61] Particular attention should also be given to considerations related to the accessibility of certain areas to emergency response vehicles and personnel. Failures to consider all of these matters may well be deemed to be negligent and substandard. The foregoing case was based on the *Restatement of the Law (Torts) Second,* Vol. 2, Sections 314 and 315. These sections of that treatise provide that there is no duty to control the conduct of a third person so as to prevent harm to another unless a special relationship exists between the property owner and the victim. Despite this apparent limitation on potential liability as enumerated by the Ohio Supreme Court in *Simpson,* at least one other case heard in Washington state may indicate some potential liability as to at least negligent injuries suffered by others in areas recommended to exercise participants to carry on relevant activity.

In this Washington state case, *Weade v. Vancouver School Dist. 37,*[62] a student was hit by an automobile and injured while running off campus pursuant to instruction provided by his physical education teacher. He suffered a severe head injury and thereafter instituted suit claiming the school was negligent "in allowing teachers to require their students to run off campus and through city streets as part of school activities." Care also needs to be given to recommending activity to be carried out where other "natural" conditions may expose exercisers to danger.[63] Consideration needs to be given to all of these issues, which are addressed in a number of other sources.[64-69] Health/fitness facilities should consider the use of informational alerts or warnings related to such potentialities such as the warning shown in Figure 10-2.

The use of park lands or other property used for recreational purposes might well afford benefits to some programs because of so-called state recreational immunity statutes or even the limited duties owed to park users.[70] Under these enactments, lands made available for recreational use without charge to the user or compensation to the landowner are subject to special rules that provide immunity from suit to the landowner or occupier. In some states, these statutes provide protection for both private as well as governmental landowners. Programs that provide access to such lands without charge may well be able to claim the benefits of the enactments in the event of participant injury.[11,71] However, claims related to prescription, supervision (or the lack thereof), failure to monitor or provide proper emergency response, and so on, may still be available as separate and distinct claims.

WARNING!
APPROACH OFF-PREMISE EXERCISE
ACTIVITIES WITH CAUTION

Exercise activities such as jogging which are carried on off premises should be carefully considered. Not only should exercisers undergo preparticipation health screening, proper warm-up, and professional prescription for activity, care should be given to the selection of the actual area where activity is to be carried out. While consideration must be given to environmental factors such as heat, humidity, and other weather-related matters, concern must also be directed at the area to be used for exercise/activity. Answers to the following questions should be provided before beginning activity: Is the area in a high-crime locale? If so, avoid it. If you don't know, avoid it until you find out. The police department is your best source of information for this purpose. If you can't find out, don't use the area. Is the area properly illuminated at night? If not, avoid it. Is a public telephone in the immediate area? If not, avoid it. Is the ground surface in good condition? If not, avoid it. Is the area in a remote location or interspersed with hiding places for assailants? If so, avoid it.

Helpful Hints:
➢ Exercise in pairs.
➢ Carry and be prepared to use a whistle if needed to obtain attention.
➢ Carry mace or keys in fist to use if attacked.
➢ Carry a quarter(s) or other appropriate change for emergency telephone use.
➢ Exercise during daylight hours if possible.

FIGURE 10-2 Warning! Approach Off-Premise Exercise Activities with Caution (Adapted and reprinted with permission from: Herbert DL. Jogger's attack in high crime area leads to suit. *Exercise Standards and Malpractice Reporter.* 1991;5(2):30.[67])

Off Premises: Sponsored Events

Aside from the activities recommended for performance off the premises of a health/fitness facility, facility-sponsored events can also create risks that can at least potentially lead to liability. For example, bicycle-sponsored events have been the subject of substantial litigation. For example, in a 1997 wrongful death case, *McDonough v. National Off-Road Bicycle Assn.,*[72] McDonough collapsed during an off-road race. When he was found by a club official, he appeared to be unconscious, was breathing heavily, and was unresponsive. The official called 911 with a cellular phone and went to the start/finish area to get help. He took two people to help McDonough. They administered CPR until the ambulance arrived about 20 minutes later. The race had been generally disorganized, starting 30 minutes late with no maps of the course for participants. No water was provided and no medical personnel were on site for the unusually long race.

The court ruled that waivers such as that relied on by the defendant in this case are effective in Delaware; however, the court determined that for such waivers to be enforceable, it must appear that plaintiff understood the terms of the agreement.

Pertinent wording within the waiver was "I release. . . . NORBA and the U.S. Cycling Federation . . . from any and all liability . . . and waive any such claims . . . attributable . . . to any action . . . of any such person."[73] The court, deciding that the wording did not clearly indicate that the signer waived liability hazards created by negligent conduct, ruled that the waiver was not enforceable and thus offered no protection for the defendants.

Two older cases arose out of injuries attributed to poor supervision or organization of events. In *Staadeker v. The Emerald Health Network*,[74] a volunteer for the triathlon walked in front of Staadeker's bike in an area where bananas were being passed out to participants, causing him to swerve and run over a banana peel. The bike flipped and Staadeker was injured. The preinjury waiver failed to protect the defendants because they were unable to produce the waiver. Following a bicycle race collision in *Buchan v. U.S. Cycling Federation, Inc.*,[75] Buchan alleged poor supervision in allowing a less experienced biker in the race and not requiring the use of hard-shell protective helmets. The court ruled that the waiver barred action and protected the defendant from liability for negligence.

In three cases in which plaintiffs alleged the route selected was unsafe, the waivers signed by the participants were effective in protecting the event organizers. In *Watts v. Country Cycle Club, Inc.*,[76] the participant in a bike trip was injured when he fell crossing a steel deck bridge. He alleged sponsor negligence in choosing the route. Two cases involved the U.S. Cycling Federation as the defendant. In *Peters v. U.S. Cycling Federation*,[77] Peters was killed when his bicycle left the road while he was attempting to make a sharp turn at the bottom of a hill. A few years earlier, in *Okura v. U.S. Cycling Federation*,[78] a participant in a bicycle race was injured when he fell crossing a railroad track. Apparently, loose debris on the surface caused the fall. In all three cases, the preinjury waiver signed by the participant was ruled effective in protecting the event organizer from liability for negligence.

Event organizers in two 1991 cases were protected by preinjury waivers when accidents occurred because of the presence of automobiles on the bike route. In *Banfield v. Louis*,[79] Banfield was injured while participating in the bicycle portion of a triathlon when she was struck by a motor vehicle. She alleged the event organizers had breached their duty by failing to control traffic around the course. In *Walton v. Oz Bicycle Club of Wichita*,[80] Walton took a turn at about 30 miles per hour and was unable to avoid striking the open door of a referee's van that was parked on the street and hidden from view by the crowd on the street corner. In each case, the injured participant had signed a preinjury waiver. The *Banfield* waiver released the organizer from liability for "injuries . . . based on negligence . . . of the . . . parties." The *Walton* waiver released the organizers from "any and all damages . . . arising out of, my participation in . . . the event."

Two other organizers were not so fortunate in somewhat similar cases. In *Coles v. Jenkins*,[81] Mr. and Mrs. Coles were participating in a bicycle tour when struck by a pickup truck. Coles was killed and his wife was seriously injured. In *Bennett v. U.S. Cycling Federation*,[82] Bennett was participating in a scheduled racing event when he collided with a moving automobile. The driver had been allowed on the course by a person stationed at a barrier. Bennett expected no vehicles on the course, having seen the barriers prior to the race.

The court in the *Coles* case ruled in favor of the plaintiff, stating that "Virginia law is, and has been abundantly clear that pre-injury exculpatory clauses . . . are void as against public policy."[83] The waiver in the *Bennett* case, in contrast, would normally have protected the organizer. The court stated, "There is little doubt that a subscriber of the bicycle release at issue here must be held to have waived any hazards relating to bicycle racing that are obvious or that might reasonably have been foreseen."[84] However, because the course was supposed to be closed to automobiles, striking an automobile was not within Bennett's contemplation when he signed the waiver. It therefore didn't provide protection to the defendant from the suit.

THE PUBLISHED STANDARDS OF PRACTICE

Standards, guidelines, and industry recommendations as to facilities have been developed by many professional and independent organizations. The breadth and scope of these resources is vast and available for considerations related to the design, layout, and maintenance of facilities. These resources also deal with a number of significant topics, including facility air exchanges, heat, humidity, lighting, and a host of other subjects. Several of these published standards of practice are described as follows.

The ACSM's H/F Standards[85] include the following seven standards related to facility risks:

> #11—*Facilities, to the extent required by law, must adhere to the building design standards that relate to the designing, building, expanding, or renovating of space as presented by the Americans with Disabilities Act (ADA).*
>
> #12—*Facilities must be in compliance with all federal, state, and local building codes.*
>
> #14—*Facilities must have a system in operation that monitors the entry to and usage of the facility by all individuals, including members and users.*
>
> #15—*Facilities that offer a sauna, steam room, or whirlpool must ensure that these areas are maintained at the proper temperature and that the appropriate warning systems are in place to notify members and users of any unacceptable risks and changes in temperature.*
>
> #16—*Facilities that offer members and users access to a pool or whirlpool must ensure that the pool water chemistry is maintained in accordance with state and local codes.*
>
> #18—*Facilities must post the appropriate caution, danger, and warning signage in conspicuous locations where existing conditions and situations warrant such signage.*
>
> #19—*Facilities must post the appropriate emergency and safety signage pertaining to fire and related emergency situations, as required by federal, state, and local codes.*
>
> #20—*Facilities must post all required ADA and OSHA signage.*[86] (From American College of Sports Medicine, 2007, *ACSM's Health/Fitness Facility Standards and Guidelines*, 3rd ed., pp. 1–2. © 2007 by American College of Sports Medicine. Reprinted with permission from Human Kinetics, Champaign, IL.)

The ACSM/AHA Joint PP[87] recommends that flooring should be designed to reduce risks and that facilities should be clean, well maintained, and provide space for comfort and safety for participants. In addition, changing and shower areas should be provided, and indoor facilities should be climate controlled.

Under Equal Opportunity & Access, NSCA Standard #7.1 states, "Strength & Conditioning professionals and their employers must provide facilities, training, programs, services and related opportunities in accordance with all laws, regulations and requirements mandating equal opportunity, access and non-discrimination. . . . Discrimination or unequal treatment based upon race, creed, national origin, sex, religion, age, handicap/disability or other such legal classification is generally prohibited."[88]

The IHRSA Standards[89] contain the following three standards regarding facility risks:

> *Standard #1—The club will open its membership to persons of all races, creeds, places of national origin, and physical abilities.*[90]
>
> *Standard #6—The club will conform to all relevant laws, regulations, and published standards.*[91]
>
> *Standard #10—The club will post appropriate signage alerting users to risks involved in their use of those areas of the club that may present increased risks. The intent of this standard is twofold: (1) to assure that IHRSA facilities address basic safety issues, in part, through responsible signage; and (2) to comply, to the best of their knowledge, with local and state codes and laws regarding signage. Appropriate signage, especially in "wet" areas of the club, can greatly reduce a club's liability in the event of an injury to a patron.*[92]

The Canadian Standards[93] provide the following four standards under Fitness Environment:

Standard #2—Access to a clean drinking water supply is required at or near all physical activity areas.[94]

Standard #5—Floors in wet areas have a non slip surface with adequate drainage to prevent pooling of water.

Standard #6—Whirlpools, spas and tubs shall comply with the Recommended Standards for the Operation of Public Spas (Ministry of Health & Long term Care Act, June 2001).

Standard #7—Electrical panels shall be covered. Receptacles located in wet area of a building and associated with the pool, such as locker and change room, require ground fault circuit interrupters of the Class A type.

Standard #8—A fire alarm shall be installed in a building as determined by building code requirements (Ontario Building Code 3.2.4.1). Portable fire extinguishers shall be installed in all buildings (OBC 3.2.5.17) or existing provincial/territorial code or regulations as applicable.[95]

Standard #13 of the MFA Standards states that "A Medical Fitness Center must meet all current local code, ADA, and other accessibility and safety requirements."[96] The YMCA Recommendations[97] cover various issues related to facility risks such as: (a) Children in Adult Locker Rooms (several recommendations are provided with regard to children changing/showering in opposite gender locker rooms); (b) Use of Saunas, Steam Rooms and Whirlpools (several guidelines related to temperature/humidity, safety precautions, use by children, and signage are described); (c) Smoking and Use of Tobacco (suggestions regarding a smoke-free environment are provided as well as smoking cessation programs that meet national standards); (d) Sunlight Exposure (sun protection guidelines published by the Centers for Disease Control and Prevention and the American Academy of Dermatology are recommended and YMCAs are encouraged to educate staff and participants on the risks with overexposure and precautions that should be taken); and (e) Use of Sun Tanning Units (recommends that "the use of high-intensity light sources emitting UVA and UVB for cosmetic tanning purposes should be eliminated by all YMCAs,"[98] which is consistent with the American Academy of Dermatology's strong discouragement regarding the use of such tanning units).

STEP 2 DEVELOPMENT OF RISK MANAGEMENT STRATEGIES

The physical plant of health/fitness facilities, as well as any areas where activities are carried out off premises from such facilities or through facility sponsorship of various events, can impact the risks for participants as business invitees. This in turn can impact the legal risks for facilities and their employees. As presented earlier, the ADA is one federal law with which health/fitness facilities must comply. It is also reflected in many of the published standards of practice that are described. In addition, a variety of case law examples were described in which negligence claims were made against health/fitness personnel and facilities with regard to all types of facility risks. A number of risk management tools can be used to assist facilities in minimizing those risks associated with their facilities while also helping them to meet their duties and responsibilities to their members and guests. The following should be of benefit in this regard.

Risk Management Strategy 1: Comply with the ADA.

Facilities need to comply with the requirements of the ADA. Title III addresses architectural barriers as well as provision of programs and services for persons with disabilities. Individual legal consultation should be obtained in this regard to ensure that facilities and programs are made available in compliance with the law and regulations.

At least one particularly good guide has been developed by the North Carolina Office on Disability and Health that is specifically geared toward health/fitness facilities. The publication "Removing Barriers to Health Clubs and Fitness Facilities: A Guide for Accommodating All Members, Including People with Disabilities and Older Adults" is available online at www.fpg.unc.edu/~ncodh/pdfs/rbfitness.pdf. It provides clear and very useful guidance on the steps health/fitness facilities need to take to comply with the law. In addition, health/fitness professionals should consider obtaining the specialty certification offered by the ACSM and the National Center on Physical Activity and Disability (NCAPD). The NCAPD also regularly publishes an informative newsletter. See the NCAPD website for more information (www.ncapd.org).

Risk Management Strategy 2: Establish a check-in system to monitor facility access.

To determine who is on the premises and for what purpose, facilities should develop a check-in system and establish access rules. Such a system can distinguish members and guests from others on the premises and allow for only "authorized" individuals to enter the building. One method to safeguard entrance into the building is to have everyone show their membership card to a staff member at the front desk. The card can contain a photo and be scanned to help ensure proper authorization. Such a system can also help protect participants from anyone entering the building who might commit crimes such as theft and sexual assault. In addition to a check-in system, health/fitness facilities should take other steps to protect against such crimes within the facility, such as providing proper lighting, security cameras, and so on, in potential danger zones inside and outside the facility.

Risk Management Strategy 3: Follow facility design and construction specifications.

There are numerous design/construction specifications that health/fitness facilities should follow, and only a few of these are discussed here. As mentioned at the beginning of this chapter, *Facility Design and Management for Health, Fitness, Physical Activity, Recreation and Sports Facility Development*[1] is an excellent resource in this regard. Of particular importance are floor surfaces. As shown in Table 1-2 in Chapter 1, slip-and-fall liability claims are quite common. The first step to minimize these types of injuries and subsequent negligence claims is to install the proper floor surfaces. A variety of factors should be considered for wet areas (e.g., locker/shower areas, steam rooms, etc.), as well as areas such aerobic/exercise facilities, racquetball courts, strength training areas, and so on.[1] Some of these factors are point-elastic versus area-elastic flooring, resilience, and rolling load.[1] Because the selection of floor surfaces is important from a risk management perspective, health/fitness facilities should consult with qualified manufactures and have installers who are recommended by the manufacturer.

Activity areas that require electrical power need to be properly equipped with grounded electrical outlets and, in areas where wet or perspiring participants will come in contact with electrically powered devices, such devices must be equipped with ground-fault circuit interrupters. Likewise, exclusive use of electrically powered equipment fitted with heavily insulated and grounded power cords and larger plugs need to be standard in all facilities. For example, see Appendix 10 (p. 1–1) for important voltage information and grounding instructions for the Cybex 750T Treadmill.

Additional design and construction specifications also need to be followed and include, but are not limited to, the following:

- Hot tubs, whirlpools, and steam rooms
- Changes in elevation, passageway widths, height of electrical switches and water fountains, and those other design and construction issues necessary for ADA requirements
- Signage and floor space issues
- Compliance with various codes
- Air circulation and temperature
- Activity and other space allocations
- Lighting requirements
- Noise levels

Risk Management Strategy 4: Develop and implement regular facility inspection schedules.

To meet the duty owed to facility business invitees, facilities should establish and carry out a regular facility inspection schedule and assign specific areas to particular employees for inspection. Such inspections should be of essentially all facility areas—inside and outside—and should be completed in accordance with manufacturer specifications as well as other published standards and guidelines.

Given the recent case law on facility physical plant issues and appreciating the duties owed to health/fitness facility members and other similarly situated persons, it is necessary to have a risk management plan in place to deal with these risks. Such a plan must begin with a complete initial survey of a facility's physical plant to determine the status of the facility. Such determinations also need to be performed thereafter on a regular basis—which might be as short in duration as after every use of an area, or on a daily, weekly, monthly, quarterly, or as long as yearly schedule for other issues. Industry standards and guidelines in this regard can be of importance and serve as a valuable resource for health/fitness professionals.

Risk Management Strategy 5: Develop and implement maintenance and cleaning schedules.

Regular cleaning and maintenance schedules for health/fitness facilities need to be developed to ensure that the standard of care owed to business invitees is met by facilities. Such maintenance and cleaning schedules need to be established in accordance with manufacturer specifications as well as other published standards and guidelines and address all areas of the facility—inside and outside.

Because of the increased risks that facilities such as hot tubs, steam rooms, and whirlpools present, it is critical that proper maintenance and cleaning strategies are in place to help minimize injuries associated with using such facilities. As indicated from the case law and several of the published standards of practice presented in this chapter, maintaining proper temperature is critical along with appropriate warning systems. Maintaining proper pool chemistry levels is also essential.

Risk Management Strategy 6: Post and maintain facility signage.

Facility signage needs to be developed and maintained in accordance with the needs of the facility and its participants and in compliance with the law (e.g., ADA), standards of practice published by professional organizations, and manufacturers of facilities such as saunas, steam rooms, hot tubs, and so on. Professional assistance may be needed to ensure that the signage is appropriate and consistent with these requirements and recommendations. In addition, signs should be posted in locations where participants can easily see them and use appropriate symbols and word messages so they are properly understood and interpreted.

Risk Management Strategy 7: Plan carefully for outdoor and off-premise activities.

Facility recommendations for the performance of outdoor and off-premise activities by participants need to be carefully thought out because away-from-facility activities can involve multiple risk management issues. These include area concerns such as those related to environmental issues, potential criminal activities of third parties, dangers and concerns presented by wild animals, motor vehicles, and other hazards, as well as those issues dealing with instruction, supervision, and emergency response. It is important to warn participants of these potential risks. See Figures 10-1 and 10-2.

For sponsored events, for example, a bicycle race or triathlon, organizers need to prepare for and plan each event carefully. Organizers should select routes with care, and select courses that are safe. Organizers must also effectively control courses from entry by motor vehicles. Finally, organizers should use waivers that are carefully written and meet the requirements in their state. However in this regard, waivers should be broadly written so the contemplated activity will be within the contemplation of the signer.

Still, even with well-written waivers, event organizers should not rely completely on waivers for protection. This is illustrated by the fact that the same waiver was used in three of the cases cited in this chapter. In two cases, *Buchan*[75] and *Okura*[78], the waiver was upheld and protected the defendant from liability. The same waiver, however, was not upheld in *Bennett*[82] because the court felt the presence of an automobile on the course was not within the contemplation of Bennett when he signed the waiver.

Risk Management Strategy 8: Keep records of all facility installations, inspections, and maintenance and cleaning schedules.

Records of all facility installations, regular inspections, and maintenance and cleaning schedules need to be maintained in documented form for a period of time to conform to the applicable statutes of limitation for personal injury/wrongful death actions and based on advice from facility legal counsel. These records should be kept in a secure location.

✓ PUT INTO PRACTICE CHECKLIST 10-1

Rate your phase of development for each of the following risk management strategies related to facility risks:

	Developed	Partially Developed	Not Developed
1. Complying with the ADA.			
2. Establishing a check-in system to monitor facility access.			
3. Following facility design and construction specifications.			
4. Developing and implementing regular facility inspection schedules.			
5. Developing and implementing maintenance and cleaning schedules.			
6. Posting and maintaining facility signage.			
7. Planning carefully for outdoor and off-premise activities.			
8. Keeping records of all facility installations, inspections, maintenance, and cleaning schedules.			

SUMMARY

Health/fitness facilities need to be properly designed, constructed, and maintained to minimize those risks to business invitees in the use of those facilities. Facilities have an obligation to make their premises reasonably safe for their business invitees and to warn of those risks that they know or could be reasonably discovered. As presented in this chapter, a variety of liability exposures exist related to the use of health/fitness facilities, both inside and outside the facility as well as any off-premises activities. Compliance with the requirements of federal and state laws and regulations, including the ADA, should minimize the legal exposures presented by such laws to facilities. Adhering to published standards of practice and manufacturer specifications regarding installation, inspection, maintenance and cleaning, and signage will also minimize those risks associated with the physical plant of such facilities.

RISK MANAGEMENT ASSIGNMENTS

1. Develop a list of those potential risks associated with the physical plant of a typical health/fitness facility.

   _____

   _____

   _____

   _____

2. Prepare an entry/check-in, check-out plan to identify who may be in health/fitness facilities at any given time, and be prepared to discuss why that information is important—at least potentially.

   _____

   _____

   _____

   _____

3. Consider the possible risks (and identify risk management strategies to address each risk) that might occur as to a specific off-premise activity (e.g., personal training in a client's home or a sponsored event like a triathlon).

   _____

   _____

   _____

   _____

4. Design a facility inspection, maintenance, and cleaning schedule for a particular area of a facility.

   _____

   _____

   _____

   _____

5. Decide and plan for facility compliance in its physical plant for the ADA compliance.

   _____

   _____

   _____

   _____

KEY TERMS

Business invitees   Licensee   Trespasser

REFERENCES

1. Sawyer TH, ed. *Facility Design and Management for Health, Fitness, Physical Activity, Recreation and Sports Facility Development.* 11th ed. Champaign, Ill: Sagamore Publishing; 2005.
2. *Bertrand v. Palm Springs and European Health Spa, Inc.,* 257 Or. 532 (Or., 1971).
3. *Bertrand v. Palm Springs and European Health Spa, Inc.,* 257 Or. 532 (Or., 1971):535.
4. *Bertrand v. Palm Springs and European Health Spa, Inc.,* 257 Or. 532 (Or., 1971):536.
5. *Brown v. Racquetball Centers, Inc.,* 369 Pa. Super. 13 (Pa. Super. Ct., 1987).
6. *Woolsey v. Holiday Health Clubs and Fitness Centers, Inc.,* 820 P.2d 1201 (Colo. Ct. App., 1991).
7. *Leenen v. Ruttgers Ocean Beach Lodge, Ltd.,* 662 F.Supp. 240 (S.D., Fla., Miami Div., 1987).
8. *Leon v. Family Fitness Center,* 61 Cal. App. 4th 1227 (Cal. Ct. App., 1998).
9. *Hoffman v. New Life Fitness Centers, Inc.,* 116 Ohio App.3d 737 (Ohio Ct. App., 1996).
10. *Hutto v. Gold's Gym, Inc.,* 703 S0.2d 974 (Ala. Civ. App., 1996), and *Peterson v. Summit Fitness, Inc.,* 920 SW 2d 928 (Mo. Ct. App., 1996).
11. Herbert DL, Herbert WG. *Legal Aspects of Preventive, Rehabilitative and Recreational Exercise Programs.* 4th ed. Canton, Ohio: PRC; 2002.
12. Herbert DL, Herbert WG. *Legal Aspects of Preventive, Rehabilitative and Recreational Exercise Programs.* 4th ed. Canton, Ohio: PRC; 2002:227–228.
13. *Montalvo v. Radcliffe,* 167 F.3 873 (4th Cir., 1999).
14. *Montalvo v. Radcliffe,* 528 U.S. 813 (U.S., 1999).
15. *Montalvo v. Radcliffe,* 528 U.S. 813 (U.S., 1999):875.
16. *Montalvo v. Radcliffe.* Analyzed in: Herbert DL. Barring individuals from activity—Defending against ADA claims. *Exercise Standards and Malpractice Reporter.* 1999; 13(2):25–26, 25.
17. *Montalvo v. Radcliffe,* 528 U.S. 813 (U.S., 1999):875–876.
18. *Montalvo v. Radcliffe.* Analyzed in: Herbert DL. Barring individuals from activity—Defending against ADA claims. *Exercise Standards and Malpractice Reporter.* 1999;13(2): 25–26, 25–26.
19. *Montalvo v. Radcliffe,* 167 F.3 873 (4th Cir., 1999):874.
20. *Montalvo v. Radcliffe.* Analyzed in: Herbert DL. Barring individuals from activity—Defending against ADA claims. *Exercise Standards and Malpractice Reporter.* 1999;13(2):25–26, 26.
21. *Kuketz v. Petronelli,* 443 Mass. 355 (Mass., 2005).
22. *Kuketz v. Petronelli,* 443 Mass. 355 (Mass., 2005):355.
23. *Kuketz v. Petronelli,* 443 Mass. 355 (Mass., 2005):356–357.
24. *Kuketz v. Petronelli,* 443 Mass. 355 (Mass., 2005):357–359.
25. *Kuketz v. Petronelli,* 443 Mass. 355 (Mass., 2005):359–360.
26. *Kuketz v. Petronelli,* 443 Mass. 355 (Mass., 2005):360.
27. *Kuketz v. Petronelli,* 443 Mass. 355 (Mass., 2005):361–362.
28. *Kuketz v. Petronelli,* 443 Mass. 355 (Mass., 2005):362.
29. *Kuketz v. Petronelli,* 443 Mass. 355 (Mass., 2005):365–366.
30. *Claveloux v. Downtown Racquet Club Assoc.,* 691 A. 2d 1112 (Conn. App. Ct., 1997). Analyzed in: Paralyzed racquetball player's action to proceed against club. *Exercise Standards and Malpractice Reporter.* 1997;11(5):69.
31. *Weithofer v. Unique Racquetball and Health Clubs, Inc.,* 621 N.Y.S.2d. 384 (N.Y. App. Div., 1995). Analyzed in: Suit against health club dismissed. *Exercise Standards and Malpractice Reporter.* 1998;12(2):24.
32. *Jacobsen v. Holiday Health Club* (Civil Action No. A85, CV 1249, Arapaho County, Colo., 1986). Analyzed in: Rabinoff MA. An examination of four recent cases against fitness instructors. *Exercise Standards and Malpractice Reporter.* 1988;2(3):43–47.
33. Richie DH. Medical legal implications of dance exercise leadership: The aerobic dance floor surface. *Exercise Standards and Malpractice Reporter.* 1988;2(6):87–88.
34. Richie DH. Medical legal implications of dance exercise leadership: The role of footwear. *Exercise Standards and Malpractice Reporter.* 1989;3(4):60–63.

35. *Goynias v. Spa Health Clubs, Inc.,* 148 N.C. App. 554 (N.C. Ct. App., 2002).
36. *Goynias v. Spa Health Clubs, Inc.,* 148 N.C. App. 554 (N.C. Ct. App., 2002):555.
37. *Goynias v. Spa Health Clubs, Inc.,* 148 N.C. App. 554 (N.C. Ct. App., 2002):555–556.
38. *Goynias v. Spa Health Clubs, Inc.,* 148 N.C. App. 554 (N.C. Ct. App., 2002):556–557.
39. Herbert DL. Equipment deficiencies and improper instruction. *Fitness Manage.* January 1989:12–19.
40. Herbert DL, Herbert WG. Frequent claims and suits in equipment related injuries. *Fitness Manage.* July 1988:22.
41. Rabinoff MA. An examination of four recent cases against fitness instructors. *Exercise Standards and Malpractice Reporter.* 1988;2(3):43–47.
42. Herbert DL. Legal aspects of water based fitness activities. *Fitness Manage.* March 1988:37.
43. *Leenen v. Ruttgers Ocean Beach Lodge, Ltd.,* 662 F.Supp. 240 (S.D., Fla., Miami Div., 1987). Analyzed in: Superheated hot tub leads to significant claim and suit. *Exercise Standards and Malpractice Reporter.* 1988;2(1):11–12.
44. Herbert DL. Superheated hot tub case resolved for substantial settlement. *Exercise Standards and Malpractice Reporter.* 1989;3(2):23–25.
45. *Simon v. Eaton Corp., et al,* Case No. 88-CV-1835, El Paso County District Court, El Paso, Colo., affirmed and remanded, 876 P.2d 10 (Colo. Ct. App., 1993).
46. *Tirella v. American Properties Team, Inc.,* 535 N.Y.S. 2d 252 (N.Y. App. Div., 1988).
47. *Woolsey v. Holiday Health Clubs and Fitness Centers, Inc.,* 820 P.2d 1201 (Colo. Ct. App., 1991). Analyzed in: Whirlpool death claim results in verdict in favor of health club. *Exercise Standards and Malpractice Reporter.* 1992;6(2):23.
48. Two corporate challenge series participants die. *Exercise Standards and Malpractice Reporter.* 1988;2(6):94.
49. *Gehling v. St. George University School of Medicine,* 698 F. Supp. 419 (E.D. N.Y., 1988).
50. *Hoffman v. New Life Fitness Centers, Inc.,* 116 Ohio App.3d 737 (Ohio Ct. App., 1996). Analyzed in: Can tanning beds facilitate transmission of herpes virus? Substantial award to health club patron overturned on appeal. *Exercise Standards and Malpractice Reporter.* 1998;12(2):25.
51. *State Farm and Casualty v. Scandinavian,* 104 Ohio App.3d. 582 (Ohio Ct. App., 1995). Analyzed in: Herbert DL. Action for theft of member's property not barred by health club release. *Exercise Standards and Malpractice Reporter.* 1996;10(3):38–39.
52. Koeberle BE. Outdoor training: A trainer's duty to inspect and warn. *Exercise Standards and Malpractice Reporter.* 1990;4(2):21–22.
53. Herbert DL. Selected liability considerations of prescribed but unsupervised cardiac rehabilitation activities. *Exercise Standards and Malpractice Reporter.* 1988;2(6):89–94.
54. Kenney WL. Considerations for preventive and rehabilitative exercise programs during periods of high heat and humidity. *Exercise Standards and Malpractice Reporter.* 1989;3(1):1, 4–8.
55. *Wight v. Ohio State University,* 112 O.Misc.2d 13 (Ohio Ct. Cl., 2001) and Heat stress at police academy. *Exercise Standards and Malpractice Reporter.* 1989;3(1):8.
56. 'Inflexible' rule results in death due to heat stress. *Exercise Standards and Malpractice Reporter.* 1991;5(4):62.
57. Herbert DL. Another heat stroke race victim. *Exercise Standards and Malpractice Reporter.* 1995;9(5):73.
58. Good risk management advice for joggers from the American Running Association. *Exercise Standards and Malpractice Reporter.* 1999;13(6):91.
59. *Davis v. City of Miami,* 568 S0.2d 1301 (Fla. Dist. Ct. App., 1990).
60. Club not liable for criminal attack. *Exercise Standards and Malpractice Reporter.* 1998;12(3):37.
61. *Simpson v. Big Bear Stores,* 73 Ohio St. 3d 130 (Ohio, 1995), 135. Analyzed in: Herbert DL. Business owner's liability for third party criminal attacks defined in Ohio—Implications for fitness professionals. *Exercise Standards and Malpractice Reporter.* 1995;9(5):71.
62. *Weade v. Vancouver School Dist. 37,* 93–2-04062–1 (Supreme Court, Clark County, Washington), reported in: Verdicts and Settlements. The National Law Journal, Monday, August 21, 1995, p. A9. Analyzed in: Liability may exist for recommended off-premises activities. *Exercise Standards and Malpractice Reporter.* 1995;9(5):72.
63. California hunting mountain lion that ambushed jogger. *The Repository* [Canton, Ohio]. April 28, 1994:A-11.
64. Can health/fitness facilities be liable for third-party criminal attacks on patrons? *Exercise Standards and Malpractice Reporter.* 1994;8(4):60.

65. One injured jogger recovers damages while another's suit results in defense verdict. *Exercise Standards and Malpractice Reporter.* 1992;6(3):39–40.

66. Cities not liable for alleged negligence in park activities. *Exercise Standards and Malpractice Reporter.* 1991;5(6):93–94.

67. Herbert DL. Jogger's attack in high crime area leads to suit. *Exercise Standards and Malpractice Reporter.* 1991;5(2):29–30.

68. Herbert DL. An examination of litigation related to runners' deaths. *Exercise Standards and Malpractice Reporter.* 1990;4(3):42–45.

69. Provider's alleged advice to ski may result in liability. *Exercise Standards and Malpractice Reporter.* 1990;4(1):13–14.

70. *Dennis v. City of Tampa,* 581 S0.2d 1345 (Fla. Dist. Ct. App., 1991), and *Prunier v. City of Watertown,* 936 F.2d 677 (2nd Cir., 1991). Analyzed in: Cities not liable for alleged negligence in park activities. *Exercise Standards and Malpractice Reporter.* 1991;5(6):93–94.

71. Herbert DL. Recreational user statutes: Are they serving their purpose? *Sports, Parks and Recreation Law Reporter.* 1987;1(1):10–13.

72. *McDonough v. National Off-Road Bicycle Assn.,* 1999 WL 309503 (D. Del., 1997).

73. *McDonough v. National Off-Road Bicycle Assn.,* 1999 WL 309503 (D. Del., 1997):6.

74. *Staadecker v. The Emerald Health Network,* 1993 WL 526679 (Ohio Ct. App., 1993).

75. *Buchan v. U.S. Cycling Federation. Inc.,* 277 Cal. Rptr. 887 (Cal. Ct. App., 1991).

76. *Watts v. Country Cycle Club, Inc.,* 1997 N.Y. App. Div. LEXIS 2349 (N.Y. App. Div., 1997).

77. *Peters v. U.S. Cycling Federation,* 779 F.Supp. 853 (E.D. Ky., 1991).

78. *Okura v. U.S. Cycling Federation,* 231 Cal. Rptr. 429 (Cal. Ct. App., 1986).

79. *Banfield v. Louis,* 589 S0.2d 441 (Fla. Dist. Ct. App., 1991).

80. *Walton v. Oz Bicycle Club of Wichita,* 1991 WL 257088 (D. Kan., 1991).

81. *Coles v. Jenkins,* 1997 WL 820959 (W.D. Va., 1997).

82. *Bennett v. U.S. Cycling Federation,* 193 Cal. App.3d 1485 (Cal. Ct. App., 1987).

83. *Coles v. Jenkins,* 1997 WL 820959 (W.D. Va., 1997):3.

84. *Bennett v. U.S. Cycling Federation,* 193 Cal. App.3d 1485 (Cal. Ct. App., 1987):1490.

85. Tharrett SJ, McInnis KJ, Peterson JA, eds. ACSM's *Health/Fitness Facility Standards and Guidelines.* 3rd ed. Champaign, Ill: Human Kinetics; 2007.

86. Tharrett SJ, McInnis KJ, Peterson JA, eds. ACSM's *Health/Fitness Facility Standards and Guidelines.* 3rd ed. Champaign, Ill: Human Kinetics; 2007:2.

87. American College of Sports Medicine and American Heart Association Joint Position Statement. Recommendations for cardiovascular screening, staffing, and emergency policies at health/fitness facilities. *Med Sci Sports Exerc.* 1998;30:1009–1018.

88. *NSCA Strength & Conditioning Professional Standards & Guidelines.* May 2001. Available at: http://www.nscalift.org/Publications/standards.shtml. Colorado Springs: National Strength and Conditioning Association (NSCA) Accessed September 2, 2007:15.

89. IHRSA Club Membership Standards. In: *IHRSA's Guide to Club Membership & Conduct.* 3rd ed. Boston: International Health, Racquet & Sportsclub Association (IHRSA); 2005.

90. IHRSA Club Membership Standards. In: *IHRSA's Guide to Club Membership & Conduct.* 3rd ed. Boston: International Health, Racquet & Sportsclub Association (IHRSA); 2005:2.

91. IHRSA Club Membership Standards. In: *IHRSA's Guide to Club Membership & Conduct.* 3rd ed. Boston: International Health, Racquet & Sportsclub Association (IHRSA); 2005:3.

92. IHRSA Club Membership Standards. In: *IHRSA's Guide to Club Membership & Conduct.* 3rd ed. Boston: International Health, Racquet & Sportsclub Association (IHRSA); 2005:5.

93. *Canadian Fitness Safety Standards & Recommended Guidelines.* 3rd ed. 2004. Available at: http://www/oases.on.ca/safety/safetyStdsCurrent.htm. Ontario, Canada: Ontario Association of Sport and Exercise Sciences (OASES). Accessed September 2, 2007.

94. *Canadian Fitness Safety Standards & Recommended Guidelines.* 3rd ed. 2004. Available at: http://www/oases.on.ca/safety/safetyStdsCurrent.htm. Ontario, Canada: Ontario Association of Sport and Exercise Sciences (OASES). Accessed September 2, 2007:2.

95. *Canadian Fitness Safety Standards & Recommended Guidelines.* 3rd ed. 2004. Available at: http://www/oases.on.ca/safety/safetyStdsCurrent.htm. Ontario, Canada: Ontario Association of Sport and Exercise Sciences (OASES). Accessed September 2, 2007:3.

96. *The Medical Fitness Model: Facility Standards and Guidelines,* Richmond, Va: Medical Fitness Association (MFA); May 2006:13.

97. *Medical Advisory Committee Recommendations: A Resource Guide for YMCAs.* Chicago: YMCA of the USA; February 2007.

98. *Medical Advisory Committee Recommendations: A Resource Guide for YMCAs.* Chicago: YMCA of the USA; February 2007:116.

APPENDIX 10

The following information has been reprinted from the Owner's Manual of the Cybex 750T Treadmill:

Chapter 1 – Safety (Pages 1-1 to 1-6)

Reprinted, with permission, from the Owner's Manual of the Cybex 750T Treadmill, Rev C, Copyright, 2007. Cybex International Inc., 10 Trotter Drive, Medway, MA 02053.

Cybex 750T Treadmill Owner's Manual

1 - Safety

IMPORTANT: Read all instructions and warnings before using the treadmill.

Important Voltage Information

Before plugging the power cord into an electrical outlet, verify that the voltage requirements for your area match the voltage of the treadmill that you have received. The power requirements for the Cybex 750T Treadmill include a grounded, dedicated circuit, rated for one of the following:

- 100 VAC, 50/60 Hz, 20A
- 115 VAC, 60 Hz, 20A
- 220 VAC, 60 Hz, 15A
- 230 VAC, 50 Hz, 15A
- 230 VAC, 50 Hz, 13A

See the serial number decal for the exact voltage requirements of your treadmill.

! WARNING: Do not attempt to use this unit with a voltage adapter. Do not attempt to use this unit with an extension cord.

! WARNING: Do not plug more than one unit into a single circuit.

Grounding Instructions

This treadmill must be grounded. If it should malfunction or break down, grounding provides a path of least resistance for electric current to reduce the risk of electric shock. This product is equipped with a cord having an equipment-grounding conductor and a grounding plug. The plug must be plugged into an appropriate outlet that is properly installed and grounded in accordance with all local codes and ordinances.

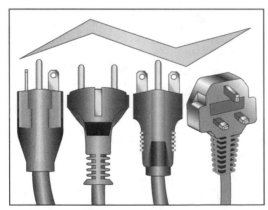

115 VAC   Euro Plug   220 VAC   UK
NEMA 5-20   CEE 7/7   NEMA 6-15   230 VAC

! DANGER: Improper connection of the equipment-grounding conductor can result in a risk of electric shock. Check with a qualified electrician or service provider if you are in doubt as to whether the treadmill is properly grounded. Seek a qualified electrician to perform any modifications to the cord or plug. Cybex is not responsible for injuries or damages as a result of cord or plug modification.

This treadmill is for use on a grounded, dedicated circuit. Make sure that the treadmill is connected to an outlet having the same configuration as the plug. Do not use a ground plug adapter to adapt the power cord to a non-grounded outlet.

Cybex 750T Treadmill Owner's Manual

Important Safety Instructions

(Save These Instructions)

! DANGER: **To reduce the risk of electric shock, always unplug this treadmill from the electrical outlet immediately after using it and before cleaning it.**

! WARNING: **Serious injury could occur if these precautions are not observed. To reduce the risk of burns, fires, electric shock, or injury:**

User Safety Precautions

- Obtain a medical exam before beginning any exercise program.
- Stop exercising if you feel faint, dizzy, or experience pain and consult your physician.
- Obtain instruction before using.
- Read and understand the Owner's Manual and all warnings posted on the unit before using.
- Read and understand emergency stop procedures.
- **DO NOT** wear loose or dangling clothing while using the treadmill.
- Keep all body parts, towels, water bottles and the like free and clear of moving parts.
- Place your feet on the two top steps when starting or stopping the treadmill.
- Use the treadmill handrails for support and to maintain balance.
- Keep children away from the treadmill. Teenagers and disabled persons must be supervised while using.
- **DO NOT** use the unit if you exceed 400 lbs. (181 kg). This is the rated maximum user weight.
- Report any malfunctions, damage or repairs to the facility.
- Replace any warning labels if damaged, worn or illegible.
- Stop and place the treadmill at 0 degrees incline (level) after each use.
- Disconnect power before servicing.

Facility Safety Precautions

- Instruct all users on how to clip the e-stop clip onto their clothing and carefully test it prior to using the treadmill.
- Instruct all users to use caution when mounting and dismounting the treadmill.

Cybex 750T Treadmill Owner's Manual

- Use a dedicated line when operating the treadmill. *NOTE: A dedicated line requires one circuit breaker per unit.*

- Connect the treadmill to a properly grounded outlet only.

- **DO NOT** operate electrically powered treadmills in damp or wet locations.

- Keep the running belt clean and dry at all times.

- **DO NOT** leave the treadmill unattended when plugged in and running. *NOTE: Before leaving the treadmill unattended, always wait until the treadmill comes to a complete stop and is level. Then, turn all controls to the STOP or OFF position and remove the plug from the outlet. Remove the e-stop key from the treadmill.*

- Immobilize the treadmill (when not in use) by removing the e-stop key.

- Inspect the treadmill for worn or loose components before each use. Do not use until worn or damaged parts are replaced.

- Maintain and replace worn parts regularly. Refer to "Preventive Maintenance" section of Owner's Manual.

- **DO NOT** operate the treadmill if: (1) the cord is damaged; (2) the treadmill is not working properly or (3) if the treadmill has been dropped or damaged. Seek service from a qualified technician.

- **DO NOT** place the cord near heated surfaces or sharp edges.

- **DO NOT** use the treadmill outdoors.

- **DO NOT** operate the treadmill around or where aerosol (spray) or where oxygen products are being used.

- Read and understand the Owner's Manual completely before using the treadmill.

- Ensure all users wear proper footwear on or around all Cybex equipment.

- Set up and operate the treadmill on a solid, level surface. Do not operate in recessed areas or on plush carpet.

- Provide the following clearances: 19.7 inches (0.5 m) at each side, 79 inches (2.0 m) at the back and enough room for safe access and passage at the front of the treadmill. Be sure your treadmill is clear of walls, equipment and other hard surfaces.

- **DO NOT** attempt repairs, electrical or mechanical. Seek qualified repair personnel when servicing. If you live in the USA, contact Cybex Customer Service at 888-462-9239. If you live outside the USA, contact Cybex Customer Service at 508-533-4300.

- Use Cybex factory parts when replacing parts on the treadmill.

- **DO NOT** modify the treadmill in any way.

- **DO NOT** use attachments unless recommended for the treadmill by Cybex.

- Ensure all User and Facility Safety Precautions are observed.

Cybex 750T Treadmill Owner's Manual

- Carefully read and understand the following before using the 750T treadmill:

  - Warning Decals
  - Caution Decals

To replace any worn or damaged decals do one of the following: Visit www.cybexinternational.com to shop for parts online, fax your order to 508-533-5183 or contact Cybex Customer Service at 888-462-9239. If you live outside of the USA, call 508-533-4300. For location or part number of labels, see the parts list and exploded-view diagram. This information can be found in the *Service* chapter in this manual or on the Cybex web site at www.cybexinternational.com.

Warning Decals

Warning decals indicate a potentially hazardous situation, which, if not avoided, could result in death or serious injury. The warning decals used on the Cybex 750T are shown below.

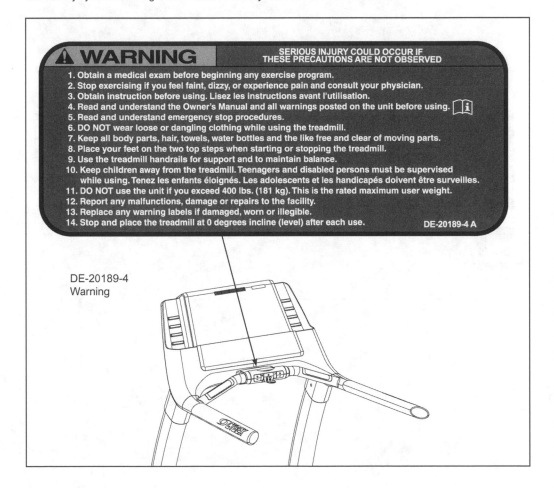

DE-20189-4
Warning

Cybex 750T Treadmill Owner's Manual

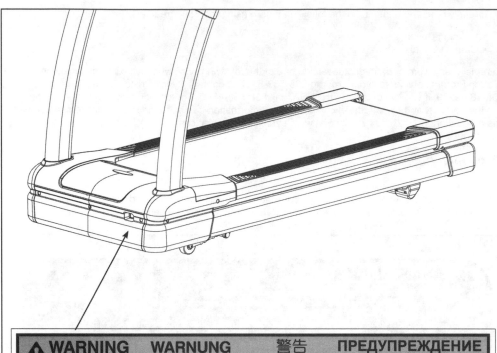

⚠ **WARNING   WARNUNG   警告   ПРЕДУПРЕЖДЕНИЕ**
AVERTISSEMENT   ADVERTENCIA   VARNING

DISCONNECT POWER BEFORE SERVICING.	DÉBRANCHEZ L'ALIMENTATION AVANT DE FAIRE L'ENTRETIEN	VOR SERVICEAR-BEITEN NETZSTECKER ZIEHEN.	CORTE LA ENERGIA ELECTRICA ANTES DE REPARAR.	修理点検の前に電源を切って下さい。	KOPPLA IFRÅN STRÖMMEN INNAN SERVICE UTFÖRS.	ОТКЛЮЧИТЕ ПИТАНИЕ, ПРЕЖДЕ ЧЕМ ПРИСТУПАТЬ К ОБСЛУЖИВАНИЮ.

DE-16928

DE-16928
Warning Motor
Cover

Cybex 750T Treadmill Owner's Manual

Caution Decals

Caution decals indicate a potentially hazardous situation, which if not avoided, may result in minor or moderate injury. There are no caution decals used on this unit. However, there are caution statements listed in Chapters 5 and 6 of this manual. See Chapters 5 and 6.

Emergency Stop Key (e-stop)

The e-stop key functions as an emergency stop. In an emergency situation, the e-stop key disengages from the console and the treadmill will come to a stop. Before using the treadmill, clip the e-stop key as described below.

1. Compress the spring and clip the e-stop clamp to your clothing. Ensure the clip engages enough clothing so it does not fall off in an emergency situation. See Figure 1. *NOTE: Be sure the string is free of knots and has enough slack for you to workout comfortably with the e-stop key in place.*

2. Without falling off the treadmill, carefully step backward until the e-stop pulls out of the console. See Figure 2. *NOTE: If the e-stop clip falls off your clothing then the test has failed. Reclip the e-stop clip to your clothing and repeat this step.*

3. Replace the e-stop key. See Figure 2.

4. The treadmill is now ready to be used. *NOTE: Ensure the the e-stop clip is secured to your clothing at all times during use.*

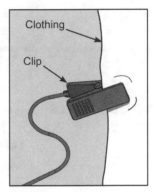

Figure 1

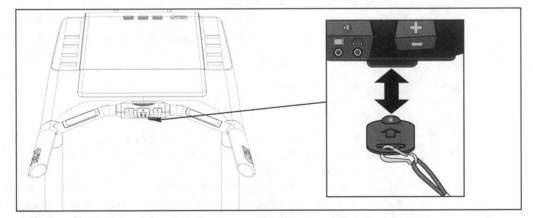

Figure 2

5. After use, remove the e-stop key from the treadmill.

NOTE: The e-stop key shall be removed to help prevent unauthorized use. Refer to the Stopping the Treadmill section in the Operation chapter for more information about the e-stop key.

CHAPTER 11

Medical Emergency Action Plans

LEARNING OBJECTIVES After reading this chapter, health/fitness students and professionals will be able to:

1. Understand the laws that apply to medical emergency action planning in health/fitness facilities.

2. Appreciate the professional and legal need to plan and practice appropriate and legally sufficient responses for medical emergencies.

3. Describe the various published standards of practice applicable to medical emergency action planning in health/fitness facilities.

4. Understand the major elements of a medical emergency action plan (EAP).

5. Develop risk management strategies related to medical emergency action planning in health/fitness facilities.

This chapter describes the professional and legal need to plan and practice for medical emergencies in health/fitness programs. As presented in Chapter 1, medical emergencies can occur because of **health risks**, for example, medical conditions and/or risk factors that can lead to problems such as a cardiac arrest, stroke, or an insulin reaction, and **injury risks,** for example, conditions or situations that can lead to problems such as a back injury, fractured bone, or cut/abrasion that causes bleeding. Health/fitness personnel have a legal obligation to render and/or secure the appropriate emergency care when situations due to either of these risks arise. This chapter describes administrative, statutory, and case law as well as published standards of practice as they relate to medical emergency action planning. Finally, risk management strategies are presented to guide health/fitness professionals and their risk management advisory committees in the development of their own risk management strategies related to medical emergency action planning.

Although this chapter focuses on planning for and responding to medical emergencies, prudent health/fitness facility managers/owners, professionals, and risk management committees also need to plan for a wide range of other potential emergencies. These may include but are not limited to plans for dealing with a violent person, bomb threat, terrorist activity, fire, major power failure, and environmental emergencies such as a flood, tornado, or hurricane. It is recommended that health/fitness facility owners and operators work with local authorities to develop such plans, which in several of these cases involve developing and practicing an evacuation plan.

In January 2002 there were 17,807 commercial health clubs in the United States.[1] By January 2005, this number increased to 26,830[2] with club memberships totaling 41.3 million.[3] In 2006, there were more than 2,600 YMCAs in the United States serving over 20 million people.[4] Furthermore, these data do not reflect the proliferation of many other health/fitness facilities, such as corporate, university/college, hospital-based, government, and retirement settings. As the number of health/fitness facilities and participants continues to increase, so do the chances for medical emergencies. In addition to the rising number of facilities and participants, member demographics have also changed. For example, the percentage of members 55 years and older has greatly increased and remains one of the fastest growing segments of new health/fitness program population. Furthermore, members past the historically typical retirement age often use their memberships more frequently than younger members.[5]

The American Heart Association (AHA) estimates that one in three adult men and women in the United States have some form of cardiovascular disease.[6] Although regular exercise reduces the risk of cardiovascular disease and death, the chance of a cardiovascular event occurring during exercise among people with cardiac disease is estimated to be at least 10 times more than that among apparently healthy individuals.[7] Because of the increase of participation in health/fitness activity, particularly by those in older age groups and/or those with known cardiovascular disease and/or cardiovascular risks, health/fitness professionals must plan and prepare for medical emergencies such as **sudden cardiac arrest (SCA)**, the occurrence of which must be said to be clearly foreseeable. In addition to being prepared for such potentially life-threatening cardiovascular events, health/fitness personnel also need to be prepared to handle other potentially serious injuries such as fractured bones, back injuries, and so on, as well as those less serious, such as a sprained ankle. Both of these types of medical emergencies occur in health/fitness facilities with some regularity as pointed out in the many case law examples described throughout this book. And, unfortunately, the legal liability claims that result can be quite costly (see Table 1-2 in Chapter 1). Therefore, health/fitness facilities must have a well thought-out, written, medical emergency action plan that addresses all types of legally foreseeable medical emergencies.

Although many injuries sustained during participation in health/fitness programs are relatively minor, potential serious and life-threatening emergencies can be unpredictable and sometimes occur without warning. The short- and long-term effects of a medical emergency largely depend on whether an adequate plan exists to handle the emergency. Those involved in providing health/fitness activities must not only try to prevent medical emergencies (through **loss prevention** strategies), they must also plan and practice for them to mitigate the events (through **loss reduction** strategies) when they do occur.

STEP 1 ASSESSMENT OF LEGAL LIABILITY EXPOSURES

Although it is very important to plan and prepare for medical emergencies from a legal and risk management perspective, several studies suggested that many health/fitness facilities may not be doing so adequately. A 1997 survey of health/fitness facilities in Massachusetts[8] revealed that approximately half of the programs that responded to the survey did not practice their medical emergency action plans in accordance with published standards of practice. Another study,[9] conducted in 2000, suggested that the majority (53%) of the Ohio clubs that responded to that survey did not have a written emergency response plan, and 92% failed to conduct quarterly medical emergency drills as recommended by the ACSM/AHA Joint PP (see Published Standards of Practice later).

The study also revealed that 72% of the respondents either never practiced or did not have a emergency medical action plan, and that only 18% of the respondents were familiar with the ACSM/AHA Joint PP recommendations.

A national study[10,11] conducted in 2001 involving more than 400 health/fitness facilities found that 79% of them had a written emergency action plan but only 61% had taken steps to ensure that staff members fully understood how to implement it. When these data were compared by type of facility, only 37%, 51%, 52%, and 71% had taken these steps among private for profit, community nonprofit, government, and university settings, respectively. The results for clinical and corporate settings were higher with 91% and 83%, respectively.[11] Another study[12] conducted in 2004 involving college/university-based health/fitness facilities found that although 92% had a written emergency response plan, only 50% posted it, and only 27% did the recommended quarterly emergency drills.

Additional data from some of the studies just cited are also relevant to emergency action plans. The 2000 study[9] and the 2004 study[12] reported 17% and 27%, respectively, of facilities had one or more cardiovascular emergencies (e.g., SCA or sudden cardiac death) occur within these facilities during the previous 5 years. It also appears from these studies that the number of health/fitness facilities that have an automated external defibrillator (AED) has increased dramatically from earlier time periods. The 2000 study reported only 3% of health/fitness facilities had an AED, whereas the 2004 study reported that 73% of facilities had an AED. As to the effectiveness of AEDs in health/fitness facilities, a year-long study of 76 health clubs in Great Britain found that out of eight people who suffered an SCA, an AED along with CPR saved the lives of 75% of them, at least in the short term.[13]

The Law

This section describes administrative and statutory laws and presents several case law examples that apply to emergency medical action plans. Key elements of one federal law—OSHA's Bloodborne Pathogens (BBP) Standard—are presented first, followed by an examination of applicable state laws (immunity statutes and recent state statutes that require health/fitness facilities to have an AED). Next, several case law examples are described to help health/fitness professionals understand and appreciate the many types of negligence claims made by plaintiffs who have experienced a medical emergency and subsequently filed suit predicated on such an issue.

OHSA's Bloodborne Pathogens (BBP) Standard

As described in Chapter 2, numerous administrative agencies—specialized bodies created by legislation at all governmental levels—are granted rule-making power by such legislation to regulate specific activities. Administrative agencies exist at the federal, state, and local level. These agencies investigate problems within their respective jurisdictions; enact rules and regulations that have the force and effect of law; and resolve disputes, similar to court trials, to determine if their rules have been violated and, if so, what sanctions should be imposed for those violations. Federal agencies such as the Occupational Safety and Health Administration (OSHA), as well as a myriad of state and local agencies, make and enforce numerous rules and regulations that impact the operations of health/fitness programs and facilities.

The purpose of OSHA is to assure the safety and health of employees in the United States by setting and enforcing standards; providing training, outreach, and education; establishing partnerships; and encouraging continual improvement in workplace safety and health. Almost all working men and women in America fall under OSHA's jurisdiction.[14] OSHA has many standards that affect the daily operations of health/fitness facilities; however, this section only discusses the Bloodborne Pathogens (BBP) Standard. In addition to the federal OSHA laws, many states administer their own occupational safety and health programs, which must adopt standards and requirements that are at least as effective as the federal OSHA requirements.

The failure to comply with any of OSHA's regulations can result in hefty fines, lawsuits, and interventions imposed by OSHA. At any time, OSHA can conduct an inspection to determine if an employer is compliant with OSHA requirements such as having written OSHA safety plans in place. In 2002, about 75% of all OSHA inspections were random, and of the 6,000 fines issued, 70% were related to an employer's failure to have written safety plans in place.[15] Although it is unknown how many health/fitness facilities have been fined for noncompliance with OHSA's BBP Standard, OSHA violations have been issued. For example, a California gym paid $37,825 for violations including improper fatality/injury reporting; a New Jersey fitness center paid $4,500 for violations including the failure to maintain a proper log of occupational injures and illnesses; and a Massachusetts health club paid $7,500 for violations including the failure to providing proper eye, face, and hand protection for its workers.[15]

The OSHA Bloodborne Pathogens Standard[16] became effective in March 1992. The purpose of the **bloodborne pathogens** standard is to eliminate or reduce **occupational exposure** to blood and **other potentially infectious materials (OPIM)** in the work environment that could lead to disease or death. Two well-known pathogens are the human immunodeficiency virus (HIV) and the hepatitis B virus (HBV). The BBP Standard affects employees in many types of occupations and is not exclusive to the medical or health care industries. OSHA, however, has not identified all occupations where exposures could occur, but rather leaves it up to employers to determine where exposure occurs.

The BBP Standard applies to all employers whose employees could be "reasonably anticipated," as the result of performing their job duties, to come in contact with blood and/or other potentially infectious materials. The occupational exposure must be reasonably anticipated. For example, the employer would reasonably anticipate that contact with blood or other potentially infectious materials would occur when a health/fitness employee, certified in first aid, is performing first-aid procedures on a bleeding client. But the employer might not reasonably anticipate that contact with blood or other potentially infectious materials would occur when a sales staff employee is providing a video-demonstrated tour of the health/fitness facility to a potential member.

In addition to being reasonably anticipated, the contact must result from the performance of an employee's job duties. An example of a contact with blood or other potentially infectious materials that would not be considered as an occupational exposure would be a Good Samaritan Act situation. For example, a sales staff employee may assist another employee who has a nosebleed. This would not be considered an occupational exposure unless the employee who provided assistance was expected to render first aid as one of his or her job duties.[16]

It is necessary for employers to know which employees may be potentially exposed so the employer can assure that all provisions of the standard are implemented. This requires that the employer examine the job duties and procedures, and determine if it can be reasonably anticipated, based on such information, that an exposure may occur. Which facility employees are subject to occupational exposure varies from program to program, but several groups may be particularly vulnerable. These may include employees who are responsible for administering first aid and cardiopulmonary resuscitation (CPR); staff who administer cholesterol (i.e., fingerstick) screenings, lifeguards, physical therapists, and athletic trainers. Other such groups may include those responsible for child care, cleaning (janitors, custodians, etc.), or handling bloody laundry, razors, or other types of potentially infectious waste. Employees such as massage therapists, whose positions require close personal contact with clients, may also be at risk of exposure to BBPs.[17]

Compliance with OSHA's Bloodborne Pathogens Standard among health/fitness facilities was investigated in the 2001 study[10,11] described earlier. Of the respondents,

74% of them reported they were compliant. However, when these data were compared among types of facilities, it was found that compliance rates were 52%, 66%, 82%, 83%, 85%, and 95% for private for-profit, community nonprofit, university, government, corporate, and clinical settings, respectively. However, this study did not determine if these facilities were compliant with all of the key elements of this law as described in the following sections. The key elements presented by no means include all the OSHA BBP Standard requirements. Health/fitness managers/owners and professionals should obtain and read a full-text copy of the actual standard, available on the OSHA website (www.osha.org).

Exposure Control Plan The BBP Standard requires employers to establish a "written" exposure control plan (ECP). The plan must outline the protective measures an employer will take to eliminate or reduce employee exposure to blood and OPIM. The exposure control plan, at a minimum, must:

- Identify job classifications, and in some cases, employee tasks and procedures where occupational exposure occurs;
- Contain the procedure for evaluating the circumstances surrounding an **exposure incident**; and
- Contain a schedule of how and when other provisions of the standard will be implemented, including methods of compliance, hepatitis B vaccination and post-exposure follow-up, communication of hazards to employees, and recordkeeping.[18]

The ECP must be accessible to all employees as well as to OSHA representatives. Employees must be able to access a copy of the plan at the workplace during a work shift. The plan may be a part of another document, such as the facility's health and safety or employee manual, as long as all components are included. If the ECP is maintained solely on computer, employees must have training to operate the computer and access the plan. The standard also requires that the ECP be reviewed annually. Additionally, when changes in duties, procedures, or employee positions influence or generate new occupational exposure, the current plan must be reviewed and adjusted accordingly.[18] In the plan, employers must document that they have solicited input from frontline employees in identifying, evaluating, and choosing engineering controls .[19]

Engineering and Work Practice Controls **Engineering controls** are devices that isolate or remove the BBP hazard from the workplace. Examples of such controls include sharps disposal containers and medical waste containers.[19] For example, a facility that offers cholesterol or glucose screenings must provide sharps containers (that are sealable, puncture resistant, leakproof, and labeled) for the disposal of sharps (fingerprick lancets, needles, etc.).

Work practice controls are procedures that reduce the likelihood of exposure by changing the way a task is performed. These include **universal precautions** or body substance isolation, appropriate **handwashing facilities** and procedures, laundry handling, sharps disposing, and contaminated material cleaning.[19]

The adoption of so-called universal precautions is OSHA's required method of control to protect employees from exposure to BBPs and OPIM. The term *universal precautions* refers to a concept of control that requires all human blood and certain human body fluids to be treated as if they were actually infected with HIV, HBV, and/or other bloodborne pathogens. Body substance isolation (BSI) is a control method that defines *all* human body fluids and other substances as infected. BSI includes not only the fluids and materials covered by the BBP Standard, but increases coverage to include all body substances. BSI is an acceptable substitute to universal precautions, provided programs using BSI follow all other provisions of the BBP Standard.[18]

Personal Protective Equipment To be compliant with the applicable requirements, employers must provide **personal protective equipment** such as latex gloves, protective eyewear, and face shields or masks (for administering CPR) at no cost to the employee. Wearing such equipment can significantly reduce health risks for workers exposed to blood and OPIM. Employers must also train employees how to use, remove, and dispose of such items properly. The protective gear must be readily accessible and available in appropriate sizes. Employers must also replace this equipment as needed.[18,20]

If an employee is expected to have hand contact with blood or OPIM (e.g., those responsible for administering first aid) or contaminated surfaces, he or she must wear protective gloves. Single-use gloves must not be washed or decontaminated for reuse. If workers are allergic to standard gloves, the employer must provide hypoallergenic gloves or similar alternatives. Employees must remove personal protective equipment and clothing before leaving the work area or when it becomes contaminated.[20]

Other protective practices include handwashing. If an employee's skin or mucous membranes come into contact with blood or OPIM, he or she is to wash with soap and water and flush their eyes as soon as feasible. Additionally, employees must wash their hands immediately or as soon as feasible after removing protective equipment. If soap and water are not immediately available, employers may provide moist towelettes or other handwashing measures; however, employees must still wash with soap and water as soon as possible.[20]

Hepatitis B Vaccination   Hepatitis B virus is a potentially life-threatening BBP. The Centers for Disease Control and Prevention (CDC) estimates that approximately 280,000 individuals are infected with HBV each year in the United States. Any person with occupational exposure to blood is at risk for contracting HBV.[21]

The HBV vaccination series must be made available at the employer's expense to employees that have occupational exposure. The vaccination must be made available within 10 days of initial assignment. The employer does not have to offer the vaccination to employees who have previously received it, who are immune as evidenced by an antibody test, or who are prohibited from receiving the vaccine because of medical reasons.[18,21]

Employees have the right to refuse the vaccination and/or any postexposure evaluation and follow-up. However, the employee needs to be properly educated regarding the benefits of the vaccine and postexposure evaluation through training. The employee also has the right to accept the vaccination at a later date if he or she chooses, and the employer must make it available at that time. If an employee declines the vaccine, the employer must ensure that the employee signs an HBV vaccine declination form. The declination's wording must be identical to that found in the BBP Standard. A photocopy of the form, found in the standard, may be used or the exact words can be typed onto a separate document.[18,21]

Reporting of Exposure Incidents and Postexposure Follow-Up   It is important to report any exposure incident right away. Early action is crucial and permits immediate medical follow-up. Employers must inform the employee what to do if an exposure incident occurs.

Employers must provide postexposure follow-up to any employee who experiences an exposure incident, at no cost to the employee. This includes conducting laboratory tests; providing confidential medical evaluation from a licensed health care professional; identifying and testing the source individual, if feasible; testing the exposed employee's blood, if he or she consents; conducting postexposure prophylaxis; offering counseling; and evaluating reported illnesses.[19,21,22]

To the extent possible by law, the employer is to determine the source individual for HBV and HIV infectivity. The employee's blood will also be screened if he or she consents. The licensed health care professional must follow the guidelines of the U.S. Public Health Service in providing treatment to the employee, including HBV vaccination. The health care professional is to give a written opinion regarding whether or not the vaccination is recommended and whether the employee received it. Only this information

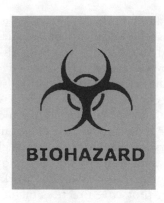

FIGURE 11-1 Biohazard Symbol (Available at: http://www.osha.gov/pls/oshaweb/owadisp.show_document?p_table=STANDARDS&p_id=10051. Accessed June 29, 2006.)

may be reported to the employer. Employee medical records and every diagnosis must remain confidential and are not to be reported to the employer.[19,21,22]

Communication of Hazards to Employees   The BBP Standard requires that employers use labels and signs to communicate hazards. A warning label that includes the universal biohazard symbol, followed by the term *biohazard*, must be affixed to containers of contaminated laundry, bags/containers of regulated waste (i.e., used first aid or cholesterol screening supplies), and other containers used to store or transport blood or OPIM. Facilities can use red bags or containers instead of labels.[16] See Figure 11-1.

Information and Training for Employees   Employers must provide their employees with regular training that covers the risks of bloodborne pathogens, preventive practices, and postexposure procedures. This training must be offered on initial assignment and then at least annually. All employees with occupational exposure, including part-time and temporary employees, must receive initial and annual training. The training must include making a copy of the standard accessible and explaining its contents, a general discussion on bloodborne diseases and their transmission, the exposure control plan, engineering and work practice controls, personal protective equipment, hepatitis B vaccine, response to emergencies involving blood and OPIM, how to handle exposure incidents, postexposure evaluation and follow-up program, and hazard communication (signs, labels, etc.). There must be opportunity for questions and answers, and the person providing the training must be knowledgeable in the subject matter and have expertise in the area of occupational hazards of bloodborne pathogens.[15,18]

Record Keeping.   The OSHA BBP Standard also requires extensive record keeping. For instance, medical records for each employee with an occupational exposure incident must be kept for the duration of employment plus 30 years. These records must be confidential and must include certain specified information. Training records, which must be kept for 3 years from the training date, must contain the dates of the training, the contents or a summary of the training, the names and job titles of everyone who attended the training, and the names and qualifications of the person(s) conducting the training.[18,19]

State Laws

It is clearly a legal duty for health/fitness professionals while on the job to render proper and timely aid to a participant who has experienced a medical emergency. However, the law does not require a health/fitness professional (or any person) to come to the aid of another outside of the facility or beyond the employment relationship. However, to encourage assisting others in peril (e.g., those who have been injured in a car accident), all 50 states have passed so-called Good Samaritan statutes that protect individuals from civil liability (e.g., liability associated with any negligence) if acting in good faith and with no expectation of compensation of any type when they respond to an emergency. In addition, their assistance must be free of any intentional, gross, willful/wanton, or reckless conduct. These statutes do not provide civil liability protection for individuals who originally caused the medical emergency. If able, these individuals generally have a duty to take appropriate action to provide reasonable assistance (e.g., soliciting help, calling 911).

All of the Good Samaritan statutes provide some immunity for individuals acting in good faith in an emergency.[23] Most Good Samaritan statutes specify protection for volunteer health care professionals (e.g., physicians) who provide assistance (e.g., voluntarily at a scene of an accident) without compensation and within the scope of their practice.[23] Most Good Samaritan laws apply to "individual" volunteers. However, in light of events such as 9/11 and Hurricane Katrina, an effort to expand this immunity to organizations and other individuals who assist in such emergencies is under way.[23] However, this effort does not include health/fitness personnel who have a legal duty to provide assistance to a participant in their facility who experiences a medical emergency. It is important that health/fitness professionals understand that these statutes do not apply to them while they are "on the job."

Similar to Good Samaritan statutes, all 50 states and the U.S. federal government have enacted laws that provide at least some degree of protection from civil liability for users of AEDs if their actions are free from any intentional, gross, willful/wanton, or reckless conduct.[24,25] The extent of immunity provided and who it applies to can vary from state to state. For example, in some states for the AED user to have liability protection, the user must have received training and/or be authorized or certified in the use of an AED. Other states extend this immunity provision to: (a) persons/entities that train individuals to use an AED in emergency situations, (b) persons responsible for the site placement of the AED or for the site where the AED is located, (c) persons providing AED-program supervision, and (d) purchasers of the AED. Whether protection is offered to other parties varies from state to state. The advice of an attorney familiar with the laws of a particular state should be sought to determine the type of immunity provided by statute in that state.

Whether or not health/fitness facilities have a legal duty to have an AED has been an issue in several legal cases in recent years (see Case Law later). Professional standards of practice and the law have changed in this area and are continuing to evolve. Many professional organizations now require or recommend health/fitness facilities have an AED (see Published Standards of Practice later), and several states have passed legislation that requires AEDs in health/fitness facilities.[26-28] However, as described in Chapter 1, compliance with such laws in at least in one state (New York) was only 34% among health/fitness facilities. Legislation in this area is rapidly developing, and health/fitness professionals and their risk management advisory committees need to stay abreast of any proposed AED laws in their states. The advice of an attorney familiar with state laws should be sought to determine possible AED statutory requirements in particular jurisdictions.

Although the requirements within these AED state statutes can vary, the following describes some of the provisions within the New Jersey law that requires health clubs, as of January 12, 2007, to have an AED. This bill requires the owner or operator of a registered health cub to:

- Acquire at least one AED . . . and store it in a central location within the health club that is known and available to the employees of the health club;
- Ensure that the AED is tested and maintained, and provide notification to the appropriate first aid, ambulance, or rescue squad or other appropriate emergency medical services provider regarding the defibrillator, the type acquired and its location;

- Arrange and pay for the training in cardiopulmonary resuscitation and the use of an AED for the employees of the health club;
- Ensure that the health club has at least one employee on site during its normal business hours who is trained in cardiopulmonary resuscitation and the use of an AED.[29]

Civil penalties are not less than $250, $500, and $1,000 for first, second, and third violations, respectively. The statute also provides immunity from liability because of any malfunctioning of an AED that has been maintained and tested by the health club based on the manufacturer's guidelines.[28]

Case Law

This section describes certain cases involving employees who feared they had been infected with bloodborne pathogens while performing their jobs. Additional cases address a variety of negligence claims made by plaintiffs after they had experienced some type of medical emergency in a health/fitness facility. These claims involve issues such as the facility's failure to have (a) a proper medical emergency action plan (EAP), (b) qualified staff members to carry out the plan in a timely fashion, and (c) an AED. Cases up to this point involving AEDs have resulted in verdicts (or settlements) for both plaintiffs and defendants. However, as state laws and published standards of practice continue to change (see Published Standards of Practice later), it is essential from a legal liability perspective that health/fitness facilities have an AED and related procedures as part of their written medical EAP and overall risk management plan.

Case Law: Bloodborne Pathogens The following two cases, *Keelean* and *Hartwig*, demonstrate the legal need to comply with OSHA's BBP Standard. In *Keelean et al. v. Department of Corrections*,[30] the plaintiffs Richard Keelean and James Wood were plumbers employed at defendant's Michigan Reformatory in Ionia. As the plaintiffs were pulling on an auger in an attempt to unplug a toilet in inmate Pluckett's cell, a full-sized bath towel, covered with clotted blood, released suddenly and launched from the toilet. The towel sprayed the men with water mixed with blood clots. The blood came from inmate Holmes's cell, which shared plumbing drains with Pluckett's cell. Inmate Holmes, who was a homosexual and known self-mutilator, flushed a blood-stained towel down the toilet. Later, a correctional officer also dumped into that clogged toilet a small container of blood he found in Holmes's cell. The plaintiffs' efforts to clear the towel from the pipes apparently drew the blood from Holmes's toilet into Pluckett's toilet, where it then sprayed onto the plaintiffs.

Both men instantly felt blood and water on their faces, mouths, eyes, inside and outside their eyeglasses, and down the front of their bodies. After the exposure, the plaintiffs used water from a sink to wash off as best as they could. They washed again using industrial soap and an iodine scrub when they returned to the maintenance shop. However, neither man rinsed out their eyes. No one gave the plaintiffs a change of clothes or told them to change their clothes. After completing employee accident reports and exposure incident investigation forms, the plaintiffs reported the incident to Frank Russell, the personnel officer at the reformatory. They asked Russell if they could go to Ionia County Memorial Hospital for blood tests and medical evaluation because of their exposure to the inmate's blood. Russell refused their request because the plaintiffs had already received their hepatitis B shots. Because the men received this news near quitting time, they went home in their still-damp, bloodstained clothing. Both of the plaintiffs' wives touched the clothing with their bare hands, included it in the family laundry, and did not use any bleach on the clothing.

The Department of Correction's own policies provided that blood-contaminated clothing must be bagged carefully and properly labeled, must not be worn home, and must be handled by workers wearing utility gloves. The policies further stated that after an employee's exposure to bloodborne pathogens, the source individual's blood must be tested and results given to the employee or employee's physician. The day following the exposure, Keelean filed a request asking for the prisoner's blood to be tested or for his blood test results and for any history of his infectious diseases. His request was denied. As a result of defendant's failure to cooperate with plaintiffs' requests for inmate Holmes's medical information and initial refusal to test plaintiffs for HIV and AIDS, the plaintiffs filed a grievance against defendant.

The plaintiffs' grievance resulted in an arbitration hearing. Both plaintiffs were very anxious to have the arbitration because they had not yet received inmate Holmes's blood test results that Kelli Corner, the plaintiffs' AIDS/HIV consultant from the Ionia County Health Department, needed to assess plaintiffs' risk factors accurately. Only after testimony began at the arbitration hearing did the defendant's labor relations representative offer to settle the grievance. The parties reached an agreement in lieu of continuing with the arbitration.

The defendant, however, persisted in its refusal to produce any medical information regarding inmate Holmes. As a result, both plaintiffs became more and more fearful that inmate Holmes was HIV positive and the defendant was attempting to hide this from them and their families. Because of defendant's failure to produce the test results despite the settlement agreement, the plaintiffs filed the suit, and the Court of Claims entered an order directing the defendant to produce inmate Holmes's blood test. Neither the plaintiffs nor the Health Department received the test results until after this order was entered. Finally, via a letter from Assistant Attorney General Allan Soros to plaintiffs' counsel, the defendant turned over Holmes's blood test results.

Because the defendants had not tested inmate Holmes before they released him, the plaintiffs remained concerned about Holmes's HIV status. Fortunately, the secretary for the plaintiffs' counsel was able to track Holmes to a morgue in Los Angeles, California, where he was tested for HIV postmortem. This test was negative.

The trial court awarded each plaintiff $85,000 and each plaintiff's wife $15,000 in past damages for, in part, (a) a breach of contract that was part of the grievance settlement that was exclusively for the purpose of providing mental solace to these employees; (b) exposure to the fresh blood of an inmate known to have engaged in homosexual acts; and (c) reasonable fear given the departmental policies and counseling providing that such exposures should be treated with extensive precautionary measures that were not taken in this case. The defendant's representatives acknowledged that the plaintiffs' concerns were reasonable. The court determined that the defendant breached the contract by (a) failing to furnish the information set forth in the settlement agreement, (b) failing to communicate that Holmes had been tested for HIV within several weeks of the exposure and that his test was negative, and (c) failing to test Holmes again before he was discharged to see if he was HIV or HIB positive. Both plaintiffs and their wives testified credibly that they suffered great fear as a result of defendant's breach of contract. The defendant appealed.

On appeal, the court noted that it took a court order and more than 2 years before defendant turned over the results of Holmes's blood test. The defendant failed to explain this delay. Furthermore, the defendant's own policy regarding the control of communicable bloodborne diseases stated that a prisoner who is a source of an exposure to blood in a manner that could transmit HIV shall be tested for HIV unless the prisoner is already known to be positive. Obviously, the defendant ignored the mandatory nature of this policy when, for over 2 years, it ignored repeated requests for Holmes's blood test results, particularly when the defendant knew this information was critical to the medical or psychological management of the plaintiffs. Therefore, the court ruled that the defendant's callous disregard for the plaintiffs' reasonable requests for Holmes's HIV information exacerbated beyond measure the plaintiffs' initial fear at the exposure, and the plaintiffs were entitled to emotional distress damages caused by defendant's noncooperation.

Sandra Keelean testified that her husband could not sleep after the exposure incident. She said that he distanced himself from his children because he feared that he had

HIV, and he panicked whenever one of them would get a cut or scrape, so the children started to avoid him. Even though his test results all came back negative, Keelean was still fearful, which affected his and his wife's physical relationship. It was only after Holmes's body was found in Los Angeles and his blood tested negative for HIV and HBV that Keelean began to relax and was able to sleep. The court believed this testimony established the mental anguish and distress that the defendant proximately caused the plaintiffs and their wives by refusing to disclose inmate Holmes's HIV status to the plaintiffs' health care provider in a timely fashion. The court therefore affirmed the Court of Claims' damage award in favor of plaintiffs and their spouses.[30]

In *Hartwig v. Oregon Trail Eye Clinic et al.*,[31] Penny Hartwig's employer, Merry Maids, entered into a contract with the clinic to provide cleaning services for its medical facility. Hartwig was assigned to clean the clinic on the first night of the contract. To gather the clinic's nonmedical waste, Hartwig carried a large trash bag from room to room, collected the small trash bags from the individual waste receptacles, and placed the small trash bags into the large trash bag. After collecting a few small trash bags, Hartwig picked up the large collector trash bag, and in doing so, it inadvertently swung against her leg. Hartwig instantly felt a stinging sensation and, looking down, observed a needle protruding from the area of the trash bag that contacted her thigh.

Hartwig informed a clinic employee that she had been stuck with a needle disposed of in the nonmedical waste. The clinic employee treated Hartwig's injury by cleaning the injured area with alcohol and placing a bandage over the puncture. Hartwig testified that the clinic employee then asked her to retrieve the needle from the trash bag. As Hartwig reached into the trash bag to obtain the needle, she was stuck by another needle. The clinic employee treated this wound in the same manner as the other. Hartwig testified that both needlesticks caused a small amount of bleeding. Hartwig finished cleaning the clinic that evening without any further problems.

A couple of days later, Hartwig received a telephone call from a registered nurse employed by Regional West Medical Center in the area of epidemiology and infectious disease control. The nurse had been told by the clinic of Hartwig's accident and phoned Hartwig so they could discuss the risks associated with needlesticks. The nurse informed Hartwig that she was at risk for HIV and HBV infections because of the needlesticks. The nurse provided Hartwig with pamphlets and other information regarding additional risks associated with a needlestick, such as the fact that sexual intercourse with her husband would place him at risk of HIV infection and that her children as well as her husband were at risk of infection through exposure to her body fluids.

To treat her possible exposure to infectious disease, Hartwig obtained four different injections over a period of time, vaccinating her against hepatitis and tetanus. Hartwig was also informed that she would have to submit to four blood tests to determine whether she had been infected with HIV. The first test was conducted immediately to determine whether Hartwig was HIV positive prior to sustaining the needlesticks at the clinic. The subsequent tests were to be performed 3 months, 6 months, and 1 year from the time of the incident. Ultimately, Hartwig did not test positive for HIV on any incident. The clinic was unable to ascertain positively the identity of the patient or patients on whom the needles were originally used. The record was not clear as to why, but the needles that caused Hartwig's injuries were never tested to determine whether they were contaminated with HIV-infected tissue, blood, or body fluid.

Hartwig filed suit against the clinic to recover damages for her physical injuries related to the needlesticks as well as the anxiety and mental suffering resulting from her fear of HIV infection. Prior to trial, the district court sustained the clinic's motion to exclude testimony concerning Hartwig's mental anguish caused by her fear that she had indeed been infected with HIV. The court concluded that to recover for such damages, Hartwig would have to prove actual exposure to HIV.

The trial court sustained Hartwig's motion for a directed verdict as to the clinic's negligence. However, regarding the issue of damages, the court instructed the jury that it might not award any damages to Hartwig for anxiety, emotional distress, or mental suffering alleged to have been sustained or incurred by her, or her husband, as the result of fear of contracting AIDS or fear or anxiety of testing positive for the presence of the HIV virus or other infectious diseases.

The jury returned a $3,000 verdict in favor of Hartwig. Hartwig motioned for a new trial, which was overruled, and she then appealed claiming that the trail court erred by (a) refusing to allow her to present evidence in regard to mental anguish and emotional distress resulting from her reasonable fear of contracting AIDS caused by the clinic's negligence; (b) instructing the jury that it could not award damages to her for anxiety, emotional distress, or mental suffering sustained by her or her husband resulting from her fear of contracting AIDS caused by the clinic's negligence; and (c) overruling her motion for new trial.

On appeal, the court noted that the question presented in the matter was purely one of law: Whether a plaintiff who sustains a minimal physical injury, caused by the defendant's negligence, may recover damages for anxiety and mental suffering occasioned by his or her fear of testing HIV positive and contracting AIDS, absent a showing of actual exposure to blood or body fluid infected with HIV? Hartwig argued that Nebraska law had long recognized that where mental suffering and anguish accompany a physical bodily injury, such mental suffering and anguish are compensable in damages. The clinic, for the most part, did not take issue with this position. However, the clinic argued that the physical bodily injury must be of sufficient severity, such that it could reasonably be expected to produce mental suffering, and that the mental suffering must directly result from the physical injury. The clinic contended that only a severe injury can reasonably cause anxiety and mental suffering sufficient for compensation. Accordingly, the clinic asserted that it is only when a plaintiff such as Hartwig is actually exposed to HIV that such plaintiff suffers a severe injury for which it is reasonable to conclude that anxiety and mental anguish are a consequence.

The court stated that it is certainly reasonable to fear AIDS if one has been exposed via a medically recognized channel of transmission to blood known to be HIV positive. Conversely, it is unreasonable to fear AIDS when one is exposed to HIV-positive blood or body fluid by means other than a medically recognized channel of transmission, or when, although exposed by a medically recognized channel of transmission, the blood or body fluid is not HIV positive. The court further stated that it is not unreasonable to fear HIV infection or AIDS when someone such as Hartwig is exposed via a medically sufficient channel of transmission to the tissue, blood, or body fluid of another and it is impossible or impracticable to ascertain whether that tissue, blood, or body fluid is in fact HIV positive.

The court recognized the fact that modern medicine treats a *potential exposure* to HIV virtually the same as it treats an *actual exposure* to HIV. When a person such as Hartwig is *potentially* exposed to HIV through a medically viable channel of transmission, the applicable standard of medical care requires that such person conduct his or her life as if they were *actually* exposed to HIV-positive tissue, blood, or body fluid until such a time that a blood test reveals, to a certain statistical level of confidence, that such person is HIV negative. The court thought it was inconsistent to suggest that during the period of time in which such a person is required by competent medical advice to conduct his or her life as though he or she were HIV infected, the law would conclude that it is unreasonable, speculative, or whimsical for such person to have a real and intense fear that he or she is indeed HIV positive and may suffer a slow, agonizing death from AIDS. Furthermore, the court could not say, as a matter of law, that one's fear of testing HIV positive and contracting AIDS was unreasonable when one suffers an injury in a manner by which medical science has concluded that HIV could be communicated.

The court therefore held that a plaintiff may adduce proof and potentially recover damages for the mental anguish of reasonably fearing AIDS resulting from a physical injury when the plaintiff may have been exposed, via a medically sufficient channel of transmission, to the tissue, blood, or body fluid of another in circumstances where the identity of the patient on whom the contaminated needle or instrument was used is unknown, and when it is impossible or impracticable to ascertain whether any such tissue, blood, or body fluid may be HIV positive. They further held that there is no reason in law, policy, or fact why Hartwig should not be allowed the opportunity to prove to a jury that, at least for a certain "window of anxiety," her fear of HIV infection and contracting AIDS was reasonable and genuine and that it resulted in mental suffering occasioned by a physical injury for which she may receive compensation.

The court noted that (a) Hartwig was potentially exposed to tissue, blood, or body fluid of other unidentified persons by being stuck by discarded hypodermic needles; (b) it was impossible or impracticable to determine whether the needles were in fact contaminated with HIV positive blood; and (c) needlesticks are a medically sufficient channel of transmission of HIV. After the needlesticks, Hartwig was informed by a medical professional to conduct her life as if she were HIV positive until a series of blood tests indicated that she was not HIV positive. The lack of severity of Hartwig's physical injury bears no relationship whatsoever to the reasonableness or genuineness of her fear of HIV infection or of contracting AIDS. Instead, the medical realities of HIV infection required Hartwig to act as though she were HIV positive until medical evidence told her otherwise and she could resume her normal life.

The court concluded that the trial court erred in excluding testimony concerning Hartwig's mental anguish occasioned by her fear that she had been infected with HIV. Thus the trial court abused its discretion when it denied Hartwig's motion for a new trial. As a result, the order of the trial court denying Hartwig's motion for a new trial was reversed and the issue of damages was remanded for a new trial.[31]

Case Law: Medical Emergencies   Several cases involving the failure to carryout proper medical emergency procedures have been presented throughout this book. A few of these cases are described again in this section to point out the many types of negligence claims that plaintiffs make and the importance of having a proper medical emergency action plan (EAP). Additional case law examples are also presented with earlier cases addressing the failure of health/fitness facilities to: (a) have an EAP in place, (b) have qualified staff members trained to carry out the plan in a timely fashion, and (c) contact emergency medical services (EMS). More recent cases focus on issues related to AEDs.

In *Vanderburg v. Spa South Corporation*,[32] the plaintiff joined the defendant health spa in 1986. He allegedly informed the health spa that he had a previous myocardial infarction. One day, after riding an exercise bike at the spa, he collapsed apparently suffering another myocardial infarction. The complaint alleged that employees, servants, and/or agents of the defendant spa contacted EMS but did nothing more than observe the plaintiff until EMS arrived 10 to 15 minutes later. The complaint also alleged that the plaintiff suffered severe brain damage because of the delay in resuscitation caused by the failure of the defendant spa to carry out duties such as the following:

(a) to prepare and arrange an individualized exercise program tailored to suit the individual needs of the patrons and guests;
(b) to explain, train, and demonstrate to patrons and guests the use and function of various equipment within its facilities;
(c) to supervise and observe patrons and guests during the course of their use of equipment within its facilities;
(d) to ensure that the staff and/or other employees of Defendant Spa were at least minimally trained in cardiopulmonary resuscitation and/or other specific safety-related programs;
(e) to ensure that a specific program and protocol for the handling of preventive and emergency procedures was promulgated and utilized at the premises of Defendant Spa;
(f) to maintain records of emergency and preventive protocols;

(g) to discern adequate and reasonable health and medical information for prospective members, with said duty continuing as medical, physical, and health conditions changed; and

(h) to take affirmative measures and to instruct the employees, servants and/or agents of Defendant Spa to prepare proper and reasonable programs for individual members who were predisposed to injury or physical harm as a result of physical conditions which the Defendant Spa knew, or should have known, through the exercise of reasonable diligence.[33]

A settlement for $500,000 for the plaintiff was completed prior to trial. Expert depositions indicated that the presence of CPR-trained personnel was mandatory at such facilities.[32]

In *Kleinknecht v. Gettysburg College*,[34] a 20-year-old college lacrosse player, Drew Kleinknecht, died from cardiac arrest while practicing with his team. On that day, neither of the two coaches supervising practice had CPR certification. Additionally, no communication devices were present on the field. The nearest telephone was approximately 200 to 250 yards away, and the shortest route to this phone required scaling an 8-foot-high fence. The coaches never discussed how they would handle an emergency during fall practices.

After Drew Kleinknecht's death, his parents filed a wrongful death action against the college. They contended that as long as 12 minutes elapsed after Drew collapsed and before CPR was administered. They also estimated that approximately another 10 minutes passed before the first ambulance arrived on the scene. The Kleinknechts alleged, among other things, that the college's negligence and that of its agents (coaches and athletic trainers) was the proximate cause of their son's death. The plaintiffs claimed that the college breached its legal duty by (a) not having a written emergency medical action plan, (b) not ensuring that the coaches present at practice were CPR certified, (c) not having student trainers or other CPR-certified trainers present at practice, and (d) not having a communication device, such as a walkie-talkie, at the practice field. The U.S. District Court entered summary judgment in favor of the college. The court held that the college had no duty to anticipate and guard against the chance of a fatal arrhythmia in a young and healthy college athlete. They also held that the actions taken by the college employees following Kleinknecht's collapse were reasonable, and therefore the college did not breach any duty that existed. The Kleinknechts appealed.

On appeal, the U.S. Court of Appeals noted that the Kleinknechts produced ample evidence that a life-threatening injury occurring during participation in an athletic event like lacrosse was reasonably foreseeable and, therefore, the college did owe Drew a duty to take reasonable precautions against the risk of death while Drew was participating in the college's lacrosse program. The court recognized that the college owed a duty to Drew to have measures in place at the lacrosse practice to provide prompt treatment in the event that he or any other team member suffered a life-threatening injury. The district court's holding that the college's duty of care did not include, before Drew's collapse, a duty to provide prompt emergency medical response while he was engaged in a school-sponsored athletic activity was reversed. Additionally, the district court's holding that the college acted reasonably and thus did not breach any duty following Drew's collapse was also reversed. The case was remanded.

In *Brown v. Bally Total Fitness Corporation*,[35] the plaintiff collapsed with cardiac complications while exercising on a treadmill at the defendant's facility and later died. After Brown collapsed, two Bally's employees and an off-duty police officer, Alex Escobar, ran to check on him. Escobar noticed that Brown had a weak pulse, was breathing, but was unresponsive to verbal commands. Frank Ramirez, a Bally's employee, who was CPR certified, also checked Brown's vital signs and told Escobar to step back, claiming that he had control of the scene.

Ramirez stated that he was trained in CPR, as did Escobar, who also identified himself as an off-duty police officer. They then, with the assistance of another Bally's employee, moved Brown off the treadmill and onto the floor. As he was providing information to a Bally's employee who was filling out an incident report, Escobar noticed several Bally's employees standing around Brown but not monitoring his vital signs. He noticed Brown was turning pale and informed the employees that they needed to monitor Brown's vital signs. Ramirez instructed Bally's staff to "get these people back."

Escobar went over to Brown a second time and checked his vitals. He observed that Brown's skin was cold, his respirations were shallow, and his pulse was weak. Bally's staff members informed Escobar that paramedics were on the way and for him to stand back. Shortly thereafter, Escobar observed that Brown was pale and appeared not to be breathing. Again, he observed Bally's employees just standing around Brown. He was told again to stand back.

At that time, Police Officer Egigian arrived on the scene and checked Brown. Escobar identified himself as an off-duty police officer and also checked Brown's vitals. He informed Egigian that Brown was not breathing and did not have a pulse. The two police officers began CPR. Shortly thereafter, Brown began to breathe and move his extremities; however, within seconds, Brown went into cardiac arrest and they began CPR again. The paramedics arrived and provided further treatment to Brown. He was transported to the hospital where further efforts to resuscitate him were unsuccessful.

An eyewitness, Rose Valdez, provided information for a police report to the effect that Bally's employees did not appear to know how to administer first aid and prevented Escobar from providing first aid. She also wanted to know why it took so long for emergency medical services to respond. During her deposition, Valdez stated, "It seemed like the Bally's staff didn't know what to do, they were unsure what they should do, and they didn't really have anybody supervising or directing the staff as to how to handle an emergency situation."[36]

The plaintiffs filed four causes of action against Bally's: "(1) negligence (wrongful death); (2) negligent employment, training, management and supervision; (3) negligent misrepresentation; and (4) fraud and deceit. Plaintiffs alleged that defendant's employees failed to check decedent's pulse, failed to administer cardiopulmonary resuscitation (CPR), and prevented a Good Samaritan, off-duty police officer Escobar, from attempting lifesaving procedures. In addition, plaintiffs alleged that defendant knew or should have known that its employees were not qualified nor able to provide emergency medical services, including CPR, and that defendant failed to properly train and manage its employees, which created an undue risk to persons such as decedent."[37]

The trial court granted the defendant's motion for summary judgment based on a waiver and release Brown had signed. On appeal, the appellate court ruled that the defendant's alleged negligence was not reasonably related to the purpose for which the release was given because the release "did not contain any express provisions purporting to release defendant from any liability if it negligently rendered first aid or negligently prevented a Good Samaritan from rendering first aid. Nowhere in the waiver and release is there any reference, even impliedly, to releasing the defendant for these alleged acts of negligence."[38]

As described in Chapter 5, in *Chai v. Sports & Fitness Clubs of America, Inc.*,[39,40] the plaintiff suffered an apparent cardiac arrest while exercising at the defendant's club ("Q" The Sports Club) and consequently was left in a vegetative state. The plaintiffs alleged, among other things, that the defendant:

- Negligently failed to have personnel adequately trained to recognize cardiac arrest and to subsequently start CPR;
- Negligently failed to have employees adequately trained in the administration of CPR, available to assist . . . [the member] when he collapsed while exercising;
- Negligently failed to have employees adequately trained in the use and operation of an automated external defibrillator, available to assist . . . [the member] when he collapsed while exercising;
- Negligently failed to have automated external defibrillators on the premises and available for use at all times;

- Negligently failed to promptly perform CPR, on . . . [the member] when he collapsed while exercising;
- Negligently failed to promptly use an automated external defibrillator, on . . . [the member] when he collapsed while exercising;
- Negligently failed to properly monitor . . . [the member] while he was exercising in the cardiovascular room;
- Negligently failed to promptly call for emergency medical assistance for . . . [the member] when he collapsed while exercising;
- Negligently failed to require prescreening of members, including . . . [the member], to assess his fitness and health, prior to his use of the Defendant's exercise facilities;
- Negligently failed to require sufficient certification or training of staff members designated to train and monitor . . . [the member] when he was using the cardiovascular exercise equipment.[39]

The case resulted in a defense verdict. However, prior to the verdict, both parties agreed that if a plaintiff's verdict was returned, no more that $7 million would be awarded to the plaintiff and if a defense verdict was returned, the plaintiff would recover a verdict of not less than $2.25 million. Therefore, the plaintiff received $2.25 million.[40]

Similarly, in *Fruh v. Wellbridge Club Management, Inc.,*[41] the plaintiff, a 52-year-old man, was exercising at the Wellbridge Health & Fitness Center when

> [H]e began to complain of discomfort and then collapsed, became pulse-less, breathless and unresponsive. Because of his condition, the complaint alleges that employees of the center began CPR and initiated 911 procedures and that some 9 minutes after the placement of the 911 call, emergency response personnel arrived with an AED and used it to eventually restore the plaintiff's heart to a normal rhythm. However, because of the passage of time from the time of the onset of the plaintiff's symptoms and the use of the AED, it is alleged that the plaintiff was left completely disabled suffering from anoxic brain damage leaving him with profound anterior retrograde amnesia, anxiety, and depression.[42]

The complaint also alleges that the fitness center advertised its programs to older adults as well as those suffering from diabetes, heart disease, and hypertension, and promised medically based programs in a safe, comfortable environment. It also promised and warranted to its members that it conformed to standards of quality such as those published by the IHRSA (see IHRSA Standards later). In addition, the complaint alleges that the "defendant facility had a duty to assess the likelihood of injuries to its customers, the seriousness of such potential injuries, and the burden of avoiding the risks of such injuries; that sudden cardiac arrest was a reasonably foreseeable risk to those patrons utilizing the defendant's facilities and that despite such knowledge, it did not have an AED on its premises at the time the plaintiff suffered his sudden cardiac arrest."[43]

The incident occurred in April 1999 and the complaint was filed in April 2002 seeking a sum of damages in excess of $75,000.[41] However, a petition for court approval of a settlement was filed on March 17, 2004, and the court approved it on March 18, 2004, for $1.8 million.[44] The defendants agreed to pay the plaintiff this amount, which is the second highest settlement involving the alleged failure to have an AED. The settlement in the *Chai* case just described is the highest thus far at $2.25 million.

On March 29, 2006, in *Tringali Mayer v. L.A. Fitness International, LLC,*[45] a Florida jury awarded the plaintiff a sum of $619,650 to compensate the family for the loss of their family member, who died while working out at the defendant fitness facility in April 2003. The plaintiffs claimed that the defendant negligently and carelessly breached its duty to render aid to Mr. Tringali once he was having a medical emergency in one or more of the following ways:

(a) by failing to properly screen the Plaintiffs Decedent's health condition at or about the time he initially joined Defendant's health club;
(b) by failing to administer cardiopulmonary resuscitation (CPR) to Mr. Tringali;

(c) by failing to have on its premises and use an Automated External Defibrillator (AED) on Mr. Tringali;

(d) by failing to properly train its employees and agents regarding the recognition, treatment of, and protocol for handling medical emergencies in its health clubs, including but not limited to the club in question;

(e) by otherwise failing to render aid to Mr. Tringali.[46]

In addition, the plaintiffs alleged that the defendant was in violation of industry standards, specifically those published by the IHRSA (see Published Standards of Practice later) "because it did not have an employee trained in CPR on it premises."[46] The plaintiffs sought loss of consortium and loss of parental consortium damages as well as damages to "recover the loss of earnings of the Deceased from the date of the injury to the date of death, loss of net accumulations beyond death, and medical and funeral expenses due to the Decedent's injuries and death."[47]

In response to the complaint, the defendants claimed that the decedent was guilty of his own negligence and that he assumed the risks associated with the activity. An expert witness for the plaintiff, Dr. VanCamp, cited the 2002 ACSM/AHA Joint PP-AEDs (see Published Standards of Practice later) that recommended the use of AEDs in health/fitness facilities. The lawyer for the plaintiff in his opening remarks stated, "Alessio Tringali died way too soon and his death was foreseeable. It was predictable and it was preventable. But because these people [the defendants] had no regard for the safety of their patrons, they didn't even have a plan when this went down, they didn't really know what to do and they didn't do anything. And calling 911 wasn't enough."[47] The defendant's lawyer, in his opening statement, claimed that in April 2003, it was not a standard for health clubs to have an AED. He stated that the airlines did not have to have AEDs at that time, other health clubs like Bally's didn't have AEDs, and that a Florida AED statute did "not require that an automated external defibrillator be placed in any building or any location, or required to be made available to premises of one or more employees trained in the device."[48] Given the statements of the defendant's lawyer in this case, it is important to remind health/fitness professionals that a defense such as "other health clubs don't have AEDs" is generally not a viable defense, but that adherence to the standard of care is a viable defense in negligence claims and lawsuits (see Chapter 2, Defenses That Don't Work).

Regarding issues related to health/fitness facilities having AEDs, the *Chai* and *Fruh* cases just described resulted in large settlements for the plaintiff. The *Tringali Mayer* case from Florida was the first case that resulted in a plaintiff's verdict. However, an earlier Florida case, *Delibero v. Q Clubs, Inc,*[49] resulted in a ruling for the defendant club. While exercising at the defendant's health club, Delibero suffered a sudden cardiac arrest. The club did not have an AED, but the employees called 911 and performed CPR. Although Delibero survived, he suffered brain damage. The plaintiff (guardian for Delibero) claimed the club was negligent because it did not have an AED available.

On appeal, the plaintiff claimed that "the trial court erred in not instructing the jury that evidence of custom in the industry does not by itself establish a standard of care."[50] The plaintiff's instruction request stated, "Evidence of what was usually done in the health club industry is not conclusive or controlling on the question of negligence and does not by itself establish a standard of care. It is only some evidence to be considered with all the evidence in determining what is reasonable."[50] The court stated,

Although we agree . . . , the evidence in this case did not require a cautionary instruction, because it did not amount to evidence of a custom or standard in the industry. The evidence in this case was that, at the time of this accident in 2000, AEDs were being considered, but there was no custom or standard of care as to whether a health club should or should not have an AED. If defendants had put on evidence that the standard or custom in the industry was not to have AEDs, we would agree with plaintiffs that the cautionary instruction should have been given. Under the circumstances in this case, however, where defendants did not assert that there was a custom or standard, the court did not err in refusing the requested instruction.[51]

The appellate court affirmed the trial court's ruling in favor of the defendants. Another AED case, *Lewin v. Fitworks of Cincinnati, LLC,*[52] also resulted in a ruling in favor of the defendants. In February 2002, Lewin joined one of the 13 defendant facilities located in Ohio and Kentucky. According to the following facts he was exercising at the Florence, Kentucky, Fitworks on July 20 of that year:

At some point, while seated on an exercise machine, he suffered a cardiac event. . . . As soon as this event was brought to the attention of Fitworks staff, 9-1-1 was immediately called and Fitworks staff assisted in removing Mr. Lewin from the machine that he was on and placed him onto the floor. CPR was promptly administered by two bystanders. The paramedics arrived a short time after being called. It took them a few minutes to assess Mr. Lewin and to defibrillate him. Mr. Lewin was transported to St. Luke's hospital where he was pronounced dead. . . . Medical testimony at trial reflected Mr. Lewin died as a result of sudden cardiac arrest.[53]

The plaintiff, the administratrix of the estate of Mr. Lewin, sued the defendant facility for wrongful death claiming, among other things, that it (a) "negligently, grossly negligently, wantonly, recklessly and/or carelessly failed to have an AED on the premises" and (b) "negligently, grossly negligently, wantonly, recklessly and/or carelessly failed to provide any training and/or adequate training to its employees to perform CPR, nor did Defendant have an employee on site capable of performing CPR."[54] The complaint sought damages in excess of $25,000 as well as punitive damages of $10 million.[52] The court, in its ruling in favor of the defendants stated,

The Court finds that the defendant acted reasonably and not in derogation of any duty owed Mr. Lewin. The evidence is clear that the defendant thru its agents were instructed in any emergency to call 9-1-1 immediately. That procedure was followed in this unfortunate situation. . . . The Court finds . . . that defendant did not violate their duty to Mr. Lewin on July 20, 2002. In support of this decision, the Court cites the following:

1. *Defendants had no other similar events in their 13 facilities which might tend to put them on notice and thereby alerting them that there may be some duty or responsibility;*
2. *Few fitness clubs in the entire country, perhaps 5%, had AEDs in July, 2002, and there was no evidence that any Kentucky or Ohio fitness club had AEDs at that time;*
3. *There were honest concerns on part of defendant that misuse of AEDs could cause serious problems and after consultation with others, a valid fear that AEDs may create liability;*
4. *There was, and is, no law requiring [AEDs in] fitness centers, other businesses or homes (where 85% of cardiac arrests occur) in Kentucky.*[55]

The final AED case to be described, *Salte v. YMCA of Metropolitan Chicago Foundation,*[56] again resulted in a ruling favoring the defendant. While using the treadmill at the defendant club, Terry Alan Salte suffered a cardiac arrest. The plaintiffs filed a complaint for negligence and loss of consortium that included the following allegations:

Defendant owned and operated a health club and extended memberships to the public for a fee. On April 29, 2003, Terry, a member of the club, was exercising on one of defendant's treadmills. At that time, defendant had on its staff a paramedic who was nearby assisting another member of the club on a different fitness machine. While using the treadmill, Terry suffered a cardiac arrest. Plaintiffs' complaint alleged that Terry's cardiac arrest was a predictable and reasonably foreseeable event. Plaintiffs alleged that defendant had a duty to equip its "paramedics and athletic or fitness trainers" with cardiac defibrillators, which plaintiffs alleged were inexpensive, easy to use, and readily available. Defendant did not have any defibrillators on its premises. Plaintiffs alleged that, as a direct and proximate result of defendant's negligent failure to equip its facility and paramedics with a defibrillator, Terry remained in cardiac arrest for eight minutes until the county paramedics arrived. Plaintiffs alleged that this delay led to his brain suffering an anoxic event, which in turn led to physical and emotional damages.[57]

In analyzing this case, the court relied on the Restatement (Second) of Torts § 314A and rulings of other courts and held that the

> *[D]efendant did not have a duty to have a defibrillator on its premises and to use the defibrillator on Terry. Defendant's duty was only to provide to its business invitee the level of aid that was reasonable under the circumstances. . . . This simply means that defendant and its staff were required to render whatever first aid that, under the circumstances, they were reasonably capable of providing to Terry. . . . This duty, however, did not require defendant to provide, or to be prepared to provide, all medical care that it could reasonably foresee might be needed by a patron. . . . Accordingly, we hold that defendant did not have a duty to have a defibrillator on its premises and that its staff did not have a duty to defibrillate Terry.*[58]

A dissenting justice in this case stated,

> *I disagree with the majority's and defendant's characterization of the issue as solely a legal question of whether defendant had a duty to provide a defibrillator. Defendant's duty, as it acknowledges, was to render reasonable first aid until professional assistance arrived. See Restatement (Second) of Torts § 314A. . . . Whether reasonable assistance encompasses the use of a defibrillator by defendant's staff paramedic is, I believe, a factual question. I further believe that a reasonable jury could find that defendant did not provide reasonable first aid to Terry when it failed to equip its paramedic with a defibrillator to use on Terry.*[59]

Since the decision in this case, Illinois, like a number of other states, has passed legislation mandating the presence of AEDs in health clubs.[60] Therefore, a similar case now in Illinois would likely result in a different outcome favoring the plaintiffs.

PUBLISHED STANDARDS OF PRACTICE

All 10 of the published standards of practice identified in Chapter 3 include standards and guidelines related to medical emergency action plans. Some of these also include standards and guidelines related to OSHA's BBP Standard and AEDs. The following is considered a summary and by no means an inclusive list of these published statements.

ACSM's H/F Standards, ACSM's Guidelines, ACSM/AHA Joint PP, and ACSM/AHA Joint PP-AEDs

The ACSM's H/F Standards[61] contain the following standards with regard to emergency action plans:

> *Standard #5—Facilities must have in place a written system for sharing information with users and employees or independent contractors regarding the handling of potentially hazardous materials including the handling of bodily fluids by the facility staff in accordance with the Occupational Safety and Health Administration (OSHA).*

Standard #6—Facilities must have written emergency response systems polices and procedures, which must be reviewed and rehearsed regularly, as well as documented. These policies must enable staff to handle basic first-aid situations and emergency cardiac events.

Standard #7—Facilities must have as part of their written emergency response system a public access defibrillation (PAD) program.[62]

(From American College of Sports Medicine, 2007, *ACSM's Health/Fitness Facility Standards and Guidelines*, 3rd ed., pp. 1–2. (c) 2007 by American College of Sports Medicine. Reprinted with permission from Human Kinetics, Champaign, IL.)

Note: Related ACSM's H/F Standards: (a) #10, and (b) #19 and #20, were listed in Chapters 7 and 10, respectively. Standard #10 described certification requirements (AED and CPR) that health/fitness staff members need to possess, and Standards #19 and #20 addressed emergency safety and ADA/OSHA signage requirements.

The ACSM's Guidelines[63] provide some key points with regard to emergency planning and management that include: (a) qualifications of personnel (e.g., CPR training) involved with exercise testing, (b) posting of emergency telephone numbers, (c) establishment of emergency plans, (d) regular rehearsal of emergency drills at least quarterly and documentation of such drills, (e) use of AEDs, and (f) two tables that describe plans for nonemergency situations and potentially life-threatening situations.

The ACSM/AHA Joint PP[64] requires staff members such as exercise specialists and exercise leaders to be trained in CPR. In addition, it states,

All health/fitness facilities must have written emergency policies and procedures that are reviewed and practiced regularly. Such plans will correspond to the type of facility and risk level of its membership outlined in Table 5. [Table 6-2 in Chapter 6 here]. All fitness center staff who directly supervise program participants should be trained in basic life support. Health/fitness facilities must develop appropriate emergency response plans and must train their staff in appropriate procedures to provide during a life-threatening emergency. When an incident occurs, each staff member must perform the necessary emergency support steps in accordance with established procedures. It is important for everyone to know the emergency plan. Emergency drills should be practiced once every 3 months or more often with changes in staff; retraining and rehearsal are especially important. When new staff are hired, new team arrangements may be necessary. Because life-threatening cardiovascular emergencies are rare, constant vigilance by staff and familiarity with the plan and how to follow it are important.

It is essential to acknowledge that emergency equipment alone does not save lives. . . . The training and preparedness of an astute professional staff who can readily handle emergencies is paramount. This issue is particularly important if persons with certain medical conditions are recruited and encouraged to exercise in a specific health/fitness facility. Such a facility has the responsibility to offer appropriate coverage by personnel as outlined . . . in Table 5. [Table 6-2 in Chapter 6 here]. Acquisition of equipment for emergency evaluation and resuscitation will depend on the risk level of participants, personnel, and medical coverage. All facilities must have a telephone that is readily accessible and available when emergency assistance is needed. It would be useful for all supervised facilities to have a sphygmomanometer and stethoscope readily available. Level 4 and 5 facilities that recruit members with known cardiovascular disease must have such equipment available . . .

The emergency plan must address transportation of victims to a hospital emergency room and must include telephone access to 911 or the local emergency unit access system. Health/fitness facility personnel should be familiar with emergency transport teams in the area so that access and location of the center are clearly identified. Staff should greet the emergency response team at the entrance of the facility so they can be promptly guided to the site of the emergency. A staff member should remain with the victim at all times.[65] (Reprinted with permission. AHA/ACSM Scientific Statement: Recommendations for Cardiovascular Screening, Staffing, and Emergency Policies at Health/Fitness Facilities [*Circulation.* 1998;97:2283–2293.] ©1998 American Heart Association, Inc.)

The ACSM/AHA Joint PP-AEDs,[66] which is a supplement to the ACSM/AHA Joint PP,[64] provides recommendations with regard to AEDs. It states, "Effective placement and use of AEDs at all health/fitness facilities . . . is encouraged."[67] In addition, this published statement includes information regarding: (a) the coordination of PAD programs with the local emergency medical system (EMS), (b) emergency drills that should include the simulated use of AEDs, (c) proper maintenance of the AED device, and (d) compliance with local or regional regulations and legislation.

NCSA Standards, IHRSA Standards, and MFA Standards

The NSCA Standards[68] include two standards and one guideline under Emergency Planning & Response as follows:

> *Standard 5.1—Strength & Conditioning professionals must be trained and certified in current guidelines for cardiopulmonary resuscitation (CPR) established by AHA/ILCOR . . . ; as well as universal precautions for preventing disease transmission established by the CDC . . . and OSHA. . . . First Aid training/ certification is also necessary if Sports Medicine personnel (e.g., MD or ATC) are not immediately available during Strength & Conditioning activities. New staff engaged in Strength & Conditioning activities must comply with this standard within six (6) months of employment.*
>
> *Standard 5.2—Strength & Conditioning professionals must develop a written, venue-specific emergency response plan to deal with injuries and reasonably foreseeable untoward events within each facility. The plan must be posted at strategic areas within each facility, and practiced and rehearsed at least quarterly. The emergency response plan must be initially evaluated (e.g., by facility risk managers, legal advisors, medical providers and/or off-premise emergency response agencies) and modified as necessary at regular intervals. As part of the plan, a readily accessible and working telephone must be immediately available to summon on-premise and/or off-premise emergency response resources.*
>
> *Guideline 5.1—The components of a written and posted emergency response plan should include: planned access to a physician and/or emergency medical facility when warranted, including a plan for communication and transportation between the venue and the medical facility; appropriate and necessary emergency care equipment on-site that is quickly accessible; and a thorough understanding of the personnel and procedures associated with the plan by all individuals.*[69]

Standard #7 from the IHRSA Standards[70] states, "The club will respond in a timely manner to any reasonable foreseeable emergency event that threatens the health and safety of its patrons. Toward this end, the club will have an appropriate emergency plan that can be executed by qualified personnel in a timely fashion."[71] The interpretation behind this standard, in part, states:

> *The key to successfully utilizing it is to understand how to provide the three critical components: (1) a timely response; (2) an appropriate plan; and (3) qualified personnel . . . Clubs should have at least one person scheduled to be on site at all times who is certified in cardiopulmonary resuscitation (CPR) by the American Red Cross, the American Heart Association, or an equivalent organization.*[71]

IHRSA Standard #6 states, "The club will conform to all relevant laws, regulations, and published standards."[72] The interpretation underneath this standard "requires clubs to comply with all local, state and federal laws . . . governing employment, membership contracts, safety, etc."[72] Therefore, this would include laws such as OSHA's BBP Standard and any state laws regarding AEDs.

MFA Standard #3 states, "The Medical Fitness Center must have a written emergency response plan that enables a timely and appropriate response to any emergency event that threatens the health and safety of facility users."[73] There are several guidelines under this standard that include recommendations such as having an adequate number of first-aid kits and AEDs, emergency drills, an incident reporting program, and a prompt/direct link to the 911 emergency response center.

MFA Standard #4 states, "With physician oversight in place, the Medical Fitness Center must have at least one AED unit that is easily accessible for use," and Guideline #1 under this standard states, "In the case of multiple story buildings or large facilities (greater that 30,000 sq. ft.), additional AEDs should be considered. AED placement should be determined by response time/distance for the AED to be brought to the victim. American Heart Association recommended response time is three (3) minutes or less."[74] A second guideline under this standard addresses CPR/AED training for staff members.

Canadian Standards, AFAA Standards, and YMCA Recommendations

The Canadian Standards[75] include the following four standards under Emergency Procedures:

Standard #1—Facilities and other environments in which fitness-related activities are offered shall have in place an Emergency Action Plan which shall be practiced twice per year and reviewed with all NEW staff at the commencement of their employment.

Standards #2—All injuries, accidents or emergencies in fitness facilities and other fitness related environments shall be documented in writing and retained.

Standard #3—A designated complement of First Aid equipment shall be readily available in fitness facilities and other fitness-related environments.

Standard #4—Immediate access must be available to in-house first aid services from qualified personnel. Contact information for external medical services (e.g. ambulance/hospital emergency phone numbers) must also be posted and phones readily accessible in all high risk/injury area (e.g. pools and fitness testing areas).[76]

The AFAA standards[77] state the following, in part, with regard to emergency response procedures: "All emergencies need to be handled in a professional manner. . . . It is recommended that all facilities establish and implement a written emergency response procedure. Instructors should have knowledge to recognize that an emergency exists and to take appropriate action. Such plan should be at least periodically rehearsed and practiced."[78] In addition, "Instructors should maintain a current nationally recognized adult-level CPR certification. Instructors may also want to complete a nationally recognized standard-level first-aid course."[79]

The YMCA Recommendations[80] state that "CPR and First Aid training and certification are necessary for most YMCA staff members and volunteers in order to provide a safe environment for YMCA members."[81] Their recommendations on CPR and first-aid training include several criteria that training programs should meet, as well as a list of nationally recognized organizations that offer CPR and first-aid certifications that are considered acceptable. In addition, the YMCA has a recommendation regarding the use of supplemental oxygen in certain medical emergencies, but several considerations are listed that YMCAs should follow prior to making it available.

The YMCA Recommendations also state that "The Medical Advisory Committee of the YMCA of the USA endorses the AHA/ACSM's position on the placement and use of automated external defibrillators, and strongly recommends that YMCAs have them available in their facilities and programs."[82] Additional guidelines address:

(a) purchasing AED equipment that meets FDA standards, (b) providing training programs and AED certification for staff members, (c) practicing and following a predetermined emergency response plan that includes the use of an AED, and (d) establishing procedures for proper maintenance of the AED equipment.

In addition, the YMCA Recommendations state that "All YMCAs are obligated to act in compliance with the Occupational Safety and Health Administration (OSHA) training and documentation regarding HIV/AIDS. They are also required to have an exposure control plan relative to HIV/AIDS and other infectious diseases."[83] Additional guidelines are also provided with regard to (a) implementing HIV/AIDS education programs, (b) accepting persons with HIV/AIDS in YMCA programs, (c) considering employees with HIV/AIDS as handicapped or disabled, and (d) encouraging use of universal precautions.

STEP **2** DEVELOPMENT OF RISK MANAGEMENT STRATEGIES

The preceding sections described administrative and statutory laws that are relevant to medical emergency planning as well as several case law examples to demonstrate the many types of negligence claims that plaintiffs have made against health/fitness personnel and facilities after they experienced a medical emergency while exercising in those facilities. In addition, standards of practice published by all 10 of the professional organizations initially listed in Chapter 3 were summarized. The fact that all 10 of these organizations have standards and guidelines pertaining to emergency planning stresses the importance of this area within the overall risk management plan of a health/fitness facility. The development of a written, well-thought-out and complete medical EAP is by no means an easy task. It takes a dedicated and concerted effort among those responsible for emergency planning within a facility to complete this process.

It is also important to note that medical EAPs should not be directly copied from an appendix in a book or from plans developed by other health/fitness facilities, but rather they must be specifically tailored for each and every facility. Each facility has unique factors that must be carefully considered when developing medical EAPs. These include but are not limited to, the nature of the health/fitness program activities, the membership size and demographics, the staff size, local emergency medical services (EMS) response time, and the facility size and layout. Despite the uniqueness of each health/fitness facility, several basic components should form the foundation of medical EAPs, which are reflected in the risk management strategies listed here.

Risk Management Strategy 1: Formulate a planning team.

The initial step in developing and writing a medical EAP is to formulate a planning team that will begin the process. The team may consist of the manager and/or other full-time professional staff members, members of the facility's risk management advisory committee (i.e., medical, legal, insurance, and risk management experts), safety personnel, and local EMS personnel. It may be a good idea to have a designated staff member who serves as the facility's EAP coordinator. Because this is a significant responsibility, it should be included in this staff member's job description and he or she should be allocated adequate time to serve in this capacity. It may also be wise to include a medical liaison on this planning team. Several of the professional organizations in their published standards of practice recommend having a medical liaison or adviser that reviews medical EAPs. For example, the ACSM/AHA Joint PP[64] recommends that the "medical liaison reviews medical emergency plans, witnesses and critiques medical emergency drills, and reviews medical incident reports" and that this individual may be "a licensed physician, a registered nurse trained in advanced cardiac life support, or an emergency medical technician."[84]

The team's initial task is to review carefully with the assistance of legal counsel all applicable federal and state laws as well as standards published by professional organizations. The team also needs to identify the types of medical emergencies that may arise within their facility. Several methods of identifying potential medical emergencies exist. These methods include consultation with outside experts, reviewing health/fitness industry trends, and studying an organization's own incident report forms. The locations where prior medical emergencies occurred, the nature of the incidents, and how they were handled will be valuable information in developing a medical EAP.

Risk Management Strategy 2: Comply with OSHA's Bloodborne Pathogens (BBP) Standard.

As described earlier under OHSA's BBP Standard, there are many requirements to this federal law, including having (a) a written Exposure Control Plan (ECP); (b) initial (e.g., upon employment) and annual training programs for employees with occupational exposure; (c) providing personal protective equipment; (d) utilizing engineering and work practice controls; (e) offering HBV vaccination at no cost to employees; and (f) reporting exposure incidents, conducting postexposure follow-up, and record keeping. Employers need to be sure that all employees responsible for carrying out the health/fitness facility's medical EAP comply with OSHA's BBP Standard (see Risk Management Strategy 5). The written ECP and related policies and procedures can be included as a section within the overall written medical EAP or included as a separate section within the Risk Management Policies and Procedures Manual (RMPPM). See Chapter 12 for more on the RMPPM and how it can be organized to be an effective staff training tool.

In addition to involving legal counsel in the development of the health/fitness facility's ECP and related policies and procedures, a variety of other resources are also available. For example, each OSHA regional office has a BBP coordinator who can answer compliance and related questions. Contact information for these regional offices is available at www.osha.gov/oshdir/region.html. These offices may also have a "Prototype BBP Exposure Control Plan" that can be used as a guide. However, it is important to realize that OSHA expects an ECP that is specifically prepared for each worksite. A health/fitness facility could be fined by OSHA for photocopying and using another facility's ECP.[15] Additional resources are available from OSHA's Office of Training and Education Training Resources. They have developed brochures, fact sheets, and a videotape on the BBP Standard. Their website is: www.osha.gov/dcsp/ote/index.html.

Risk Management Strategy 3: Comply with applicable state laws.

In addition to OSHA's federal law on BBPs, it is essential for health/fitness facilities to adhere to any state laws that may be applicable to their medical EAPs. These include AED immunity statutes as well as recent statutes that now require health/fitness facilities in certain states to have an AED. Legal counsel can research these laws in your state. Legal counsel will also be necessary to interpret these laws to help ensure that the various requirements of these laws are properly developed into the health/fitness facility's medical EAP. As mentioned earlier under State Laws, several states have passed legislation requiring health/fitness facilities to have an AED, and the law is rapidly evolving in this area. The requirements within each of these state AED statutes will vary from state to state. Therefore, it is important to obtain individualized legal advice as to these enactments and their application to particular programs.

Risk Management Strategy 4: Prepare written contingency plans for various medical emergencies.

All types of medical emergencies can occur in a health/fitness facility, such as (a) minor injuries (e.g., sprained ankle), (b) major injuries (e.g., a serious back injury, fractured bone), (c) minor/major injuries that cause bleeding, and (d) life-threatening events such as SCA. For each type of possible medical emergency, a written contingency plan should be developed that not only includes the appropriate first-aid/CPR/AED procedures but designated staff members' responsibilities (see Risk Management Strategy 5) and an appropriate communications system (see Risk Management Strategy 6).

Although these written contingency plans should be comprehensive, they also need to be written in a practical, easy-to-understand manner. If they are too detailed, it may be difficult for staff members to remember everything and may prevent flexibility when needed to carry out the plan. To help in this regard, written contingency plans should include a written flowchart or algorithm that would clearly depict the steps that staff members should follow in the medical emergency response. Many examples of these flowcharts can be found in resources published by organizations such as the ACSM,[63] the American Red Cross, and the American Heart Association. However, if used as examples, these flowcharts have to be adapted to meet the specific needs of each health/fitness facility. Another excellent resource that specifically addresses the development of AED plans, published by the YMCA of the USA and coauthored by Drs. Kyle McInnis and William Herbert,[85] provides helpful information such as conducting a facility needs assessment, developing an emergency response plan, establishing roles and responsibilities of the AED response team, and implementing staff training programs.

Risk Management Strategy 5: Determine staff qualifications and responsibilities.

As specified in many of the published standards of practice just described, health/fitness facility staff members need to have appropriate emergency training and certifications, for example, first aid, CPR, and AED. All staff members within the facility who would be responsible for responding to a medical emergency should have these certifications. These staff members would likely include, but not be limited to, managers, health/fitness directors and coordinators, personal fitness trainers, groups exercise leaders, child care workers, and front desk staff members. Staff members must keep these certifications current. Many health/fitness facilities have a staff member who is also certified as an instructor who can conduct in-service trainings (e.g., a few times a year) to recertify staff members.

As stated in Risk Management Strategy 1, it is a good idea to have a designated staff member who serves as the EAP coordinator, and who would have overall responsibility for the written medical EAP. The medical EAP should describe the responsibilities of this individual as well as other staff members who will carry out certain roles at the time of any emergency (e.g., first responder, manager on duty, front desk person, etc.). It will be necessary to designate these individuals and their responsibilities before finalizing the contingency plans described in Risk Management Strategy 4.

At all times of operation, there should be a staff member who is designated as the manager on duty (MOD). The MOD would be summoned to the location of the emergency to assist the first responder if necessary, help control the area (e.g., keeping people away) if needed, assist EMS when they arrive, and, after the incident, complete the incident report form (see Risk Management Strategy 8). Staff members selected to serve in this role need to be highly responsible and competent individuals.

Risk Management Strategy 6: Establish a communications system.

The medical EAP should include an effective communications system. For example, staff members should know the emergency communications system and who is responsible for what communications and in what order. For example, if a staff members calls 911 from an emergency phone in the lower level of the facility, his/her next step may be to call the front desk (or solicit a bystander to inform the front desk person) so this staff member is aware that EMS is on their way.

The front desk staff member then perhaps calls the MOD to summon him or her to the location of the emergency as well as calls another staff member to meet and guide EMS to the location of the emergency. The communications system should also specify who retrieves the first-aid kit and/or AED at the time of a medical emergency (e.g., how and to whom does the first responder communicate his or her need for this equipment). In addition, the written medical EAP should specify where emergency phones, first-aid kits, and AEDs are located throughout the facility. Posted next to each emergency phone should be appropriate written procedures when making an emergency telephone call. A secondary communication system (e.g., cell phone, two-way radio) should be identified in case the primary system fails.

As part of an overall communications system, some facilities may want to consider developing "code blue" procedures to be used at the time of a life-threatening situation.[86] In this scenario, a code blue announcement is made over the facility's intercom indicating the location of the emergency. This alerts all staff members to assume their roles immediately. In addition, some facilities set up emergency stations at various locations in the facility that have a red panic button, which when pressed connects directly to a separate telephone at the front desk indicating the location of the emergency. These emergency stations can also contain gloves, protective eyewear, face masks, and so on, to help comply with universal precautions. Some facilities have also included an abbreviated EAP on the back of an employee's identification badge to help remind staff members of the proper EAP procedures at a glance.[86]

Each facility needs to develop the best communications system possible, given their circumstances and any unique features (e.g., size of facility, stairs, and elevators) within their facility. It is essential, as stated earlier, to have local EMS involved in the development of the medical EAP, especially with this component addressing the communications plan. For example, a transportation route should be preestablished for EMS personnel to enter and exit the facility, and be included in the medical EAP.

The communications system should be tested and practiced during EAP trainings and drills (see Risk Management Strategy 9) to help ensure staff members are carrying out the communications system properly. It will be necessary to complete the development of the communications system before finalizing the contingency plans described in Risk Management Strategy 4.

Risk Management Strategy 7: Provide and maintain a first-aid kit(s) and AED(s).

All health/fitness facilities need to have at least one first-aid kit and one AED; however, large facilities may need to have more. Only the MFA Standards provide some guidance to help make this determination regarding the number of AEDs as follows: "In the case of multiple story buildings or large facilities (greater that 30,000 sq. ft.), additional AEDs should be considered. AED placement should be determined by response time/distance for the AED to be brought to the victim. American Heart Association recommended response time is three (3) minutes or less."[74] The medical EAP should describe the locations of all first-aid kits and AEDs. Of course, these should be located in areas of quick and easy access.

Regular maintenance of this equipment is also essential. First-aid kits should always be checked to be sure they are properly stocked with the appropriate supplies. Information regarding the contents of workplace first-aid kits (that meet OSHA's compliance regulations) as well as purchasing information can be found on the American Red Cross website at www.redcross.org/servcies/hss/resources. Regarding AEDs, they should be inspected and maintained regularly in accordance with the manufacturer's guidelines. These maintenance tasks could be included in the EAP coordinator's responsibilities.

Risk Management Strategy 8: Address post-emergency procedures.

Although standards of practice published by professional organizations address various emergency procedures, they do not provide specific post-emergency procedures that can be just as important from a legal liability perspective. As mentioned earlier, during all hours of operation, health/fitness facilities should have a staff member who is designated as the MOD. This individual may have several responsibilities when a medical emergency occurs, but one area of responsibility will probably include carrying out post-emergency procedures. Once the injured party has been sent home or to the hospital, the several procedures described here should be completed. If a participant is sent to the hospital, every effort should be made to contact a member of the victim's family right away. Note: At the time of joining, members should be asked to submit the names/contact information of two individuals who could be contacted in the case of an emergency and this information should be kept in each member's file.

First, all staff members should be trained on what to say and not to say to an injured participant. Staff members should express sympathy but not say something like "it is our fault" or "our insurance will pay for everything." Participants may rely on these comments and include them in any future legal claim(s). If the injured participant is conscious and able to speak, a designated staff member (e.g., the first responder or MOD) should ask the participant to describe the incident, including what, how, why, when, and where. These statements should then be recorded onto the Incident Report Form. This evidence may be useful because any admission on part of the participant may protect the health/fitness facility in any later litigation. If the injured party is unable to answer questions or unconscious, then witnesses to the incident (e.g., staff members, other participants) should be asked the what, how, why, when, and where and their responses recorded on the Incident Report Form. It may also be a good idea to ask the witnesses if they noticed any unusual behavior of the injured party prior to the injury (e.g., misuse of the equipment, overtraining, etc.). Contact information of witnesses should also be recorded.

The MOD should also take any photographs of any conditions present where the medical emergency occurred (e.g., wet or dry surfaces, signage posted in the area, any exercise equipment involved in the injury). If a piece of exercise equipment was involved, photos may show that the injury was possibly due to a product defect or that the equipment was working and maintained properly—evidence that may help protect the health/fitness facility from liability. The MOD should also record the name of the manufacturer and serial number of the piece of equipment. In addition, as mentioned in Chapter 9, such equipment should be inspected (and repaired/serviced if needed) before anyone uses it again. Any damaged parts should be retained.

Once all evidence is obtained, the MOD should complete the Incident Report Form properly. See Appendix 11 for a sample form. The EAP coordinator and perhaps others on the EAP planning team should work closely with the facility's legal and insurance experts in the development of this form so that the information gathered will help provide a good defense in any future litigation that might occur. It may also be a good idea to state "privileged and confidential"[87] on this form so legal counsel can then perhaps claim that this document is subject to attorney-client privilege and therefore should not be disclosed to third parties.

Once completed in a timely fashion, the MOD should submit the Incident Report Form to the manager/owner, who in turn submits it to the facility's legal and insurance representatives. A copy should be retained in a secure place within the facility for at least as long as the respective state's statutes of limitations.

After a serious medical emergency, it may be common for participants and perhaps the media to ask staff members about the incident. It will be important that staff members are trained on how to respond to these questions—what to say and not to say. But it may be necessary for management to remind staff members of the facility's policy in this regard after any such incident. For example, a response may be "the incident is being handled by experienced experts" along with a referral to the designated spokesperson for the facility when these situations occur. Also, after a medical emergency, later that day or the next day, either the MOD or manager should contact the injured party, or in the case of a serious injury, one of the victim's emergency contacts. The purpose of this follow-up would be to show concern and obtain the status of the injury. Any information obtained could be added to the Incident Report Form.

Lastly, after these procedures have been completed, the MOD and manager of the facility should evaluate how well the medical EAP was carried out. Depending on the outcome of this evaluation, changes may be needed and/or staff members may need to be retrained. A close investigation to determine how a similar incident could be avoided in the future should also be made. Note: The preceding post-emergency procedures were summarized from an article previously published.[88]

Risk Management Strategy 9: Test the medical EAP, train staff members, and conduct regular drills.

After the Medical EAP is drafted, it will be important to simulate medical emergencies to test the written EAP procedures and staff members' actions in carrying them out. Based on this initial test (or evaluation) of the draft medical EAP, it should be modified or adjusted accordingly. A final draft should be approved by the EAP planning team, the risk management advisory committee, and the medical liaison. It is then included in the RMPPM so that all staff members who have responsibility for it will have access to it.

Additionally, staff members should be trained in the EAP at the beginning of their employment and regularly thereafter. Even staff not trained in CPR/AED and first aid, and not responsible for administering emergency response, can be trained to assist in the event of a medical emergency. They may be able to ensure that EMS has been notified, retrieve first-aid supplies, or direct EMS to the exact location inside the facility.

Medical EAPs must be regularly practiced, evaluated, and updated. Announced and unannounced drills or rehearsals of the EAPs are necessary and should be conducted regularly. They should include practicing the various contingency plans in the medical EAP and proper completion/filing of the Incident Report Form. The ACSM/AHA Joint PP[64] states that emergency plans should be practiced at least once every 3 months, and more often if there are changes in staff. Documentation of such rehearsals should be carefully retained. Some administrators use standardized forms or videotape for evidence that their EAP was rehearsed.

Risk Management Strategy 10: Create EAP documentation and record-keeping procedures.

Creating procedures to document properly all key components of the medical EAP is essential, as is keeping these documents stored in a secure place for a period of time to conform to the applicable statutes of limitation. These documents may serve as helpful evidence to demonstrate that the health/fitness personnel and facilities were adhering to the standard of care in the event of a negligence or wrongful death claim or lawsuit. These include: (a) the written medical EAP; (b) the written ECP and other related requirements of OHSA's BBP Standard such as staff training sessions and any exposure incident; (c) dates of staff trainings (e.g., initially on hiring and regular drills throughout the year) and a list of staff members who attended/participated; (d) the name of the individual who conducted the staff trainings, their credentials, and the content of each training session; (e) certification (first aid, CPR, AED) records of all staff members responsible for carrying out the medical EAP; (f) inspections of first-aid kits and AEDs; and (g) Incident Report Forms and any related evidence that was gathered.

PUT INTO PRACTICE CHECKLIST 11-1

Rate your phase of development for each of following risk management strategies related to medical emergency action plans:

	Developed	Partially Developed	Not Developed
1. Formulating a planning team.			
2. Complying with OSHA's Bloodborne Pathogens (BBP) Standard.			
3. Complying with applicable state laws.			
4. Preparing written contingency plans for various medical emergencies.			
5. Determining staff qualifications and responsibilities.			
6. Establishing a communications system.			
7. Providing and maintaining a first-aid kit(s) and AED(s).			
8. Addressing post-emergency procedures.			
9. Testing the medical EAP, training staff members, and conducting regular drills.			
10. Creating EAP documentation and record-keeping procedures.			

SUMMARY

This chapter presented laws such as OSHA's BBP Standard and state laws that require health/fitness facilities to have an AED, standards practice published by professional organizations, and a variety of risk management strategies applicable to medical EAPs. After reading the chapter, health/fitness professionals should realize that this is a key component of a health/fitness facility's overall risk management plan. A common mistake that many professionals make is thinking that they, and/or their staff, will know exactly what to do in the event of a medical emergency. However, often if there is no specific plan of action—particularly one that has not been rehearsed—people may not know how to react properly, quickly, and calmly to a medical emergency. Having a written, well-thought-out, and complete medical EAP that is understood and regularly practiced by all staff members should greatly assist them in the event of an actual medical emergency, and help minimize any subsequent litigation as demonstrated in the case law examples described in this chapter.

Knowing and practicing what to do in the event of a medical emergency should rank high on the priority list for all health/fitness managers and professionals. Although serious life-threatening medical emergencies may occur infrequently at health/fitness facilities, it is absolutely essential that facility personnel are prepared to respond properly and according to the standard of care. It may mean the difference between life and death, and the difference between a satisfied participant and a lawsuit.

RISK MANAGEMENT ASSIGNMENTS

1. Locate and analyze the strength and weaknesses of several programs' Exposure Control Plans (ECPs) online. Then draft a written ECP tailored to meet your facility's needs.

   _____

   _____

   _____

   _____

2. Visit a local health/fitness facility. What jobs and tasks may expose the workers to BBP occupational exposure? What would you do to eliminate or reduce such exposure?

   _____

   _____

   _____

   _____

3. Develop an employee training program designed to cover OSHA's BBP Standard for a typical health/fitness facility.

   _____

   _____

   _____

   _____

4. Develop a list of potential common medical emergencies that could occur in a health/fitness facility and then draft contingency plans for each.

   _____

   _____

   _____

   _____

5. Develop an inspection checklist that could be used to document that certain emergency medical equipment (first-aid kit, AED, etc.) has been inspected.

   _____

   _____

   _____

   _____

6. Suppose you wanted to evaluate the staff's response to an unannounced medical EAP drill. Discuss how you would simulate a medical emergency and how you would evaluate their response.

   _____

   _____

   _____

   _____

7. Investigate several AED manufacturers to learn about the different AED models. Which model may be most effective for a typical health/fitness facility? Describe the maintenance guidelines established by the manufacturer.

_____

_____

_____

_____

8. Describe how your facility will establish procedures to help ensure that staff members who have responsibility for carrying out the medical EAP will keep their first-aid and CPR/AED certifications current.

_____

_____

_____

_____

KEY TERMS

Bloodborne pathogens
Engineering controls
Exposure incident
Handwashing facilities
Health risks
Injury risks

Loss prevention
Loss reduction
Occupational exposure
Other potentially infectious
  materials (OPIM)
Personal protective equipment

Sudden cardiac arrest (SCA)
Universal precautions
Work practice controls

REFERENCES

1. No Pain, No Gain—The Number of Health Clubs in the U.S. has Swelled 5.1 Percent to a Record 17,807 Facilities as of January 2002. Media Central, Inc. 2002. Available at: http://findarticles.com/p/articles/mi_m4021/is_2002_April_1/ai_87109757. Accessed January 11, 2008.
2. U.S. Health Club Industry Continues Strong Growth; Total Number of Health Clubs and Gyms Rose by 14% in 2004. CNET Networks, Inc. 2007. Available at: http://findarticles.com/p/articles/mi_m0EIN/is_2005_Jan_13/ai_n8690907. Accessed January 11, 2008.
3. International Health Racquet and Sportsclub Association (IHRSA).*Global Report: State of the Health Club Industry.* Boston: IHRSA; 2005.
4. YMCA. *About the YMCA.* Chicago: n.d. Available at: http://www.ymca.net/about_the_ymca. Accessed January 11, 2008.
5. International Health Racquet and Sportsclub Association (IHRSA). *Global Report: State of the Health Club Industry.* Boston: IHRSA; 2002.
6. American Heart Association (AHA). *Heart Disease and Stroke Statistics—2006 Update.* Dallas: American Heart Association; 2006.
7. Albert CM, Mittleman MA, Chae CU, et al. Triggering of sudden death from cardiac causes by vigorous exertion. *N Engl J Med.* 1999;343:1355–1361.
8. McInnis KJ, Hayakawa S, Balady GJ. Cardiovascular screening and emergency procedures at health clubs and fitness centers. *Am J Cardiol.* 1997;80:380–383.
9. McInnis KJ, Herbert WG, Herbert DJ, Herbert J, Ribisl P, Franklin B. Low compliance with national standards for cardiovascular emergency preparedness at health clubs. *Chest.* 2001;120:283–288.

10. Eickhoff-Shemek J, Deja K. Are facilities complying with ACSM standards? Part II. *ACSM's Health Fitness J.* 2002;6(2):19–24.

11. Eickhoff-Shemek J, Deja K. Are facilities complying with ACSM standards? Part I. *ACSM's Health Fitness J.* 2002;6(3):16–21.

12. Herbert WG, Herbert DL, McInnis KJ, et al. Cardiovascular emergency preparedness in recreation facilities at major US universities: College fitness center emergency readiness. *Prevent Cardiol.* Summer 2007:128–133.

13. Herbert DL. Update on AEDs in health and fitness facilities. *Exercise Standards and Malpractice Reporter.* 2004:18(2):28.

14. Occupational Safety and Health Administration (OSHA). OSHA's Mission. n.d. Available at: http://www.osha.gov/oshinfo/mission.html. Accessed June 29, 2006.

15. International Health Racquet and Sportsclub Association (IHRSA). OSHA Compliance: What It Means to Your Club. August 2003 In Brief. Available at: http://cms.ihrsa.org/index.cfm?fuseaction=Page.viewPage&pageId=15725&nodeID=15 Accessed January 13, 2008.

16. *Bloodborne Pathogens.* 29 C.F.R. § 1910.1030. Thomson/West; 2007.

17. Durkin H. OSHA standards protect health club staff from bloodborne pathogens. *ACSM's Health Fitness J.* 1998;2(1):40–41.

18. Occupational Safety and Health Administration (OSHA). Standard Interpretations. Most frequently asked questions concerning the bloodborne pathogens standard. Available at: http://www.osha.gov/pls/oshaweb/owadisp.show_document?p_table=INTERPRETATIONS&p_id=21010. Accessed June 29, 2006.

19. Occupational Safety and Health Administration (OSHA). Bloodborne Fact Sheet: An Overview of the Standard. Available at: http://www.osha.gov/OshDoc/data_BloodborneFacts/bbfact01.pdf. Accessed June 29, 2006.

20. Occupational Safety and Health Administration (OSHA). Bloodborne Fact Sheet: Personal Protective Equipment Cuts Risk. Available at: http:// http://www.osha.gov/OshDoc/data_BloodborneFacts/index.html. Accessed June 29, 2006.

21. Occupational Safety and Health Administration (OSHA). Bloodborne Fact Sheet: Hepatitis B Vaccination. Available at: http://www.osha.gov/OshDoc/data_BloodborneFacts/bbfact05.pdf. Accessed June 29, 2006.

22. Occupational Safety and Health Administration (OSHA). Bloodborne Fact Sheet: Reporting Exposure Incidents. Available at: http://www.osha.gov/OshDoc/data_BloodborneFacts/bbfact04.pdf. Accessed June 29, 2006.

23. Wood A. A Public/Private Legal Preparedness Initiative to Develop Good Samaritan Liability Protection for Business and Non-Profit Entities Assisting in Emergency Community Preparedness Activities. March 2, 2007. Available at: http://nciph.sph.unc.edu/law/Good_Sam_Background_3_02_07.pdf. Accessed January 13, 2008.

24. Connaughton DP, Spengler JO. Automated external defibrillators in sport and recreation settings: An analysis of immunity provisions in state legislation. *J Leg Aspects Sport.* 2001;11(1):50–67.

25. Spengler JO, Connaughton DP. Health/Fitness programs and AEDs: An overview of current legislation. *ACSM's Health Fitness J.* 2004;8(1):27–28.

26. Herbert DL. Health clubs and AEDs—New legislation in New York, Rhode Island and Louisiana—Bill pending in Illinois. *Exercise Standards and Malpractice Reporter.* 2004;18(4):54–59.

27. Herbert DL. California passes legislation into law on AEDs and supplements in high school athletes. *Exercise Standards and Malpractice Reporter.* 2005;19(6):81–88.

28. Herbert DL. New AED laws for health clubs in New Jersey and Michigan—one proposed in Kansas. *Exercise Standards and Malpractice Reporter.* 2006;20(2):17–25.

29. Herbert DL. New AED laws for health clubs in New Jersey and Michigan—one proposed in Kansas. *Exercise Standards and Malpractice Reporter.* 2006;20(2):17–25, 21.

30. *Keelean et al. v. Department of Corrections,* 2000 Mich. App. LEXIS 2409 (Mich. Ct. App., 2000).

31. *Hartwig v. Oregon Trail Eye Clinic et al.,* 580 N.W.2d 86 (Neb., 1998).

32. *Vanderburg v. Spa South Corporation,* Case No. 89–4267, Circuit Court, Manatee County, Florida, 1989. Analyzed in: Herbert DL. Must health clubs provide CPR for patrons? *Exercise Standards and Malpractice Reporter.* 1992;6(1):1,4–5.

33. *Vanderburg v. Spa South Corporation,* Case No. 89–4267, Circuit Court, Manatee County, Florida, 1989. Analyzed in: Herbert DL. Must health clubs provide CPR for patrons? *Exercise Standards and Malpractice Reporter.* 1992;6(1):1,4–5, 4.

34. *Kleinknecht v. Gettysburg College,* 989 F.2d 1360 (3rd Cir., 1993).

35. *Brown v. Bally Total Fitness Corporation,* 2003 Cal. App. Unpub. LEXIS 8245 (Cal. Ct. App., 2003).

36. *Brown v. Bally Total Fitness Corporation,* 2003 Cal. App. Unpub. LEXIS 8245 (Cal. Ct. App., 2003):7.

37. *Brown v. Bally Total Fitness Corporation,* 2003 Cal. App. Unpub. LEXIS 8245 (Cal. Ct. App., 2003):8.

38. *Brown v. Bally Total Fitness Corporation,* 2003 Cal. App. Unpub. LEXIS 8245 (Cal. Ct. App., 2003), 13–14.

39. *Chai v. Sports & Fitness Clubs of America, Inc.,* Case No. 98–16053 CA (05), Broward County Circuit Court, Florida, 17th Judicial District. n.d. Analyzed in: Failure to defibrillate results in new litigation. *Exercise Standards and Malpractice Reporter.* 1999;13(4):55–56.

40. *Chai v. Sports & Fitness Clubs of America, Inc.,* Case No. 98–16053 CA (05), Broward County Circuit Court, Florida, 17th Judicial District. n.d. Analyzed in: Herbert DL. Alleged failure to have AED litigation on Florida results in another defense verdict—But, plaintiff receives $2.25 million. *Exercise Standards and Malpractice Reporter.* 2000;14(4):54–55.

41. *Fruh v. Wellbridge Club Management, Inc.* Case Number 02–10689 PBS, United States, District Court, District of Massachusetts, 2004. Analyzed in: Herbert DL. Another AED case. *Exercise Standards and Malpractice Reporter.* 2002;16(6):90–91.

42. *Fruh v. Wellbridge Club Management, Inc.* Case Number 02–10689 PBS, United States, District Court, District of Massachusetts, 2004. Analyzed in: Herbert DL. Another AED case. *Exercise Standards and Malpractice Reporter.* 2002;16(6):90–91, 90.

43. *Fruh v. Wellbridge Club Management, Inc.* Case Number 02–10689 PBS, United States, District Court, District of Massachusetts, 2004. Analyzed in: Herbert DL. Another AED case. *Exercise Standards and Malpractice Reporter.* 2002;16(6):90–91, 91.

44. Herbert DL. Large settlement approved for plaintiffs in AED case. *Exercise Standards and Malpractice Reporter.* 2004;18(3):38.

45. *Tringali Mayer v. L.A. Fitness International, LLC.* Case Number 04–19840, 17th Judicial Circuit, Broward County, Florida, 2004. Analyzed in: Herbert DL. Large verdict against AED deficient health and fitness facility. *Exercise Standards and Malpractice Reporter.* 2006;20(4):49–54.

46. *Tringali Mayer v. L.A. Fitness International, LLC.* Case Number 04–19840, 17th Judicial Circuit, Broward County, Florida, 2004. Analyzed in: Herbert DL. Large verdict against AED deficient health and fitness facility. *Exercise Standards and Malpractice Reporter.* 2006;20(4):49–54, 52.

47. *Tringali Mayer v. L.A. Fitness International, LLC.* Case Number 04–19840, 17th Judicial Circuit, Broward County, Florida, 2004. Analyzed in: Herbert DL. Large verdict against AED deficient health and fitness facility. *Exercise Standards and Malpractice Reporter.* 2006;20(4):49–54, 53.

48. *Tringali Mayer v. L.A. Fitness International, LLC.* Case Number 04–19840, 17th Judicial Circuit, Broward County, Florida, 2004. Analyzed in: Herbert DL. Large verdict against AED deficient health and fitness facility. *Exercise Standards and Malpractice Reporter.* 2006;20(4):49–54, 54.

49. *Delibero v. Q Clubs, Inc.,* 956 S. 2d 1286 (Fla. Dist. Ct. App.).

50. *Delibero v. Q Clubs, Inc.,* 956 S. 2d 1286 (Fla. Dist. Ct. App.):1287.

51. *Delibero v. Q Clubs, Inc.,* 956 S. 2d 1286 (Fla. Dist. Ct. App.):1288.

52. *Lewin v. Fitworks of Cincinnati, LLC,* Case Number A0305312, Hamilton County, Ohio, 2005. Analyzed in: Herbert DL. AED case in Ohio results in judgment for defendant club. *Exercise Standards and Malpractice Reporter.* 2005;19(5):65, 68–73.

53. *Lewin v. Fitworks of Cincinnati, LLC,* Case Number A0305312, Hamilton County, Ohio, 2005. Analyzed in: Herbert DL. AED case in Ohio results in judgment for defendant club. *Exercise Standards and Malpractice Reporter.* 2005;19(5):65, 68–73, 71.

54. *Lewin v. Fitworks of Cincinnati, LLC,* Case Number A0305312, Hamilton County, Ohio, 2005. Analyzed in: Herbert DL. AED case in Ohio results in judgment for defendant club. *Exercise Standards and Malpractice Reporter.* 2005;19(5):68–73, 69.

55. *Lewin v. Fitworks of Cincinnati, LLC,* Case Number A0305312, Hamilton County, Ohio, 2005. Analyzed in: Herbert DL. AED case in Ohio results in judgment for defendant club. *Exercise Standards and Malpractice Reporter.* 2005;19(5):68–73, 72.

56. *Salte v. YMCA of Metropolitan Chicago Foundation*, 814 N.E.2d 610 (Ill. App. Ct., 2004).

57. *Salte v. YMCA of Metropolitan Chicago Foundation*, 814 N.E.2d 610 (Ill. App. Ct., 2004):611–612.

58. *Salte v. YMCA of Metropolitan Chicago Foundation*, 814 N.E.2d 610 (Ill. App. Ct., 2004):615.

59. *Salte v. YMCA of Metropolitan Chicago Foundation*, 814 N.E.2d 610 (Ill. App. Ct., 2004):617.

60. Herbert DL. Illinois appellate court rules against any requirement of AEDs in health clubs. *Exercise Standards and Malpractice Reporter.* 2004;18(5):73–76.

61. Tharrett SJ, McInnis KJ, Peterson JA, eds. *ACSM's Health/Fitness Facility Standards and Guidelines.* 3rd ed. Champaign, Ill: Human Kinetics; 2007.

62. Tharrett SJ, McInnis KJ, Peterson JA, eds. *ACSM's Health/Fitness Facility Standards and Guidelines.* 3rd Ed. Champaign, Ill: Human Kinetics; 2007:1–2.

63. Whaley MH, ed. *ACSM's Guidelines for Exercise Testing and Prescription.* 7th ed. Philadelphia: Lippincott Williams & Wilkins; 2006.

64. American College of Sports Medicine and American Heart Association Joint Position Statement. Recommendations for cardiovascular screening, staffing, and emergency policies at health/fitness facilities. *Med Sci Sports Exerc.* 1998;30:1009–1018.

65. American College of Sports Medicine and American Heart Association Joint Position Statement. Recommendations for cardiovascular screening, staffing, and emergency policies at health/fitness facilities. *Med Sci Sports Exerc.* 1998;30:1009–1018, 1016.

66. American College of Sports Medicine and American Heart Association Joint Position Statement. Automated external defibrillators in health/fitness facilities. *Med Sci Sports Exerc.* 2002;34:561–564.

67. American College of Sports Medicine and American Heart Association Joint Position Statement. Automated external defibrillators in health/fitness facilities. *Med Sci Sports Exerc.* 2002;34:561–564, 562.

68. *NSCA Strength & Conditioning Professional Standards & Guidelines.* May 2001. Available at: http://www.nscalift.org/Publications/standards.shtml. Colorado Springs, CO: National Strength and Conditioning Association (NSCA). Accessed September 2, 2007.

69. *NSCA Strength & Conditioning Professional Standards & Guidelines.* May 2001. Available at: http://www.nscalift.org/Publications/standards.shtml. Colorado Springs, CO: National Strength and Conditioning Association (NSCA). Accessed September 2, 2007:14–15.

70. IHRSA Club Membership Standards. In: *IHRSA's Guide to Club Membership & Conduct.* 3rd ed. Boston: International Health, Racquet & Sportsclub Association (IHRSA); 2005.

71. IHRSA Club Membership Standards. In: *IHRSA's Guide to Club Membership & Conduct.* 3rd ed. Boston: International Health, Racquet & Sportsclub Association (IHRSA); 2005:4.

72. IHRSA Club Membership Standards. In: *IHRSA's Guide to Club Membership & Conduct.* 3rd ed. Boston: International Health, Racquet & Sportsclub Association (IHRSA); 2005:3.

73. *The Medical Fitness Model: Facility Standards and Guidelines.* Richmond, Va: Medical Fitness Association (MFA); May 2006:8.

74. *The Medical Fitness Model: Facility Standards and Guidelines.* Richmond, Va: Medical Fitness Association (MFA); May 2006:9.

75. *Canadian Fitness Safety Standards & Recommended Guidelines.* 3rd ed. 2004. Available at: http://www.oases.on.ca/safety/safetyStdsCurrent.htm. Ontario, Canada: Ontario Association of Sport and Exercise Sciences (OASES). Accessed September 2, 2007.

76. *Canadian Fitness Safety Standards & Recommended Guidelines.* 3rd ed. 2004. Available at: http://www.oases.on.ca/safety/safetyStdsCurrent.htm. Ontario, Canada: Ontario Association of Sport and Exercise Sciences (OASES). Accessed September 2, 2007:1–2.

77. *Exercise Standards & Guidelines Reference Manual.* 4th ed. Sherman Oaks, Calif: Aerobics and Fitness Association of America (AFAA); 2005.

78. *Exercise Standards & Guidelines Reference Manual.* 4th ed. Sherman Oaks, Calif: Aerobics and Fitness Association of America (AFAA); 2005:7.

79. *Exercise Standards & Guidelines Reference Manual.* 4th ed. Sherman Oaks, Calif: Aerobics and Fitness Association of America (AFAA); 2005:6.

80. *Medical Advisory Committee Recommendations: A Resource Guide for YMCAs*. Chicago: YMCA of the USA; February 2007.

81. *Medical Advisory Committee Recommendations: A Resource Guide for YMCAs*. Chicago: YMCA of the USA; February 2007:36.

82. *Medical Advisory Committee Recommendations: A Resource Guide for YMCAs*. Chicago: YMCA of the USA; February 2007:11.

83. *Medical Advisory Committee Recommendations: A Resource Guide for YMCAs*. Chicago: YMCA of the USA; February 2007:73.

84. American College of Sports Medicine and American Heart Association Joint Position Statement. Recommendations for cardiovascular screening, staffing, and emergency policies at health/fitness facilities. *Med Sci Sports Exerc*. 1998;30:1009–1018, 1015.

85. McInnis KJ, Herbert WG. *Automated External Defibrillators (AEDs) in YMCAs: A Technical Assistance Paper*. 2nd ed. Chicago: YMCA of the USA; 2006.

86. Stoike PJ. Automated external defibrillators: Purchasing and staff training considerations. *ACSM's Health Fitness J*. 2001;5(4):20–26.

87. Herbert DL. Lawsuit prevention: 8 techniques to keep your fitness center liability free. *On-Site Fitness*. May-June 2000:36, 38.

88. Eickhoff-Shemek J. Medical emergency procedures: Minimize your liability. *ACSM's Health Fitness J*. 2006;10(3):35–37.

APPENDIX 11

The following incident report was developed by Jon Denley, Senior Vice President, Creative Agency Group, and is presented as an example only. Reprinted with permission.

HEALTH, FITNESS & RACQUET SPORTS CLUB INCIDENT REPORT
[COMPLETE FOR ALL INCIDENTS AND REPORT IMMEDIATELY – PLEASE PRINT]

Date

| Month   Day   Year | Time of Accident   A.M.   P.M. | Club Member ☐ Yes ☐ No | Club Name   Club Location |

Injured Person

FIRST   (M.I.)   LAST   AGE

NUMBER AND STREET

CITY   STATE   ZIP

BUSINESS PHONE   HOME PHONE

HOSPITAL OR FIRST AID SQUAD NOTIFIED ☐ Yes ☐ No

NAME: _____
TIME OF INITIAL CALL: _____
TIMES OF FOLLOW-UP CALLS: 1. _____
2. _____ 3. _____ 4. _____
TIME OF ARRIVAL: _____
TIME OF DEPARTURE: _____
TAKEN TO HOSPITAL? _____
NAME OF FIRST AID ATTENDANT: _____

DESCRIPTION OF ACCIDENT:

CHECK ITEMS THAT APPLY TO INJURED PERSON:

BLEEDING INJURY: ☐ YES ☐ NO   **OTHER VISIBLE INJURY:** ☐ YES ☐ NO

NO VISIBLE INJURY, BUT COMPLAINT OF PAIN: ☐ YES ☐ NO

IF EYE INJURY, WEARING EYEGUARDS? ☐ YES ☐ NO

DESCRIBE EXACT INJURY SUSTAINED:

DESCRIBE FIRST AID ADMINSTERED BY CLUB:

First Witness	Second Witness
FIRST (M.I.) LAST	FIRST (M.I.) LAST
NUMBER AND STREET	NUMBER AND STREET
CITY STATE ZIP	CITY STATE ZIP
BUSINESS PHONE HOME PHONE	BUSINESS PHONE HOME PHONE
DESCRIPTION OF ACCIDENT BY WITNESS:	DESCRIPTION OF ACCIDENT BY WITNESS:
SIGNATURE:	SIGNATURE:

HEALTH, FITNESS & RACQUET SPORTS CLUB INCIDENT REPORT
[continued]

NAME OF CLUB PERSONNEL WHO INSPECTED THE SCENE:	POSITION	DATE OF INSPECTION:

CONDITIONS FOUND: _____

_____

_____

ACTION TAKEN, IF PRACTICAL, TO AVOID RECURRENCE: _____

_____

Description of Place of Accident

☐ INTERIOR ☐ EXTERIOR ☐ WALKING AREA ☐ PLAYING SURFACE ☐ LOCKER ROOM

☐ PHY. FITNESS ROOM ☐ OTHER: _____

CONDITIONS: ☐ DRY ☐ WET ☐ SMOOTH ☐ EVEN SURFACE ☐ SLIPPERY

FOREIGN SUBSTANCE? ☐ YES ☐ NO   IF 'YES', DESCRIPTION: _____

IF INJURY TOOK PLACE OUTSIDE CLUB BUILDING, CHECK APPROPRIATE ITEMS:

WEATHER CONDITION: ☐ DRY ☐ RAIN ☐ SNOW ☐ ICE ☐ DAY ☐ NIGHT LIGHTING CONDITIONS:_____

IMPORTANT: IF INJURY TOOK PLACE ON A COURT, PROVIDE NAME, ADDRESS AND TELEPHONE NUMBER OF THOSE INDIVIDUALS WHO USED OR RENTED THE COURT DURING THE PRIOR HOUR.

_____

_____

_____

ADDITIONAL COMMENTS

_____

_____

DID POLICE INVESTIGATE?   NAME AND RANK OF OFFICER   DEPARTMENT   PHONE NUMBER
☐ YES   ☐ NO

_____

SUBMITTED BY:	SIGNATURE:	TELEPHONE:	DATE / TIME

This information is for reporting purposes only. The information provided is the responsibility of the insured and/or club.

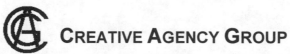

CREATIVE AGENCY GROUP

15 CREATIVE CIRCLE, ROUTE 520, HOLMDEL, NEW JERSEY 07733
800-888-8381   732-946-4000   732-946-2044 FAX

PART III

FINAL RISK MANAGEMENT STEPS, SELECTED TOPICS, AND CONCLUSION

CHAPTER 12

Implementation and Evaluation of the Risk Management Plan

LEARNING OBJECTIVES After reading this chapter, health/fitness students and professionals will be able to:

1. Describe how to implement a risk management plan.
2. Use strategic planning to implement a risk management plan.
3. Develop a Risk Management Policies and Procedures Manual (RMPPM).
4. Develop in-service staff training programs that address risk management policies and procedures.
5. Conduct both formative and summative evaluations of a health/fitness facility's risk management plan.

This chapter is divided into two major sections: implementation of the risk management plan and evaluation of the risk management plan. Implementation addresses the importance of using strategic planning to implement the many risk management strategies presented in chapters 4 through 11, organizing your written risk management strategies into a Risk Management Policy and Procedures Manual, and training staff members. The evaluation section presents both *formative evaluation* (ongoing evaluation procedures, both informal and formal) and *summative evaluation* (annual formal evaluation of the entire risk management plan).

STEP 3 IMPLEMENTATION OF THE RISK MANAGEMENT PLAN

This section describes what is meant by "comprehensive" risk management. It also presents strategic planning as a necessary approach for the two major aspects of the risk management implementation phase: developing the Risk Management Policies and Procedures Manual and conducting staff training.

"COMPREHENSIVE" RISK MANAGEMENT AND STRATEGIC PLANNING

Toward the end of Chapters 5 through 11, a Put into Practice Checklist was included so that health/fitness professionals could determine what risk management strategies had been developed, partially developed, or not developed for their facility and its programs and services. It is important that these determinations be made before beginning the next phase of the risk management process: implementing a **comprehensive risk management plan**. Comprehensive risk management involves implementing risk management strategies that reflect applicable laws (statutory, administrative, and case law) and standards of practice published by professional and independent organizations.

As discussed in Chapter 1, the health/fitness manager (i.e., the top position in the facility who has overall responsibility for the facility and programs) most often is the risk management manager and therefore ultimately responsible for risk management. Because other health/fitness professionals within the facility have significant risk management responsibilities, they too should be directly involved in all phases of the risk management process. The risk management advisory committee members also play a critical role in the risk management process, which is discussed in more detail later.

Implementing a comprehensive risk management plan involves strategic planning on part of the health/fitness manager, professional staff members, and the risk management advisory committee. A strategic plan is basically a set of decisions about what to do, why to do it, and how to do it.[1] Completing the Put Into Practice Checklists in the previous chapters was the first step in this decision-making process—it determined what needed to be done. The term *strategic planning* infers that some decisions are more important than others, and therefore sometimes involves tough decision making to prioritize the risk management strategies that a health/fitness facility needs to implement. Each facility has to determine their own priorities in implementing their risk management strategies. However, a well-established medical Emergency Action Plan (see Chapter 11) should be a top priority.

Strategic planning to implement a comprehensive risk management plan is a complex and difficult task. It takes a great deal of time and effort, but the benefits can be significant for a health/fitness facility as described in Chapter 1 and later under Evaluation of the Risk Management Plan. It appears from the research studies summarized in Chapter 1 that many health/fitness facilities are not doing an adequate job of implementing basic safety procedures (risk management strategies that are required by the law or reflected in published standards of practice) into their daily operations. As also stated in Chapter 1, there has been an increase in litigation in the health/fitness field, and this trend is predicted to continue. Although part of this is probably due to a lack of adequate education and training in the law and risk management, it is perhaps also related to health/fitness professionals thinking and acting in a more "reactive" mode rather than a "proactive" mode regarding risk management. For example, instead of thinking about how to prevent medical emergencies and potential subsequent liability (proactive thinking and acting), health/fitness professionals often just accept such risks and allow them to exist and only address them when they arise (reactive thinking and acting). As defined in Chapter 1, risk management is a proactive process that will help minimize liability losses for health/fitness professionals and the organizations they represent.

This concept is best described in Covey's book, *Fist Things First*.[2] Covey would classify implementing a comprehensive risk management plan as a Quadrant II activity. See Covey's Time Management Matrix in Figure 12-1. Covey states that the majority of our time should be spent on Quadrant II activities (important, not urgent activities) that not only help us to achieve our goals but also decrease the amount of time spent on problems that occur in Quadrant I (important, urgent activities). This concept is relevant to risk management because implementing a comprehensive risk management plan involves "planning"—a Quadrant II activity that will result in fewer "crises"—activities that occur in Quadrant I. For example, if health/fitness professionals implemented many of the risk management strategies described in Chapters 4 through 11 (a Quadrant II

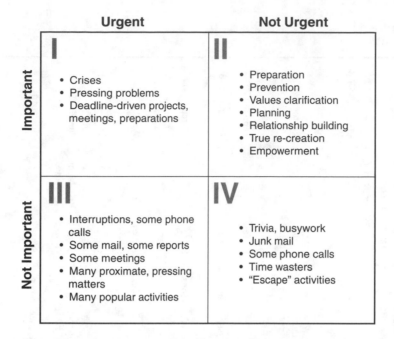

FIGURE 12-1 The Time Management Matrix (Reprinted with permission from Franklin Covey. *First Things First* by Stephen Covey, New York: Simon & Schuster; 1994.[2])

activity); it would lead to fewer medical emergencies and subsequent legal liability (crises situations in Quadrant I).

There are many strategic planning models to use when considering a strategic planning process.[3] However, a basic model applied to risk management could include the following steps:

1. Identify mission,
2. Select goals,
3. Identify objectives,
4. Identify specific risk management strategies,
5. List specific action steps for each risk management strategy,
6. Specify persons responsible and the applicable timeframe, and
7. Evaluate.

Steps 1 and 2 are discussed in the next section under Risk Management Policies and Procedures Manual and Step 7 is presented under Evaluation of the Risk Management Plan. Steps 3 through 6 are presented in the Risk Management Strategic Planning Template in Figure 12-2. This template is only an example. Many health/fitness facilities may have their own strategic planning model they use for other planning purposes that could be used or adapted for risk management planning. The template in the figure provides an example of steps 3 through 6 for implementing a risk management plan for "selected" risk management strategies involving pre-activity health screening procedures. By no means does this example describe all of the pre-activity health screening strategies described in Chapter 6 that should be considered. The written document, like the example in Figure 12-2, reflects the "implementation" phase of the risk management planning process. This document should be considered a "working document" that can be updated or changed as needed.

As indicated in Figure 12-2, it is best for professional staff members to initially take the lead in developing the risk management strategies and actions steps. They should draft written procedures and then have them reviewed by the other professional staff members in the facility. Then a second draft (if needed) is prepared to be reviewed

Objective	Risk Management Strategy	Action Steps	Person(s) Responsible	Timeframe
To implement pre-activity health screening procedures	Select the pre-activity health screening device to use or develop own.	Review applicable laws and published standards of practice as well as existing pre-activity screening devices.	Health/Fitness Director and Personal Trainer Coordinator	January 2010
	Develop written physician clearance procedures.	Establish criteria from the pre-activity health screening device that warrants physician clearance using published standards of practice.	Same	February 2010
		Decide "who" in the facility has authority to interpret data and make decisions regarding physician clearance.	Same	February 2010
		Develop a physician clearance form.	Same	February 2010
		Establish instructions on "how" physician clearance will be obtained.	Same	February 2010
	Develop written procedures for participants who refuse to complete pre-activity health screening procedures.	Review the ADA law. Establish guidelines for staff members to follow when this occurs.	Same	March 2010
	Develop a written draft describing the above risk management strategies— to be reviewed by all health/fitness professionals in the facility.	Set up a staff meeting for discussion and feedback on the "draft" procedures.	Same and all professional staff	April 2010
		Revise draft based on feedback.	Same	May 2010
	Obtain approval of above procedures from Risk Management Advisory Committee.	Send final draft to committee; set up meeting for Advisory Committee to discuss and approve.	Same and Risk Mgm. Advisory Committee	June 2010
	Include above procedures into the facility's Risk Management Policies and Procedures Manual (RMPPM) and train staff.	Insert the procedures into the appropriate section of the RMPPM.	Same	July 2010
		Conduct an in-service training for staff.	Same	July 2010

FIGURE 12-2 Risk Management Strategic Planning Template: Sample Using "Selected" Pre-Activity Health Screening Strategies

again by the professional staff members. When the draft is finalized, it should then be sent to the Risk Management Advisory Committee for their review and approval. The health/fitness manager should determine when the draft is ready for review by the Risk Management Advisory Committee. It is important to not waste the time of your experts on the committee. Therefore, it is best to have the written procedures well thought out and developed as much as possible prior to sending them to the committee members. It is also time efficient if they can address procedures for more than one area of risk management at the same meeting.

Considering all the risk management strategies that will probably need to be addressed, it can take a long time to implement a comprehensive risk management plan. If a health/fitness facility has very few professional staff members, it may take longer to do so than a facility that has a lot of professional staff members. Those facilities with a large number of professional staff members can divide up the responsibilities and can perhaps complete the risk management efforts more quickly. However, those with a large number of professional staff members may also have larger facilities and numerous programs and services, which may add time and complexity to the risk management efforts. As the written risk management procedures are approved by the Risk Management Advisory Committee, they should be included in the facility's Risk Management Policies and Procedures Manual.

Risk Management Policies and Procedures Manual (RMPPM)

Preparing a Risk Management Policies and Procedures Manual (RMPPM) is an important step in the implementation of the risk management plan. A policy is defined as "a definite course or method of action selected from among alternatives and in light of given conditions to guide and determine present and future decisions," and a procedure is defined as "a particular way of accomplishing something" or "a series of steps followed in a regular definite order."[4] An example of a policy statement could be something like "It is the policy of this health/fitness facility to have a written Emergency Action Plan (EAP) that reflects the standard of care." The procedures would then be the related written action steps that describe what staff members need to do when a medical emergency occurs. When preparing written risk management procedures that will be inserted into the RMPPM, they should be written so they are (a) in a concise sequence that makes sense, (b) easily understood by staff members, and (c) do not reflect too much detail. The last point can result in staff members having to remember too much, and it can also minimize flexibility given any unique situation that may come up. Therefore, when preparing written risk management procedures, it is important to maintain a balance between being "complete and thorough" and providing too much written detail that may add confusion or misunderstanding. It may be a good idea, where applicable, to write the risk management procedures using a sequential step approach including a brief description below each step.

Once written risk management strategies are completed and approved by the facility's Risk Management Advisory Committee, they should be inserted into the facility's RMPPM in an organized fashion (see Figure 12-3). For example, all the procedures related to compliance with OSHA's Bloodborne Pathogen Standard could be inserted behind a tab labeled OHSA's Bloodborne Pathogen Standard, procedures involving the Pre-Activity Health Screening process could be inserted behind a tab labeled Pre-Activity Health Screening, and so on. It is a good idea to have all risk management policies and procedures in this manual. This manual can then be used as an effective staff training tool (discussed later) and staff members can also reference it easily at any given time. In addition to having hard copies available in the health/fitness facility, it may also a good idea to have the RMPPM available electronically.

The RMPPM should represent the comprehensive risk management plan of the facility. It should also include an introduction or preface where step 1 (Identify mission)

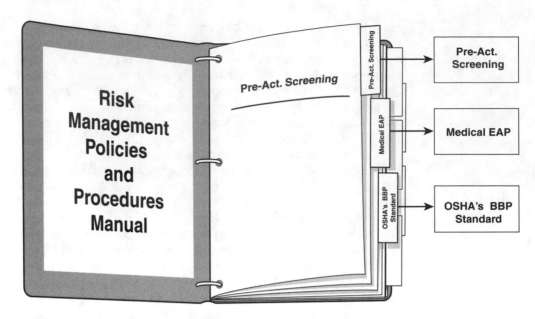

FIGURE 12-3   Risk Management Policies and Procedures Manual

and step 2 (Select goals) of the risk management strategic planning process are described. An example of a mission statement could be similar to the following:

> *The Risk Management Plan represented in this Risk Management Policies and Procedures Manual reflects the mission of _____ (name of health/fitness facility) to provide reasonably safe programs and services to our participants. We consider the safety of our participants our most important responsibility. We believe that these efforts also result in the delivery of high quality programs/services that will lead to increased satisfaction and retention among our valued participants.*

Here are some examples of selected goals (also referred to as benefits of risk management in Chapter 1):

1. To reduce legal liability exposures.
2. To enhance the quality of programs/services offered to participants.
3. To increase operational efficiency.

The next section in the introduction or preface should describe the "why." As mentioned earlier, strategic planning involves describing what to do, why to do it, and how to do it. The policies and procedures within each section of the RMPPM describes the "what" and "how" but may not include the "why." To help staff members comply with the risk management policies and procedures, they must understand "why" it is critical these are carried out properly. This section could include the "why," for example, how these policies and procedures reflect the facility's potential legal duties (standards of care) owed to participants, how they reflect applicable laws and published standards of practice, and how they (the employees) could be liable as well as the facility under the legal principle of *respondeat superior* if they do not carry out the policies and procedures properly. Lastly, it is important to explain to staff members (and to include a statement on the title page in the front of RMPPM) that the RMPPM is an internal copyrighted document. It should only be used by the staff members within the facility, and no part of it should be reprinted or given to anyone without obtaining appropriate permission. It is also important for facilities and professionals to appreciate that once the RMPPM is put into place, it may be discovered and reviewed in litigation involving the facility. As a consequence, the plan needs to be carefully developed and implemented and, most importantly, followed once adopted. A failure to follow a plan may well lead to substantial claims of negligence in the event of suit.

Staff Training

According to Mathis and Jackson, training is a "process whereby people acquire capabilities to aid in the achievement of organizational goals" and it "provides employees with specific, identifiable knowledge and skills for use in their present jobs."[5] The major goal of risk management for health/fitness professionals and facilities is to provide reasonably safe programs and services to participants. This is best accomplished by having well-trained employees who know, understand, and appreciate the importance of carrying out the comprehensive risk management plan that is represented in the facility's RMPPM.

Health/fitness managers and professionals who have responsibility for risk management should understand that many of their heath/fitness staff members probably have had little or no training or education in the law and risk management, as previously described in Chapter 1. Therefore, staff training programs in this area will have to include some basic background in these areas. Health/fitness managers and professionals may need to obtain the necessary education before they feel comfortable in leading the training efforts for their staff members. Of course, that is the main purpose of this book: to provide this education for health/fitness professionals.

The major cost associated with staff training will be staff time (salaries) as shown in Figure 12-4. However, the benefits of staff training (also shown in the figure) will often outweigh the costs. One lawsuit can cost a health/fitness facility a lot of money (e.g., hundreds of thousands, if not millions of dollars), not to mention the costs associated with any negative publicity that might also occur. Because staff training is essential in the successful implementation of a facility's comprehensive risk management plan, it is

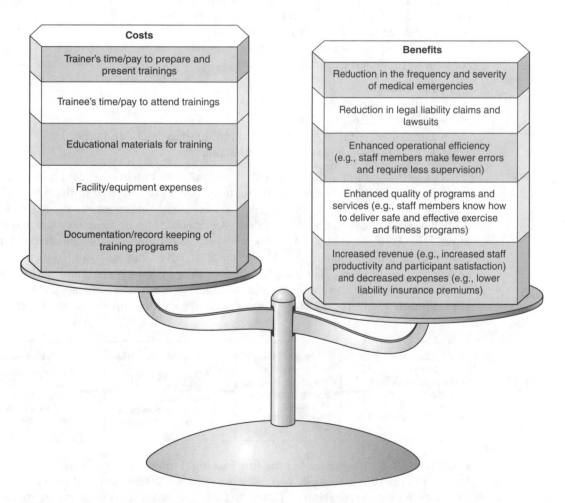

FIGURE 12-4 Weighing the Potential Costs and Benefits of Risk Management Staff Training

important to discuss the types of staff training, timeframe for staff training, and documentation of staff training.

Types of Staff Training   Three major types of staff training include internal, external, and e-learning.[6] Internal training is probably the most common type of training used in health/fitness facilities and involves both informal training and on-the-job training (OJT). Informal training occurs "through interactions and feedback among employees."[7] Examples of informal training include: (a) an employee asks his or her supervisor a question regarding a particular risk management procedure and then the supervisor answers that question, and (b) a supervisor notices an employee who did not implement a certain risk management procedure correctly then provides some retraining on the spot for the employee.

Unlike informal training, OJT (also referred to as in-service training) should be well planned and follow a logical progression of stages (see Figure 12-5). Because OJT is conducted by health/fitness managers and professionals, it is essential that they be able to effectively "teach" employees how to implement the risk management strategies in the RMPPM. It will be important to make the OJT sessions interesting for employees (see the first stage in Figure 12-5). Just describing all the risk management steps in the RMPPM they need to follow may be a boring approach. Starting with a relevant legal case that includes the issues (liability exposures) that apply to the risk management strategies presented in the training session may make the training more meaningful and interesting. The many cases presented in this book can be used for this purpose. In addition, having the employees perform/practice the tasks (see the third stage in Figure 12-5) related to the risks management strategies presented in the RMPPM will actively engage them in the learning process.

When designing in-service training programs, it is also important to prevent common errors[8] that include:

- Presenting too much information at one time,
- Telling without demonstrating,
- Lack of patience,
- Lack of preparation and failure to build in feedback, and
- Failure to reduce tension within the audience.

The first common error, essentially "feeding" too much information at one time, is essential to address. The entire risk management plan reflected in the RMPPM will be quite complex and will cover a lot of different risk management strategies. It will probably be necessary to break down the in-service trainings by various risk management topics. For example, a risk management in-service training session on the pre-activity health screening procedures should perhaps just cover this area and not attempt to address any other areas. The fourth common error lack of preparation and failure to build in feedback, also is important to address with risk management training. Health/fitness mangers and professionals, who are conducting the in-service trainings

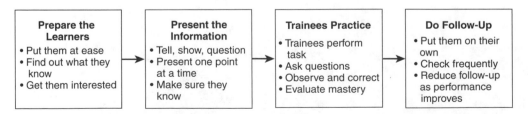

FIGURE 12-5 Stages for On-the-Job Training (From Human Resource Management, 10th edition, by MATHIS/JACKSON. 2003. Reprinted with permission of South-Western, a division of Thomson Learning: www.thomsonrights.com. Fax 800 730-2215[6].)

should have pre-established learning objectives for each training session, and a written lesson plan that includes specific learning activities that will meet the learning objectives. Employees who participate in the training should also have the opportunity to provide feedback (e.g., completing a short questionnaire to evaluate the training) so that this feedback can be used to make any improvements in future training sessions.

External training[6] may also be an option to consider when providing risk management training. This involves bringing in outside resources (outsourcing) to provide the training. Because the risk management strategies in the RMPPM will be specifically tailored to each individual health/fitness facility, it will perhaps be difficult to outsource the risk management training involving the facility's comprehensive risk management plan. However, health/fitness facilities may want to have some of their experts on their risk management advisory committee be involved periodically in risk management training. They should be familiar with most aspects of the RMPPM and can bring in different perspectives that not only help stress the importance of carrying out the risk management strategies correctly, but will help reinforce what health/fitness managers and professionals are trying to accomplish. External training could also involve officials from federal, state, and local governments. For example, when conducting a training session on OSHA's Bloodborne Pathogen Standard, a government official from OSHA could be invited to kick off this training session. When appropriate, using outside experts to address the many topic areas covered in the RMPPM can help add interesting and enjoyable dimensions to the educational process.

According to Mathis and Jackson, "e-learning is defined as the use of the Internet or an organizational intranet to conduct training on-line."[9] Using the Internet and an organization's intranet should be considered when planning risk management training. The many Internet sites listed as resources in this book provide excellent information that can be used when establishing the content of in-service training programs. In addition, employees can be referred to these sites to enhance their own learning or in preparation of an in-service training. Intranet training may be an ideal option for health/fitness facilities for their risk management training because it can be set up so it restricts access to only authorized users such as the employees. In addition to posting the RMPPM on the health/fitness facility's intranet, various online training modules could be designed and implemented. For example, a training module could be designed that addresses the procedures related to the facility's emergency action plan (EAP). Employees would read through the EAP information and then answer questions covering that information, which would then be submitted to their supervisor for evaluation and feedback. This type of online training may also be beneficial to help prepare employees for an in-service training session that they will be required to attend.

An example of a risk management training program conducted by an organization with multiple sites and including the use of its intranet is MediFit's Safety Call Program.[10] This program involves MediFit employees participating in monthly safety calls addressing emergency scenarios and training. Many of these employees represent sites in MediFit's Southwest region that only have one employee at each site, thus making staff training quite challenging compared to larger sites with several employees. During the calls, emergency scenarios (actual or hypothetical) are discussed along with strategies that could lead to a reduction in accidents or medical emergencies. The calls rotate among the sites, and the site that moderates the call is responsible for taking notes and sending a summary to all the other sites. The information addressed in these calls is then posted on MediFit's intranet so all employees can benefit from the information and training that occurred during the calls. Between 2004 and 2005, the Safety Call Program resulted in an 8% reduction in incidents and accidents and a reduction in OSHA-recordable accidents each year.

Finally, when considering the type of staff training, it is also important to consider how it will be delivered. Staff training can be done individually, in small groups (e.g., all personal trainers who are newly hired), or large groups (e.g., all staff members). The approach selected (individual, small group, or large group) will be determined largely by the specific risk management training objectives. For example, when providing training related to the facility's pre-activity health screening process, those staff members who attend should have "direct" responsibility for any of the steps involved with these procedures. If this involves only two to six staff members, all of them could attend one training session. If this applies to a large number of employees, it may be necessary to have two or three training sessions so there are not too many in any one session. Again, in each training session, the employees should be able to perform/practice the procedures (perhaps by using role playing/mock scenarios) and receive feedback from the instructor regarding their performance. An individual training may be necessary for a newly hired employee who will have responsibilities for pre-activity screening procedures. A different staff training session regarding the facility's pre-activity health screening procedures may also be necessary for those staff members who do not have direct responsibilities for pre-activity health screening, but who do need training to understand and support these procedures if ever asked by participants. This type of training could be offered to a large number of employees.

Timeframe for Staff Training   Health/fitness managers and professionals should be conducting OJT or in-service risk management trainings for their staff members several times throughout the year. Obviously when a new staff member is hired, orientation training will be needed with regard to his or her risk management responsibilities. Again, because the RMPPM covers a lot of areas, the training needed for a new employee should perhaps be divided into several training sessions and prioritized based on the employee's responsibilities. For example, a new fitness floor supervisor will first need to learn his or her risk management responsibilities with regard to supervising participants while using exercise equipment in the fitness floor area as well as the facility's emergency action plan (EAP). A newly hired personal trainer may need first to learn how to properly implement the pre-activity health screening procedures established by the facility and the facility's EAP. Once the priority training sessions have been completed, the supervisor of the employee should establish a plan so the remaining risk management training sessions are also completed in a timely fashion. Of course, it is the supervisor's responsibility to follow up by observing the performance of each new employee (see stage 4 in Figure 12-5) after training to be sure the facility's risk management procedures are being carried out properly. If they are not being carried out appropriately, retraining would be necessary.

Many of the risk management procedures in the RMPPM reflect tasks done on a daily or regular basis by staff members, for example, pre-activity health screening, health/fitness testing and prescription, instruction/supervision, and equipment/facility inspections and maintenance. Therefore, once staff members responsible for these procedures are trained and their supervisors have followed up to help ensure these procedures are being carried out properly; additional training should not be needed. However, some risk management procedures are not carried out daily, such as the EAP, which is implemented only when a medical emergency occurs. Although all staff members should be well-trained on how to implement the EAP upon hiring, it is something staff members could easily forget. Therefore, it should be the policy of all health/fitness facilities to provide EAP training on a regular basis, periodically throughout the year. The ACSM/AHA Joint PP[11] recommends the EAP be reviewed and practiced at least four times per year. These regular trainings should include mock emergency situations, perhaps some announced and some unannounced. In addition, follow-up EAP procedures (e.g., how to complete the incident report form correctly) need to be reviewed and practiced.

Training may also be necessary after performance appraisals are conducted. Performance appraisals are completed to evaluate employee performance and are usually done after an employee's probationary or introductory period, and then annually thereafter. See Chapter 8 for an example performance appraisal tool for group exercise leaders. How well the employee is carrying out his or her risk management responsibilities should be included in the performance appraisal process. If it is determined that an employee has not adequately performed his or her risk management responsibilities, follow-up training must be provided and then a reassessment of performance after a given timeframe.

Finally, staff training will be needed if, at any time, changes or revisions are made with the risk management strategies in the RMPPM (see Evaluation of the Risk Management Plan later). For example, if changes are made to the equipment/facility inspection procedures, these changes must be made in all copies (hard and soft) of the RMPPM first. Then, all those staff members directly involved in carrying out these procedures would need to attend a training session to learn and practice the newly changed/revised procedures. In addition, it will be likely that some changes with the facility's risk management plan will occur at least annually after the formal review and evaluation of the entire plan (see Summative Evaluation later). Obviously, when this occurs, staff members need to be retrained so they are well informed of the changes.

Documentation of Staff Training   As possible defendants, health/fitness managers and professionals may need to provide proof that they did indeed provide staff training. For example, a plaintiff may claim that his or her injury was caused by the facility's failure to provide proper training of its employees. Several of the cases presented in this book involved these types of allegations made by plaintiffs. For example, see *Chai v. Sports & Fitness Clubs of America Inc.,*[12] as well as *Capati v. Crunch Fitness International et al.*[13] and *Makris v. Scandinavian Health Spa, Inc.*[14]

Documentation is important to prove that proper training did occur. First, it will be important to document the dates when the training sessions were held and the staff members who attended each training session. It may also be a good idea to document the content covered in each training session—another good reason to have a written lesson plan for each training session. Documentation is also important for internal purposes. As employees attend and participate in staff training sessions, it should be documented in their personnel files. Their participation and compliance with the facility's required risk management trainings should be an issue that is addressed and documented during performance appraisals. In addition, documentation can help keep track of the staff members who have completed staff training and those who have not, therefore making it easier to follow up with those who still need to attend certain training sessions.

STEP 4 EVALUATION OF THE RISK MANAGEMENT PLAN

Evaluation of a health/fitness facility's risk management plan is conducted to determine if the risk management plan has met its goals and objectives. For example, each of the three major goals of a risk management plan (described later) could be evaluated using summative evaluation approaches. Most health/fitness professionals are familiar with both **formative evaluation** and **summative evaluation** models when it comes to evaluating their programs.[15,16] Formative evaluation is carried out throughout the planning and implementation of a program to identify any adjustments or changes that are needed. Summative evaluation, however, is conducted at the end of the program to determine if the program should be continued and/or modified before it is offered again, as well as to determine if the program was effective (e.g., did participants change their behavior and/or reduce their health risks, was the program cost effective, etc.). Although the risk management plan for a health/fitness facility is not considered a health/fitness program *per se,* it does reflect a "proactive administrative process" that can be evaluated using both formative and summative approaches.

FORMATIVE EVALUATION

Formative evaluation of the risk management plan could involve various aspects during the development and implementation phases. As risk management strategies are being reviewed, polished, and finalized by the health/fitness managers, professionals, and members of the Risk Management Advisory Committee, they are in essence being evaluated. For example, before the written risk management strategies are included in the RMPPM, questions to evaluate their purpose/effectiveness should be answered. These may include: (a) Do they reflect current law and published standards of practice? and (b) Are they written in a concise and succinct manner so that staff members will easily understand them? Formative evaluation should also occur after each risk management OJT or in-service training program. Feedback from employees regarding the training can be very helpful. It may be determined at a training that the written risk management procedures are not clear or easily understood by employees and therefore may need revision. Employees can also provide feedback on the effectiveness or helpfulness of the training and any suggestions for improvements for the next time it is offered.

Formative evaluation also occurs when a health/fitness supervisor observes the incorrect performance of an employee and then provides feedback to help the employee correct his or her performance. This can happen informally on a regular basis (e.g., a staff member is not completing the daily exercise equipment inspection logs correctly) or formally on an annual basis (e.g., performance appraisals). Informal feedback for a new employee can be particularly effective when it comes to risk management responsibilities because it can help the new employee obtain good working habits that are reinforced, which then, ideally, are continued.

Formative evaluation is especially important after a medical emergency has occurred. The health/fitness manager and professionals should review what happened and determine if the EAP was carried out properly by staff members, including the completion of the incident report form. In addition, it will be important to obtain answers to questions such as these: (a) Could the medical emergency have been prevented? (b) Is there an existing risk or danger in the facility that needs to be addressed? (c) Are changes needed with any of the risk management procedures? and (d) Do staff members need to be retrained on any of their risk management responsibilities? This type of formative evaluation may result in fewer medical emergencies and any subsequent liability in the future.

SUMMATIVE EVALUATION

Summative evaluation of the risk management plan involves two major approaches: (a) a formal review of the entire risk management plan, and (b) the measurement of outcomes, for example, have the goals of the risk management plan been met? At least annually, the health/fitness manager and professionals along with their risk management advisory committee should review the entire risk management plan and determine if any revisions or updates are needed. Revisions will be needed if laws and published standards of practice have changed. As previously mentioned in this book, the law is always evolving and it is critical to keep up with any new laws or changes to current laws. For example, several states have recently passed legislation (or are proposing legislation) that require health/fitness facilities to have an AED, and it is likely this trend will continue to expand to other states.[17] In addition, professional and independent organizations may have published new and/or updated versions of their standards of practice. Therefore, it will be important to revise the risk management strategies in the RMPPM to reflect these changes so the risk management plan remains current and is compliant with the law and the standard of care.

The summative evaluation process should also measure whether or not the risk management plan has met or is working toward achieving its goals. One way to measure if a health/fitness facility has met one of the main goals of risk management—a reduction in liability exposures—is to review all the incident report forms in the past year and ask questions such as these: (a) Have there been fewer and less severe medical emergencies in the past year when compared to the previous year? and (b) Have there been fewer negligent claims and lawsuits in the past year when compared to the previous year? If the answer is "yes" to these questions, it could be related to the health/fitness facility's risk management efforts. It is a good idea to track these types of data and to share outcomes not only with staff members, risk management advisory committee members, and others who also have vested interests in the facility (e.g., owners, CEOs, board of directors, etc.), but also with the facility's insurance provider. The insurance provider may value this effort by lowering the annual liability insurance premium for the facility. As mentioned in Chapter 1, some insurance companies are now providing this type of financial incentive if an organization has an active risk management plan.[18]

Another goal of risk management—to enhance the quality of programs/services offered to participants—can also be measured. A key component of risk management is to have qualified, competent, and well-trained employees who make every effort to teach and provide the safest and most effective programs/services possible. This effort will result in high-quality programs/services provided to participants, which, in turn, will not only help keep participants satisfied, but will help meet another primary goal of most facilities—to retain their participants. The quality of programs and services can be measured in a variety of ways, but obtaining feedback from participants through questionnaires, surveys, and so on, is an excellent way to determine if participants are satisfied with programs and services such as group exercise and personal fitness training.

Finally, a risk management goal to increase operational efficiency is an important one for health/fitness managers and professionals. Individuals in these positions have numerous responsibilities; risk management is just one area of responsibility. Therefore, one goal of health/fitness managers and professionals should be to increase daily operational efficiency; for example, spending less time putting out fires (crises activities in Quadrant I) and more time on activities that focus on continued improvement and expansion of programs and services, Quadrant II activities (see Figure 12-1). An individual's productivity is often determined by how he or she spends time and is usually measured at the time of an employee's performance appraisal. Mathis and Jackson define productivity as "a measure of the quantity and quality of work done, considering the cost of the resources used."[19] Following the basic principles presented here with regard to developing and implementing a comprehensive risk management plan (e.g., strategic planning, staff training, etc.) in all areas of operations can lead to high employee productivity. Although procedures related to all aspects of daily operations take time upfront to develop and implement, in the long run they will lead to time being spent on important issues that lead to increased efficiency and productivity, and decreased job stress.

SUMMARY

This chapter described the implementation and evaluation of a health/fitness facility's risk management plan. This chapter addressed the implementation of a comprehensive risk management plan that incorporates applicable laws and published standards of practice. This involves strategic planning, the development of a Risk Management Policies and Procedures Manual (RMPPM), and staff training. Once implemented, a health/fitness facility's risk management plan should be evaluated to determine if it is meeting its goals and objectives. Strategies on how to conduct both formative and summative evaluations were presented.

RISK MANAGEMENT ASSIGNMENTS

1. Describe the strategic planning steps your health/fitness facility will use to implement a comprehensive risk management plan.

   _____

   _____

   _____

   _____

2. Develop a table of contents for a health/fitness facility's RMPPM.

_____

_____

_____

_____

3. Develop a lesson plan for an internal (on-the-job) staff training program for any risk management area (e.g., emergency action plan, pre-activity health screening, equipment inspection/maintenance, etc.). Be sure to include specific learning objectives, the content covered, and a description of training activities that will help employees learn the risk management procedures in the RMPPM.

_____

_____

_____

_____

4. Describe how employee performance will be evaluated (formatively) after an internal staff training that covered the facility's EAP.

_____

_____

_____

_____

5. Design a summative evaluation strategy that will determine how effective a comprehensive risk management plan has been in reaching its goals.

_____

_____

_____

_____

KEY TERMS

Comprehensive risk
management plan

Formative evaluation

Summative evaluation

REFERENCES

1. Alliance for Nonprofit Management. Frequently asked questions. What is strategic planning? Available at: http://www.allianceonline.org/FAQ/strategic_planning/what_is_ strategic_ planning.faq. Accessed October 27, 2006.
2. Covey SR. *First Things First*. New York: Simon & Schuster; 1994.
3. McNamara C. Basic Overview of Various Strategic Planning Models. Available at: http:// www .managementhelp.org/plan_dec/str_plan/models.htm. Accessed October 27, 2006.
4. Merriam-Webster Dictionary. Available at: http://www.m-w.com/dictionary. Accessed October 28, 2006.
5. Mathis RL, Jackson, JH. *Human Resource Management*. 10th ed. Mason, Ohio: Thomson South-Western; 2003:172.

6. Mathis RL, Jackson, JH. *Human Resource Management*. 10th ed. Mason, Ohio: Thomson South-Western; 2003.

7. Mathis RL, Jackson, JH. *Human Resource Management*. 10th ed. Mason, Ohio: Thomson South-Western; 2003:289.

8. Sawyer TH, Smith O. *The Management of Clubs, Recreation and Sport: Concepts and Applications*. Champaign, Ill: Sagamore; 1999.

9. Mathis RL, Jackson JH. *Human Resource Management*. 10th ed. Mason, Ohio: Thomson South-Western; 2003:291.

10. Scanlin A. MediFit-Nokia wellness center. *Fitness Management Winning Innovations*. March 2006:18-19.

11. American College of Sports Medicine and American Heart Association Joint Position Statement. Recommendations for cardiovascular screening, staffing, and emergency policies at health/fitness facilities. *Med Sci Sports Exerc*.1998; 30:1009–1018.

12. *Chai v. Sports 7 Fitness Clubs of America, Inc.* Analyzed in: Failure to defibrillate results in new litigation. *Exercise Standards and Malpractice Reporter*. 1999;13(4):55–56.

13. *Capati v. Crunch Fitness International et al.* Analyzed in: Herbert DL. Update on litigation—*Capati v. Crunch Fitness*. *Exercise Standards and Malpractice Reporter*. 2001;15(4):56.

14. *Makris v. Scandinavian Health Spa, Inc.*, Ohio App. LEXIS 4416 (Ohio Ct. App., 1999.)

15. Grantham WC, Patton RW, York TD, Winick, ML. *Health Fitness Management*. Champaign, Ill: Human Kinetics; 1998.

16. Simons-Morton BG, Greene WH, Gottlieb NH. *Introduction to Health Education and Health Promotion*. 2nd ed. Prospect Heights, Ill: Waveland Press; 1995.

17. Herbert DL. New AED laws for health clubs in New Jersey and Michigan—one proposed in Kansas. *Exercise Standards and Malpractice Reporter*. 2006;20(2):17, 20–25.

18. Appenzeller H., ed. *Risk Management in Sport. Issues and Strategies*. 2nd ed. Durham, NC: Carolina Academic Press; 2005.

19. Mathis RL, Jackson JH. *Human Resource Management*. 10th ed. Mason, Ohio: Thomson South-Western; 2003:31.

CHAPTER 13

Selected Topics

LEARNING OBJECTIVES   After reading the chapter, health/fitness students and professionals will be able to:

1. Understand music copyright issues that can apply to health/fitness facilities.
2. Identify potential discrimination claims that participants could make related to eating disorders, single-gender facilities, and couples' memberships.
3. Develop a policy to address cellular phone use in health/fitness facilities.
4. Understand and appreciate the unique risks associated with unsupervised health/fitness facilities.
5. Describe how the final HIPAA rules and workers' compensation laws can impact employer-sponsored health/fitness programs.
6. Understand specific steps that should be taken after receiving a summons.
7. Understand how to select a lawyer and how a lawyer's fees are determined.
8. Identify a lawyer's role in the risk management process.
9. Understand the concept of attorney–client privilege.

This chapter is divided into three major sections. The first addresses some liability exposures that health/fitness professionals should be aware of that were not covered in the other chapters in this book, the second addresses liability exposures that are applicable to unsupervised health/fitness facilities and employer-sponsored health/fitness programs, and the third includes suggestions on what a health/fitness professional should do if ever named as a defendant in a lawsuit, considerations related to the selection and compensation of a lawyer, and attorney–client privilege.

SELECTED TOPICS: PART I

This section addresses copyright laws as well as potential discrimination claims that participants could make related to eating disorders, single-gender health/fitness facilities, and couples' memberships. Specific issues related to cellular phones are also included.

Copyright Law and Music Copyright Issues

In 1909, Congress enacted the U.S. Copyright Act that was designed to protect the work of artists (e.g., authors, composers of music, and others) from unauthorized uses of their creative materials and to provide financial incentives for artists. In 1976, this law was completely revised and has undergone several additional revisions in recent years to reflect changing technology and the Internet.[1] Canada has a similar law called the Canadian Copyright Act.

To obtain copyright protection under the U.S. law, the work must be original and in some tangible form that can be reproduced (17 U.S.C. § 102). It is not necessary for artists to register their copyrighted work. However, no claim or lawsuit can take place for unauthorized use until the copyrighted work has been registered with the federal government.[1] Copyright protection begins as soon as the work is in a tangible form and it lasts for 70 years after the death of the author.[1]

Although many health/fitness professionals are aware that the Copyright Act exists, its complexity and specific requirements are often not fully understood. Health/fitness professionals should consult with a lawyer who specializes in this area to address any copyright issues regarding their programs and services. The following discussion reflects general education information that briefly describes one of the major copyright issues facing health/fitness facilities: music copyright.

These are the three music licensing organizations in the United States and one in Canada:[2]

- Broadcast Music, Inc (BMI); www.bmi.com
- The American Society of Composers, Authors, and Publishers (ASCAP); www.ascap.com
- The Society of European Stage Authors and Composers (SESAC); www.sesac.com
- The Society of Composers, Authors and Music Publishers of Canada (SOCAN); www.socan.ca

These licensing organizations have the power to enforce the copyright law involving any music that is played within a health/fitness facility (e.g., background radio music played over a public address system, music used in fitness classes, etc.) as well as in other private or public establishments. Health/fitness facilities that do not obtain a licensing agreement with these organizations can face severe penalties, for example, paying damages ranging from $500 to $100,000 per infringement plus court costs and attorneys' fees.[2]

For health/fitness facilities in the United States, it may be necessary to purchase licensing agreements with all three of the licensing organizations because it would be difficult to determine and monitor whose music you are playing at any given time because of continual changes that occur with each licensing organization's song lists.[2] The licensing fees, which are based on a variety factors such as number of participants, square footage, and number of speakers, can be found on the organizations' websites.

Some health/fitness facilities may be exempt from paying music licensing fees under the Fairness in Music Licensing Act of 1998. This act, which was incorporated into the Copyright Act, allows some commercial businesses to use radio, television, and cable transmission on a limited basis (e.g., entertainment) without infringement.[1] In addition, the "home-use" exemption that was included in the revision of the Copyright Act in 1976 may apply to some health/fitness facilities if the equipment used to transmit the music is similar to the type of equipment used in private homes.[1] Additional requirements must also be taken into consideration for these two types of exemptions to apply to health/fitness facilities. However, it is important to realize that if any exemptions do apply, they generally would not apply to music used in group exercise classes. Health/fitness facilities often purchase tapes (e.g., "Muscle Mixes Music") to use in their group exercise program.[2] Although copyright fees are paid by the companies who produce these tapes, it does not cover the health/fitness facility's obligation to pay the music licensing fees.[2] Additional exemptions may also exist (e.g., if the music performance is used solely for nonprofit, charitable purposes[1]).

Health/fitness facilities that show movies using home videocassettes or DVDs may also be violating the Copyright Act.[2] Such products are designed for home use only. If they are shown outside the home (e.g., in a health/fitness facility's child care area), a public performance license must be obtained from the Motion Picture Licensing Corporation.[2]

Generally, unless exemptions apply, music (or any home videocassettes or DVDs) used in most health/fitness facilities is considered a "public performance" of an artist's work. Therefore, it will be necessary for health/fitness facilities to pay for the appropriate licensing fees to avoid any infringement of the Copyright Act.

ADA Issues: Eating Disorders

As presented previously in this book, two titles of the Americans with Disabilities Act (ADA) apply to health/fitness facilities. These are Title I—Employment and Title III—Public Accommodations and Services Operated by Private Entities. Previous chapters did not specifically address eating disorders, which can be considered a disability under the ADA. Therefore, this discussion focuses on what health/fitness facilities can do to help avoid violating Title III when providing programs and services to participants with covert eating disorders or suspected of having such an eating disorder.

Because individuals with eating disorders (e.g., anorexia or bulimia) often exercise excessively to lose weight, they often become members of health/fitness facilities. Health/fitness staff members may suspect that certain participants may have an eating disorder, but what should they do knowing that these individuals are often in denial that they have such a condition—and to prevent a potential discrimination violation of Title III of the ADA? There is no easy answer to this question, but the following suggestions can be considered.

First, it is recommended to educate and train health/fitness staff members about eating disorders. This includes providing information on how to recognize someone who may have an eating disorder via their behaviors (e.g., excessive exercise) and/or appearance (e.g., extreme thinness). In addition, staff members must understand that such an eating disorder can be considered a disability under the ADA (e.g., see *Shalbert v. Marcincin*, 2005 U.S. Dist. LEXIS 16564). Therefore, there are limitations as to what actions staff members can take.

Next, the health/fitness facility should have written policies and procedures on what staff members should do when they suspect a participant has an eating disorder. For example, once suspected, perhaps a staff member should first inform his or her supervisor confidentially before anything is said to the participant. Once agreed by two or more staff members that the participant may have an eating disorder, the health/fitness facility may want to have an established procedure in which a staff member (perhaps a health/fitness professional or a staff member the participant likes and respects) talks to the participant directly in private. IHRSA[3] recommends the following approaches: The staff member might begin by saying, "I don't want to offend you or appear to be prying into your private life, but I am concerned about your health." A direct approach (taken from "Out of the Dark," *IDEA Today*, March 1991) may be: "Mary, I've become concerned about you in the past few weeks. I've noticed that you have lost a lot of weight and appear to be pushing yourself very hard in class. I'm worried about your health."[4]

Health/fitness professionals are not counselors or therapists so any such discussion must remain within the proper scope of practice. However, health/fitness professionals can provide help to someone who they may suspect may have an eating disorder by talking to him or her in a discreet and respectful way and by referring them to a community resource(s). Health/fitness facilities should have established referral resources, not just for eating disorders but in other areas as well. Because an eating disorder may be considered a disability under the ADA, health/fitness facilities should not deny programs, services, or revoke the membership of anyone who they suspect of having an eating disorder. It may also be a good idea, after a conversation has occurred and a referral provided to the participant, to record/document these events in the participant's file.

In addition to the policy and procedures just discussed, it may also be wise to educate participants about eating disorders.[3] This can be done in a variety of ways (e.g., provide educational literature to new members upon joining, have personal trainers and group exercise leaders educate their participants, provide information on bulletin boards, etc.). This proactive educational approach (along with the policies and procedures just stated) may help shield some liability if a participant with an eating disorder becomes ill or dies because of the disorder.[3] In addition, it will be important to be sure that all participants, prior to participation, sign some type of an assumption of risk document and/or waiver (see Chapter 4) that informs them of the risks of exercise and that the health/fitness facility is not responsible for any illnesses or deaths caused by any medical conditions a participant may have.

One issue that often arises with regard to eating disorders (and other sensitive medical conditions such as HIV/AIDS) is whether or not the existence of these conditions should be included in the pre-activity health screening process. None of the sample screening devices provided in Chapter 6 include these particular, specific conditions. There are no published standards of practice that require or recommend that these conditions be included on these instruments. However, if a participant voluntarily discloses he or she has one of these conditions on a screening device (or in some other way), it will be up to the health/fitness professionals and their risk management advisory committees to develop policies and procedures on how to handle this situation properly. For example, would someone who self-disclosed an eating disorder on a pre-activity health screening device be required to obtain physician clearance as individuals with certain other medical conditions would be? A variety of factors should be considered before implementing policies and procedures in this area so these individuals are not discriminated against. It is also important to remember that once a participant does disclose any medical condition(s), this information must be kept confidential, private, and secure to be compliant with HIPAA and any state privacy laws that may apply.

SINGLE-GENDER HEALTH/FITNESS FACILITIES AND COUPLES' MEMBERSHIP ISSUES

Legal liability issues related to single-gender health/fitness facilities and couples' memberships can involve federal (e.g., Title VII of the Civil Rights Act), state, and local antidiscrimination laws. For example, in *LivingWell (North), Inc. v. Pennsylvania Human Relations Commission,*[5] the Pennsylvania Human Relations Commission filed a complaint against LivingWell (Elaine Powers Figure Salons) alleging that they violated the Pennsylvania Human Relations Act by refusing to admit men to their all-women health club facilities.

In this case, LivingWell had to show that their policy to offer women-only clubs did not violate Pennsylvania's antidiscrimination law by proving that (a) admitting men would undermine its business operation, (b) their female customers have a legitimate privacy interest in need of protection, and (c) no reasonable alternative existed to protect its female members' privacy interests while at the same time accommodating male members.[5] During the presentation of the case, the court determined that LivingWell met this three-prong test successfully. The court concluded that certain settings warrant the exclusion of opposite sex memberships, and a women's health club is one of these settings, primarily because of privacy rights. Privacy interests involved in exercise such as putting oneself in a compromising body position and self-consciousness about one's own body override any potential public policy issue that would involve the inclusion of men. Therefore, the court ruled that gender-based discrimination in this situation was not a violation of Pennsylvania's state antidiscrimination law because LivingWell "established that a legitimate privacy interest exists and if disallowed would undermine its business operations and there would be no practical way to ameliorate its impact."[6]

Some states have exempted health/fitness facilities from their antidiscrimination laws that generally prohibit gender-based discrimination in public accommodations.[7]

Individuals may conclude that these exemptions allow women-only clubs to discriminate but they do not allow men-only clubs to discriminate. However, courts may consider many factors in determining whether or not a policy of excluding one gender from joining a club (or exclusion from programs/services) is illegal discrimination. Men-only clubs are not necessarily in violation of antidiscrimination laws. However, cases in Massachusetts have occurred in which women have successfully won their discrimination lawsuits against private golf clubs where they claimed the club violated the state's antidiscrimination statute.[8] Because courts use a variety of factors to determine if a club violated any state or local antidiscrimination laws, and because state/local laws in this area can vary, it is best for health/fitness professionals to discuss any applicable laws in this area with their risk management advisory committees including legal counsel before providing any single-gender memberships, programs, or services.

Health/fitness facilities also face another potential legal liability exposure involving state and local antidiscrimination laws: couples' memberships. Several state and city governments have enacted laws that prohibit discrimination on the basis of sexual orientation.[8] Also, some states have passed laws that allow same-sex couples to marry, form a civil union, or register formally as a domestic partnership.[8] The primary issue for health/fitness facilities related to this matter involves discounted memberships.

IHRSA's published brief on Couples' Membership Discounts[9] describes a case in which a health club sold discounted memberships to heterosexual couples but not to homosexual couples. This practice was determined to be a violation of Philadelphia's Fair Practices Ordinance that bans this type of discrimination in public accommodations. Based on this finding, the club did away with all discounted couples memberships. IRHSA[10] provides the following suggestions, which some clubs implement when offering discounts to couples purchasing memberships:

- Any two people with the same address (proof may be requested);
- Any two people with the same last name (proof may be requested);
- Any two people who join at the same time;
- Any two people with a state or government-issued union certificate; and/or
- Any two people with documented proof of an official union (e.g., domestic partnership, civil union, marriage, etc.) regardless of whether it is recognized by the state.

As with single-gender issues, policies and procedures related to discounted memberships for couples also should include careful review of any state/local laws and a formal discussion with the health/fitness facility's risk management advisory committee including legal counsel.

CELLULAR PHONES IN HEALTH/FITNESS FACILITIES

Because many people use cellular phones, many public places have adopted policies regarding their use. Health/fitness facilities should consider adopting policies related to cellular phones (and pagers) for legal liability reasons such as helping to ensure the safety of members and protecting their privacy.[11] It is best to have a policy that does not allow participants to use their cellular phones while exercising. Participants who talk on the phone while exercising can easily be distracted, and the distraction could lead to an injury.[11]

In addition, it is important to ban the use of camera phones (especially in locker rooms) to protect the privacy of members.[11] According to Los Angeles attorney Anthony Ellrod, "a club operator who knows, or in the exercise of reasonable care should know, that camera phones are being used on its premises, could be liable to those surreptitiously photographed."[12] IHRSA[11] recommends that health/fitness facilities adopt a policy dealing with this issue and then communicate that policy in various ways (e.g., in the membership contract, posting signs in the facility, etc.). IHRSA[13] provides the following sample policy:

Please refrain from using cell phones or pagers in any area of the club except in the lobby . . . When in these areas, please keep the devices on "vibrate" or a very quiet ring, and keep conversations as short and as quiet as possible. If family or friends need to reach you due to an emergency, they may call the club and we will page you over the intercom and/or make every effort to locate you. If your occupation requires you to be 'on call' for medical, military, police, fire or related purposes, please inform the front desk staff upon entering the club. To protect the privacy of all members, camera-phones are not allowed in any areas of the facility. Anyone who violates this policy may have his or her membership privileges revoked.

SELECTED TOPICS: PART II

This section addresses two areas: unsupervised health/fitness facilities and employer-sponsored health/fitness programs. These areas present some unique liability exposures that are important for health/fitness professionals to understand and appreciate.

UNSUPERVISED HEALTH/FITNESS FACILITIES

Unsupervised health/fitness facilities are sometimes provided in the workplace, in hotels, apartment complexes, and even in traditional settings, particularly at some operational times in facilities that provide continuous 24-hour access by members. The standard of care applied in negligence claims/lawsuits may be different in unsupervised settings when compared with professionally supervised settings. For example, in *Smith v. AMLI Realty Co.*,[14] described in Chapter 3, the court used the *reasonable person standard of care* to evaluate these liability claims. When applying this standard, the courts consider two factors: (a) the defendant's burden of taking precautions and (b) the magnitude of the risks (gravity and probability) that are created. In *Smith,* a child was injured on a piece of exercise equipment in an unsupervised fitness center of an apartment complex. AMLI was found liable for the child's injury because the court ruled that the defendant's burden of taking precautions (installing a lock on the fitness center door and providing tenants with keys) was a very minor burden in comparison with the possibility of weights injuring children.

Health/fitness facilities that are professionally staffed would likely be held not to the reasonable person standard of care, but to the *professional standard of care.* As a consequence, the professional standards described throughout this book need to be used to meet the duties owed by professionals to their participants to help minimize their liability and to protect the individuals they serve. Although not always recommended, some professionally staffed facilities allow their participants to access their facilities at times when there is no staff supervision. Before making a decision to have a facility open for use with no supervision, managers/owners need to consult with their legal counsel and insurance provider with regard to whether or not they should allow such use of the facility and, if so, what special or unique precautions they should take.

Unsupervised facilities present a number of risks that are different from and to some degree enhanced when compared with supervised or staffed facilities. In these settings, various documents, including specialized releases/waivers, written warnings, and signage are very necessary to provide a facility that is as safe as possible given the circumstances of operation. In addition, those settings that provide both supervised and unsupervised hours of operation should provide their participants with a very thorough facility orientation before allowing them use of the facility during unsupervised hours.

Claims and lawsuits arising in this setting have not been as prevalent, however, as some would think, especially given the enhanced and increased risks associated with such facilities. Some claims and lawsuits dealing with unsupervised sports activities have arisen at the high school level;[15] others have dealt with claims related to the lack of adequate supervision while individuals have engaged in rehabilitative exercise activities.[16] Still others have focused on the differing duties that may be associated with the provision of just facilities as opposed to services. For example, in this regard, a 1986 case from Michigan[17] held that in the absence of special circumstances, a facility that merely rents space for a particular activity owes no duty to those using the space to supervise its use. This particular court of appeals decision dealt with the renting of court space for a wallyball game activity. The case might well have resulted in a different finding if, for example, exercise equipment and machinery had been provided along with the facility. In this regard, in *Thomas v. Sport City, Inc.,*[18] a court of appeals determined that "members of health clubs are owed a duty of reasonable care to protect them from injury while on the premises" and "this duty includes a general responsibility to ensure that their members know how to properly use gym equipment."[19]

One of the most serious concerns with unsupervised facilities is the lack of facility staff to provide any emergency response when needed—which is an obvious and inherent risk in these settings. When there are no qualified staff members present (e.g., no one with CPR/AED and first-aid certifications), emergency response when needed may be delayed or even not provided. Managers/owners of all unsupervised facilities need to give this issue serious consideration and take necessary steps to help prevent these types of scenarios.

Published standards of practice have provided some recommendations in this regard. For example, the ACSM/AHA Joint PP[20] specifies that level 1 (unsupervised) facilities (see Table 6-2 in Chapter 6) need to have an emergency plan and a telephone and signs in the room. According to the ACSM/AHA Joint PP-AEDs,[21] all health/fitness facilities are encouraged to have effective placement and use of AEDs. In level 1 facilities "such as those that might be in hotels, apartment complexes, or office buildings, the AED should be part of the overall PAD [public access to defibrillation] plan for the host facility."[22] The ACSM's H/F Standards[23] contain one guideline that recommends appropriate signage to communicate to participants that facilities are unsupervised, while highlighting the inherent risks associated with using unsupervised facilities and delineating those steps users should take in emergency situations.

None of these published standards of practice describe specifically what these steps in an emergency situation might entail. Obviously, having a phone with emergency phone numbers posted next to it is a good idea. But a person who is working out alone in this type of facility may not be able to get to or use the phone in a medical emergency situation. Therefore, some facilities have (a) encouraged a buddy system, (b) used emergency calling devices, and/or (c) provided remote video surveillance.[24] None of these options, however, equate to having a qualified staff member present to attend immediately and properly to an emergency situation.

In addition to the preceding, the following recommendations should also be considered:

- Having all participants sign a specialized waiver and assumption of risk document(s) (e.g., see Form 4-7 in Appendix 4, prior to authorizing use of the facility).
- Posting of a pre-activity health screening device, e.g., see Figure 6-1 (PAR-Q & YOU) and Figure 6-2 (AHA/ACSM Health/Fitness Facility Preparticipation Screening Questionnaire) in Chapter 6. Participants should be informed that it is their responsibility to follow the recommendations provided on these "self-guided" forms (e.g., need for consultation with health care provider before engaging in exercise).
- Posting of instructional placards and warnings on each piece of exercise equipment as well as the ASTM Facility Safety Sign (see Chapter 9).
- Posting of all facility safety policies that includes a policy regarding children such as "Children under the age of 14 are *not* permitted to be in the facility at any time; children between 14 and 17 years of age must have adult supervision."
- Posting general safety guidelines associated with exercise (e.g., warm-up, cooldown, signs/symptoms of overexertion) and including heart rate and rate of perceived exertion (RPE) charts.

Unsupervised facilities that contract with third parties to provide programs and services such as personal fitness training, group exercise, and so on, should be sure the properly written independent contracts are used (see Chapter 5). Health/fitness professionals that provide programs/services as independent contractors in these types of settings should develop and implement the risk management strategies presented throughout this book.

EMPLOYER-SPONSORED HEALTH/FITNESS PROGRAMS

A variety of legal liability exposures exist that are unique to employer-sponsored health/fitness programs. For a recent review of federal laws that can impact employer-sponsored programs, see "Regulatory and Tax Issues for Worksite Wellness Programs."[25] This article addresses laws such as the ADA, Health Insurance Portability and Accountability Act (HIPAA), Age Discrimination in Employment Act (ADEA), Consolidated Omnibus Budget Reconciliation Act (COBRA), and Employee Retirement Income Security Act (ERISA). Another article, "Preventing Legal Liability in Worksite Fitness Programs: A Proactive Risk Management Approach,"[26] discusses whether or not injuries resulting from participation in company-sponsored programs are compensable under workers' compensation. The following discussion focuses on the Final HIPAA Rules regarding program incentives as well as issues related to workers' compensation.

Final HIPAA Rules

Incentive programs are widely used in worksite health promotion programs as a strategy to encourage health behavior change among employees. Sometimes these incentives have been linked to the employer's health plan by providing lower premium contributions, reduced copayments, and lower deductibles for employees who reach a pre-established goal(s) associated with the incentive program. The initial HIPAA regulation of 1996 (P.L. 104–191) established "provisions that prevent discrimination against insurance beneficiaries arising from the application of a 'health status related factor' that affects coverage or cost to the individual under the health plan."[27] In other words, incentives related to the company's health plan could not be based on individual health factors such as cholesterol, blood pressure, smoking status, weight, etc., unless the company's incentive program met four requirements to be designated a "bona fide wellness program."[28] However, it appeared from this initial HIPPA regulation that "participation" in company-sponsored wellness programs could be used to provide employees with incentives linked to the health plan.

On December 13, 2006, three federal agencies (the Internal Revenue Service, the Employee Benefits Security Administration, and the Centers for Medicare & Medicaid Service) issued the Final HIPAA Rules in the Federal Register,[29] which now provide employers a clear set of requirements to establish their incentive programs to help ensure compliance with HIPAA. The term *bona fide* was dropped, and two types of health plan-linked wellness programs were designated: participation only and standard based.[25] Participation-only programs do not need to meet any of the final HIPAA regulations. However, those designated as standard-based wellness programs—those that link incentives to an employer's health plan such as by offering lower employee premium contributions, reduced copayments, lower deductibles, and so on, or surcharges based on an employee's health factor(s) (e.g., cholesterol, blood pressure, etc.)—must meet the following five requirements:

- *The first requirement limits the maximum allowable reward or total of rewards to a maximum of 20% of the cost of employee-only coverage under the plan (with additional provisions related to rewards that apply also to classes of dependents). The magnitude of the limit is intended to offer plans maximum flexibility while avoiding the effect of denying coverage or creating an excessive financial penalty for individuals who cannot satisfy the initial standard based on a health factor.*
- *The second requirement provides that wellness programs must be reasonably designed to promote health or prevent disease.*

- *The third requirement is that the program give individuals eligible for the program the opportunity to qualify for the reward at least once per year.*
- *The fourth requirement provides that rewards under wellness programs must be available to all similarly situated individuals. Rewards are not available to similarly situated individuals unless a program allows a reasonable alternative standard or waiver of the applicable standard, if it is unreasonably difficult because of a medical condition or medically inadvisable to attempt to satisfy the otherwise applicable standard.*
- *The fifth requirement provides that plan materials describing wellness program standards disclose the availability of reasonable alternative standards.*[30]

Employers should discuss these requirements with their legal counsel to help ensure they are meeting them before implementing any standard-based incentive programs as part of their overall employee wellness program. Compliance to these final HIPAA rules does not assure compliance with other laws such as the ADA or state insurance laws. Therefore, other laws also need to be carefully analyzed before any such program is implemented.[31]

Workers' Compensation

If an employee is injured while participating in an employer-sponsored health/fitness program, he or she may recover damages under **workers' compensation** statutes and regulations. Workers' compensation pays a fixed amount of damages for employment-related injuries that "arise out of and in the course of employment."[26] State workers' compensation laws establish a fixed amount, which generally includes only economic damages (e.g., medical expenses and a portion of lost wages).

Workers' compensation is a form of strict liability in which no fault is attributed to the employer or the employee. If workers' compensation applies, the employee cannot bring a negligence claim/lawsuit against the employer. Therefore, workers' compensation protects the employer from potentially high costs associated with negligence claims/lawsuits. The employee also benefits because he or she receives some compensation for the injury without the inconvenience and possible risk of not winning a negligence lawsuit against the employer.

To determine whether or not workers' compensation applies in employer-sponsored health/fitness programs, employers and health/fitness professionals should consider various factors that courts have used to make these types of decisions. For example, in *Price v. Industrial Claim Appeals Office*,[32] the Colorado Supreme Court established the following five factors after analyzing two applicable appellate court cases[33,34] dealing with employer-sponsored fitness programs. If any one of these factors is present, the injury would be compensable under workers' compensation.

1. Whether injury occurred during working hours
2. Whether injury occurred on employer's premises
3. Whether employer initiated employee's exercise program
4. Whether employer exerted any control or direction over employee's exercise program
5. Whether employer stood to benefit from employee's exercise program[35]

In its analysis of both appellate court cases, the Colorado Supreme Court ruled that the employers in these cases did not have sufficient control of the exercise programs and therefore the injuries were not compensable under workers' compensation. In both cases, the employees were exercising at off-premises locations. The plaintiff in *Price v. Industrial Claim Appeals Office*,[33] a prison guard at the Colorado Department of Corrections, was injured while exercising at home. He claimed his supervisor informed him that to retain his job, he had to lose some weight and therefore sought compensation via workers' compensation. The plaintiff in *City of Northglenn v. Eltrich*,[34] a police officer, suffered injuries while riding her bicycle in the vicinity of her home. She claimed that she feared losing her job if she could not pass a cardiovascular fitness test and therefore began riding her bike during off-duty hours. All police officers were required to pass a battery of fitness tests to demonstrate maintenance of certain fitness levels. The Supreme Court concluded that, in both cases, the injuries were not compensable under workers' compensation because they did not "arise out of" or were not "in the course of" employment—factors 1 and 2 above. The court gave greater weight to these factors "because these indicia of time and place of injury are particularly strong indicators of whether injury arose out of and in course of employee's employment."[36]

Employers and health/fitness professionals directly involved in employer-sponsored health/fitness programs should consult with a knowledgeable lawyer in the area of workers' compensation and determine policies and procedures consistent with state workers' compensation laws. In an effort to potentially protect against worker's compensation claims, one issue that needs careful consideration is whether or not an employee-signed waiver would be available for employer use to avoid such claims. However, because the laws vary from state to state, waivers may not be reasonable in these settings in some states to protect against these claims.

For example, in a case from Ohio, *Jones v. Multi-Color Corp.*,[37] an employer had its employees sign a waiver of workers' compensation benefits prior to participation in activities provided during an employer-sponsored fitness day. During a foot race that day, Jones suffered a heart attack and died. The family sought death benefits under workers' compensation. Prior to this event, the Ohio legislature enacted statutes allowing employers to have their employees sign a waiver that would waive their workers' compensation benefits for an injury or disability that could occur during voluntary participation in company-sponsored recreation or fitness programs. The waiver in *Jones* stated "waives and relinquishes all rights to workers' compensation benefits . . . for injury or disability"[38] but did not specify anything about dependents' death benefits. The appellate court held that the Jones could not, based on the state statutes, waive his dependents' death benefits, and that the family was free to proceed to make their death benefits claim under workers' compensation laws in Ohio.

An interesting question arises from the *Jones* case: If employers are allowed by a state statute(s) to have employees waive their workers' compensation benefits via a waiver for employer-sponsored health/fitness programs, would employees then be allowed to sue their employer for negligence? If so, this seems to defeat one of the main purposes of workers' compensation, which is to protect employers for potentially costly negligence claims and lawsuits. Again, it is important for employers and health/fitness professionals to consult with a knowledgeable lawyer regarding any state laws applicable to workers' compensation and employer-sponsored health/fitness programs.

SELECTED TOPICS: PART III

This section provides important information regarding the steps that health/fitness professionals should take if they ever receive a summons notifying them of the filing of a lawsuit against them, how to select a lawyer, and how legal fees are determined. In addition, how lawyers can assist in the risk management process and the concept of attorney—client privilege and confidentiality are also presented.

YOU RECEIVED A SUMMONS: NOW WHAT DO YOU DO?

A health/fitness professional's receipt of a **summons**—a notice that he or she has been served with a legal complaint and a notification of what must be done to answer or respond to it–can be an emotionally charged process. However, the summons and complaint and the process associated with the receipt of these filings must be addressed logically and in accordance with applicable rules and time limits for response. Although the rules surrounding this process vary somewhat from state to state, such service formally commences the adversarial judicial process.

Some individuals may attempt to avoid the service of a summons and complaint, but this generally is not a good idea. Ultimately, most judicial summons are served no matter how good a defendant or other litigant may be at attempting to avoid service. Moreover, the service process in many states is to attempt certified mail or personal service, and on a failure of such service, to then submit ordinary mail service to satisfy the process. Even though mail service in the United States is very good and there is a legal presumption that what is mailed is received, there is always a chance of nondelivery of regular mail or misplacing or losing such mailed documents somehow in the process. As a consequence, if the recipient does not actually receive the summons by ordinary mail, he or she may not be able to comply with the process or to answer the complaint and address the litigation in a timely manner. As a consequence, service by certified mail or personal service in litigation involving health/fitness facilities and personnel should probably always be accepted so the recipient actually receives the complaint, knows and appreciates the complaint, and can thereafter address the matter in a timely manner.

Once a summons and complaint is received, the recipient needs to note the actual date and method of delivery, review the documents, and notify his or her supervisor, if any, or someone in the business or corporate structure, if anyone, who is designated for notice of the filing. Thereafter and within a timeframe that would allow an answer or other responsive pleading to the complaint to be prepared by a lawyer and in situations where there is no supervisor or corporation/business involved, a lawyer must be secured and retained to defend the lawsuit.

How to Select a Lawyer for Litigation

Often many health/fitness organizations, particularly larger entities, have a lawyer or a law firm on an ongoing retainer who is the person to notify of the service of the complaint. In other situations, the agent from whom liability insurance coverage has been secured will be the contact person to notify as to the filing of the complaint. In this case, once negotiated by the agent, the insurance carrier will select a lawyer/law firm to defend against the complaint and notify the health/fitness facility and its personnel of that retention. If the facility or professional does not have a lawyer or insurance coverage, a lawyer needs to be selected directly and retained to defend the filing. Other industry sources, trade organizations, or even local bar associations can assist in the process for referrals to lawyers. Such professionals need to be selected on the basis of their trial defense knowledge and experience, their familiarity with the health/fitness profession, and their willingness to undertake the matter. Information sources like A.M. Best and Martindale Hubble—both directories for lawyers—can be used to locate experienced lawyers. Both companies publish hard copy directories of lawyers located in all areas of the United States and both maintain websites for these reference purposes: http://www.ambest.com/sales/AttorneyAdjuster/default.asp and http://lawyers.martindale.com/marhub.

Legal Fees

Most lawyers charge clients one of three ways for the services rendered: a flat fee for handling a particular matter that varies widely depending on that matter, its expected time demands, and other factors; an hourly rate, which can vary from $100 to $500 per hour or even more; and, lastly, a contingency fee, applicable in most plaintiff personal injury, wrongful death, and malpractice actions, which can vary from 25% of what is recovered to perhaps as much as 50% of any such recovery. For larger cases involving substantial sums that can be recovered, the percentages can be less and set by reference to ranges of recovery. Sometimes such fees are subject to court approval. Generally in all three situations, clients are also typically responsible for the costs and expenses involved in litigation.

For facilities that must defend against a personal injury/wrongful death/malpractice action, attorney's fees are almost always based on an hourly rate or sometimes a flat fee. In large metropolitan areas or with very experienced counsel, the hourly fee will be on the higher end of the hourly fee rates. Typically, most lawyers enter into a written agreement with clients to provide representation and to define the relationship. Lawyers may require a retainer—a deposit—to start representation on a case. Such a retainer is generally held by the lawyer in trust—pending the lawyer's actual provision of services when such fees are earned and paid from that deposit. Some law firms apply retainers to the services as they are first rendered; others hold the retainer for the last billing on a case. Hourly paid lawyers generally bill monthly, quarterly, or on some other similar basis. Monthly billings may be preferable for clients who want to be kept abreast of the fees and costs of litigation as a matter proceeds.

LAWYERS INVOLVED IN RISK MANAGEMENT

Lawyers can also be of assistance in the risk management process for facilities in efforts to reduce their risks of claim occurrence, claim assertion, and litigation. As stated previously, it is recommended to have a competent lawyer serve on the facility's risk management advisory committee. Most lawyers look at risk management as a process that might be defined for this purpose as follows:

> *Risk management is an ongoing process used to manage and reduce the risk of claim and suit in the provision of . . . [various] services. Risk management is comprised of several parts designed to:*
>
> 1. *identify relevant risks;*
> 2. *eliminate those risks which are readily correctable;*
> 3. *reduce perceived risks which cannot be eliminated . . . ; and*
> 4. *transfer those risks which cannot be eliminated, through the mechanism of . . . liability insurance.*[39]

For lawyers to participate in any health/fitness facility risk management plan, they must be familiar with a variety of issues, including the facility/equipment used in the field; applicable personnel matters; the use of releases, waivers, and assumption of risk documents; liability insurance; and published standards of practice. A number of lawyers are active in the health/fitness field and can be identified in applicable industry publications, including *The Exercise Standards and Malpractice Reporter, Fitness Management, Fitness Business Pro,* and other similar resources.

LAWYERS AND PRIVILEGE

The conversations between lawyers and their clients as to matters which are the subject of representation are privileged and confidential. Like the communications that take place between physicians and patients and clergy practitioners and parishioners, such communications are protected by the legal system from disclosure to third parties. It is therefore very important and beneficial to all attorney–client relationships that frank and ongoing conversations take place to solve the myriad of problems that can occur within health/fitness facilities. As a consequence, written communications between a client and lawyer should be labeled "Privileged and Confidential" to help protect such matters from third-party review. Although there are some exceptions to the privilege which may require disclosure of communications by a lawyer, such as where a client discloses that he or she is about to conduct a criminal act, or where client communications are made by the client in the presence of non-client, third parties, the **attorney–client privilege** should protect ongoing communications between lawyers and clients.

SUMMARY

This chapter addressed several selected topics that have provided information regarding additional legal liability exposures for health/fitness facilities. Part I addressed music copyright issues, potential ADA discrimination claims related to eating disorders, and issues related to cellular phone use. Part II covered liability issues that are unique to unsupervised health/fitness facilities and employer-sponsored health/fitness programs. Part III presented some basic information such as what to do if ever presented with a summons, how to select a lawyer, and the importance of the lawyer–client privilege.

RISK MANAGEMENT ASSIGNMENTS

1. Develop a PowerPoint presentation that could be used to educate your staff members about eating disorders and your facility's policies/procedures for dealing with participants suspected of having an eating disorder.

   _____

   _____

   _____

   _____

2. Develop a policy for your facility addressing cellular phone use and describe how it will be communicated to staff members and participants.

   _____

   _____

   _____

   _____

3. Describe your health/fitness facility's policy on couples' memberships.

   _____

   _____

   _____

   _____

4. Create a list of the types of signs that should appear in an unsupervised fitness facility and the content that each would include.

   _____

   _____

   _____

   _____

5. For health/fitness professionals directly involved with employer-sponsored programs, set up a consultation with a competent lawyer to discuss both the HIPAA final rules regarding incentive programs and any issues related to your state's workers' compensation laws.

_____

_____

_____

_____

6. Describe what you should do if you are ever served a summons and how you would go about selecting a lawyer to defend you.

_____

_____

_____

_____

KEY TERMS

Attorney–client privilege	Summons	Workers' compensation

REFERENCES

1. Moiseichik M. Copyright and patent law. In: Cotten DJ, Wolohan JT, eds. *Law for Recreation and Sport managers.* 4th ed. Dubuque, Iowa: Kendall/Hunt; 2007.
2. Music Licensing: An IHRSA Briefing Paper. International Health, Racquet & Sportsclub Association, Available at: http://cms.ihrsa.org/IHRSA/viewPage.cfm?pageId=927, September 2003. Accessed October 22, 2006.
3. Eating Disorders: Anorexia & Bulimia: An IHRSA Briefing Paper. International Health, Racquet & Sportsclub Association, Available at: http://cms.ihrsa.org/IHRSA/viewPage.cfm?pageId=912, January 2001. Accessed October 22, 2006.
4. Eating Disorders: Anorexia & Bulimia: An IHRSA Briefing Paper. International Health, Racquet & Sportsclub Association, Available at: http://cms.ihrsa.org/IHRSA/viewPage.cfm?pageId=912, January 2001:3–4. Accessed October 22, 2006.
5. *LivingWell (North) v. Pennsylvania Human Relations Commission,* 606 A.2d 1287 (1992 Pa. Commw. LEXIS 287).
6. *LivingWell (North) v. Pennsylvania Human Relations Commission,* 606 A.2d 1287 (1992 Pa. Commw. LEXIS 287):1294.
7. The Legal Implications of Women-Only Health Clubs: An IHRSA Briefing Paper. International Health, Racquet & Sportsclub Association. Available at: http://cms.ihrsa.org/IHRSA/viewPage.cfm?pageId=965, May, 2003. Accessed October 22, 2006.
8. Moorman AM. Private clubs in sport and recreation, In: Cotten DJ, Wolohan JT, eds. *Law for Recreation and Sport Managers.* 4th ed. Dubuque, Iowa: Kendall/Hunt; 2007.
9. 'Couples' Membership Discounts: IHRSA Tip. International Health, Racquet & Sportsclub Association, Available at: http://cms.ihrsa.org/IHRSA/viewPage.cfm?pageId=1427, June 2004. Accessed October 22, 2006.
10. 'Couples' Membership Discounts: IHRSA Tip. International Health, Racquet & Sportsclub Association, Available at: http://cms.ihrsa.org/IHRSA/viewPage.cfm?pageId=1427, June, 2004:2. Accessed October 22, 2006.
11. Cellular Phones in Health Clubs: IHRSA Tip. International Health, Racquet & Sportsclub Association, Available at: http://cms.ihrsa.org/IHRSA/viewPage.cfm?pageId=1104, February 2005. Accessed October 22, 2006.
12. Cellular Phones in Health Clubs: IHRSA Tip. International Health, Racquet & Sportsclub Association, Available at: http://cms.ihrsa.org/IHRSA/viewPage.cfm?pageId=1104, February 2005:2. Accessed October 22, 2006.

13. Cellular Phones in health Clubs: IHRSA Tip. International Health, Racquet & Sportsclub Association, Available at: http://cms.ihrsa.org/IHRSA/viewPage.cfm?pageId=1104, February 2005:2–3. Accessed October 22, 2006.

14. *Smith v. AMLI Realty Co.,* 614 N.E.2d 618 (Ind. App. 1993).

15. *Kahn v. East Side Union High School,* 31 Cal. 4th 990 (Cal., 2003).

16. *Rehabilitative Care System of America v. Davis,* 43 S.W. 3d 649 (Tex. Ct. App., 2001).

17. *Dillon v. Keatington Racquetball Club,* 151 Mich. App. 138 (Mich. Ct. App., 1986).

18. *Thomas v. Sports City, Inc.,* 738 So. 2d 1153 (La. App. 2 Cir., 1999), Analyzed in: Herbert DL. New judicial ruling: A failure to inspect/supervise equipment use can be breach of duty. *Exercise Standards and Malpractice Reporter.* 2000;14(3):41–42.

19. *Thomas v. Sports City, Inc.,* 738 So. 2d 1153 (La. App. 2 Cir., 1999):1157.

20. American College of Sports Medicine and American Heart Association Joint Position Statement. Recommendations for cardiovascular screening, staffing, and emergency policies at health/fitness facilities. *Med Sci Sports Exerc.* 1998;30:1009–1018.

21. American College of Sports Medicine and American Heart Association Joint Position Statement. Automated external defibrillators in health/fitness facilities. *Med Sci Sports Exerc.* 2002;34:561–564.

22. American College of Sports Medicine and American Heart Association Joint Position Statement. Automated external defibrillators in health/fitness facilities. *Med Sci Sports Exerc.* 2002;34:561–564, 563.

23. Tharrett SJ, McInnis KJ, Peterson JA, eds. *ACSM's Health/Fitness Facility Standards and Guidelines.* 3rd ed. Champaign, Ill: Human Kinetics; 2007.

24. Herbert DL, Herbert WG. *Legal Aspects of Preventive, Rehabilitative and Recreational Exercise Programs.* 4th ed. Canton, Ohio: PRC; 2002.

25. Chapman LS. Regulatory and tax issues for worksite wellness programs. *Am J Health Promotion: The Art of Health Promotion.* May/June 2007:1–12.

26. Eickhoff-Shemek J, Forbes, F. Preventing legal liability in worksite fitness programs: A proactive risk management approach. *Am J Health Promotion: The Art of Health Promotion.* 2001;5(3):1–12.

27. Chapman L. Update on another kind if legal risk: HIPAA. In: Eickhoff-Shemek J, Forbes, F. Preventing legal liability in worksite fitness programs: A proactive risk management approach. *Am J Health Promotion: The Art of Health Promotion.* 2001;5(3):1–12, 8.

28. Chapman L. Update on another kind if legal risk: HIPAA. In: Eickhoff-Shemek J, Forbes, F. Preventing legal liability in worksite fitness programs: A proactive risk management approach. *Am J Health Promotion: The Art of Health Promotion.* 2001;5(3):1–12.

29. 71 Fed. Reg. 75,013 (Dec. 13, 2006) (to be codified at 26 C.F.R. pt 54, 29 C.F.R. pt. 2590, 45 C.F.R. pt. 146).

30. 71 Fed. Reg. 75,013 (Dec. 13, 2006) (to be codified at 26 C.F.R. pt 54, 29 C.F.R. pt. 2590, 45 C.F.R. pt. 146), 75,021–75,022.

31. Simon TM, Traw K., McGeoch B, Bruno F. How the final HIPAA nondiscrimination regulations affect wellness programs. *Benefits Law J.* 2007;20(2):40–44.

32. *Price v. Industrial Claim Appeals Office,* 919 P.2d 207 (Colo., 1996).

33. *Price v. Industrial Claim Appeals Office,* 908 P.2d 136 (Colo. Ct. App., 1995).

34. *City of Northglenn v. Eltrich,* 908 P.2d 139 (Colo. Ct. App., 1995).

35. *Price v. Industrial Claim Appeals Office,* 919 P.2d 207 (Colo., 1996):210–211.

36. *Price v. Industrial Claim Appeals Office,* 919 P.2d 207 (Colo., 1996):211.

37. *Jones v. Multi-Color Corp.,* 108 Ohio App. 3d. 388 (Ohio Ct. App., 1995).

38. *Jones v. Multi-Color Corp.,* 108 Ohio App. 3d. 388 (Ohio Ct. App., 1995): 391–392.

39. Herbert DL. What is risk management? *Risk Management Reporter.* 1993;1(1):2,

CHAPTER 14

Conclusion

LEARNING OBJECTIVES After reading the chapter, health/fitness students and professionals will be able to:

1. Summarize the key topics addressed in this book.
2. Describe the Risk Management Pyramid.

This chapter is divided into two major sections. The first section is a summary of the book, highlighting the key topics. The second section presents the Risk Management Pyramid, a figure that depicts the layers of defenses to protect against not only acts of negligence but claims and lawsuits predicated on such concepts as asserted or filed against service providers.

BOOK SUMMARY

The major purpose of this book is to educate health/fitness students and professionals about the law, legal liability exposures, and risk management strategies they can implement to help minimize legal liability. The first chapter established the need for this book and also described (a) the types of risks (e.g., health risks and injury risks) that can occur to participants in health/fitness facilities and how these risks can lead to litigation, and (b) possible reasons for claims and lawsuits in the health/fitness field. In addition, risk management was defined as "a proactive administrative process that will help minimize liability losses for health/fitness professionals, and the organizations they represent." The following four risk management steps incorporated throughout the book were also presented:

Step 1: Assessment of Legal Liability Exposures—involves the assessment of programs and activities when evaluated against applicable laws and published standards of practice;

Step 2: Development of Risk Management Strategies—involves the development of administrative procedures that address the law and published standards of practice;

Step 3: Implementation of the Risk Management Plan—involves the implementation of a comprehensive risk management plan, using strategic planning and the development of a Risk Management Policies and Procedures Manual (RMPPM), as well as staff education and training; and

Step 4: Evaluation of the Risk Management Plan—involves formative (e.g., informal, continual review) and summative (e.g., formal, annual review) evaluation of the risk management plan.

Chapter 2 introduced health/fitness students and professionals to the law and legal system as well as many legal concepts and terms. This information is critical to fully understand and appreciate the information covered in subsequent chapters. Although many types of law are applicable to the health/fitness field, principles of tort and contract law are probably the most important for health/fitness students and professionals to appreciate and understand. Therefore, a fairly detailed description of both tort and contract law was provided. Negligence (one of three levels of fault under tort law) claims and lawsuits are common in the health/fitness field as demonstrated by the many cases included throughout this book. It is essential that health/fitness students and professionals understand the four elements that plaintiffs have to prove (duty, breach of duty, causation, and damages/harm) to win a negligence lawsuit, and it is especially important to understand how courts determine duty, which is covered in Chapter 3. In addition, health/fitness professionals use numerous types of contract documents (e.g., membership contracts, employment contracts, waivers, and informed consents) when carrying out the daily operations in a health/fitness facility, and therefore they need to be cognizant of the various aspects related to contract law so their contracts will be legally enforceable.

Chapter 4 presented common defenses (assumption of risk and waivers) that health/fitness professionals and facilities have available to defend themselves if they are ever named in a negligence lawsuit. These defenses can generally protect health/fitness professionals and facilities from costly negligence claims and lawsuits. This chapter described how these defenses work and provided many examples (e.g., sample assumption of risk and waiver documents) that may be helpful in the development of a facility's own documents. Of course, these are only examples and require legal review by competent lawyers within the jurisdiction (the state) where they will be used so application of any specific laws within that jurisdiction can be made before their implementation.

It is impossible for any book to identify and address all of the liability exposures that exist in the health/fitness field. However, throughout the majority of this book (Chapters 5–11), we have introduced the major liability exposures that health/fitness professionals and the facilities they represent can face. The topics covered in Part II of this book, (a) employment issues (Chapter 5), (b) the pre-activity health screening process (Chapter 6), (c) health/fitness assessment and prescription (Chapter 7), (d) instruction and supervision (Chapter 8), (e) exercise equipment (Chapter 9), (f) facility risks (Chapter 10), and (g) medical emergency actions plans (Chapter 11), were purposely selected to describe these major liability exposures and to provide related risk management strategies that health/fitness professionals can implement to help minimize these liability exposures.

Chapter 12 addressed the implementation and evaluation of a comprehensive risk management plan. Health/fitness professionals should realize, after reading this chapter along with all the others in this book, that not only is risk management one of their major responsibilities, but it takes a great deal of knowledge about the law to apply it properly through risk management practices. We hope that we have adequately provided such basic and needed knowledge in this book. In addition, the development and implementation of a comprehensive risk management plan takes good strategic planning skills, a great deal of time and effort, and a genuine desire of all parties involved to be successful. These individuals include health/fitness staff members, professionals, managers, and the facility's risk management advisory committee. Evaluating the risk management plan on an ongoing basis is also important because the law and published standards of practice are always evolving. Therefore, a dedicated effort to keep abreast of these changes is necessary to update/revise the risk management plan.

Chapter 13 covered a number of selected topics to help health/fitness professionals further understand and appreciate other areas of liability exposures, such as copyright laws, potential ADA issues including those related to eating disorders, issues related to single gender facilities and couples' memberships, and the need for policies related to cellular phones. It also addressed liability exposures that are unique to unsupervised health/fitness facilities and employer-sponsored health/fitness programs. Lastly, helpful tips were provided regarding what to do if ever presented with a summons, how to select and retain a lawyer, and how to understand the attorney–client privilege.

THE RISK MANAGEMENT PYRAMID

This book has presented a variety of liability exposures related to the violation of statutory and administrative laws (e.g., OHSA's Bloodborne Pathogens Standard, HIPAA, ADA, etc.). However, the major focus of the book has targeted negligence principles. Most of the case law examples described reflect the types of negligence claims and lawsuits that plaintiffs have brought against defendants: health/fitness professionals and facilities. The case law examples have demonstrated that sometimes the defendants were not found liable for negligence (i.e., they were able to defend/refute the negligence claims made against them) and sometimes they were held liable (i.e., they were not able to successfully defend/refute the negligence claims made against them). Health/fitness students and professionals must understand what they need to do to defend against negligence claims and lawsuits. Figure 14-1 presents the Risk Management Pyramid, which demonstrates the "layers of defenses" that health/fitness professionals and facilities can use to minimize their legal liability related to negligence.

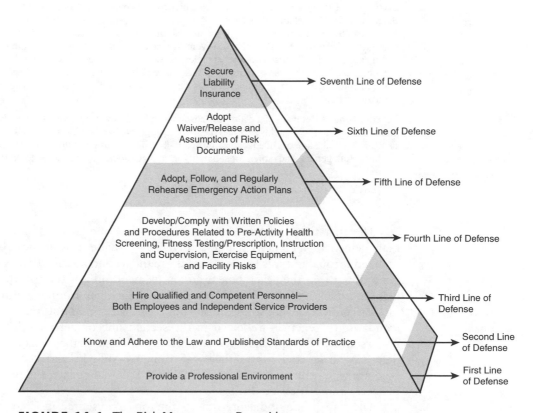

FIGURE 14-1 The Risk Management Pyramid

First Line of Defense: Risk managers and liability insurance company executives and underwriters have known for many years that a genuinely friendly, caring, and professional environment will minimize not only the occurrence of incidents that can lead to claims and suits but the actual assertion of claims and suits as well! As a starting point, such an environment should be created—not just for liability reasons but for business and professional reasons as well.

Second Line of Defense: Sadly, it appears that a significant number of health/fitness professionals do not know, understand, appreciate, or adhere to the law and published standards of practice. Health/fitness facilities must adhere to the law and should comply with published standards of practice. These standards are the established benchmarks of expected behavior for the profession and will be used to evaluate and judge the care that is provided in the event an incident which results in claim and suit may occur. Familiarity with such standards is clearly the starting point for compliance with the standard of care.

Third Line of Defense: Because all programs and services in any health/fitness facility are provided through personnel, the basic core for any facility's service delivery system will always be evaluated through those persons. Only qualified and competent personnel—be they employees or independent contractors—should be permitted to deliver service. Education, training, and certification and/or "national board" testing should serve as the basic starting point for all facility personnel.

Fourth Line of Defense: Based on the law and published standards of practice, all health/fitness facilities should adopt written policies and procedures dealing with pre-activity health screening, health/fitness assessment and prescription, and instruction and supervision provided to participants, as well as a variety of issues related to exercise equipment and the fitness facility. Compliance with these policies and procedures not only helps to prevent medical emergencies in the first place, but can also help defend successfully against any negligence claim/lawsuit by being able to demonstrate that no legal duties were breached.

Fifth Line of Defense: If a medical emergency does occur, it is important that a written emergency action plan (EAP) be in place to be properly carried out by staff members to meet the standard of care. Follow-up procedures such as completing an incident report are also important. To help make sure that these steps are properly carried out, staff members should practice all aspects of the EAP periodically throughout the year and possess current certifications related to the process (e.g., CPR/AED and first aid). Written and practiced EAPs can help mitigate a medical emergency and minimize any subsequent liability that may occur.

Sixth Line of Defense: If a court rules that a participant's personal injury or wrongful death was caused by the negligence of a health/fitness facility or its personnel, a properly written and administered release/waiver can protect the health/fitness facility from any liability for "ordinary" negligence in most states. If it is determined that a participant's untoward event was caused by the inherent risks of the activity (not based on negligence or in those jurisdictions where releases/waivers are barred or not recognized), an assumption of risk document (e.g., express assumption of risk, agreement to participate, informed consent) can help strengthen the assumption of risk defense for a health/fitness facility, which also helps to protect the facility from any liability.

Seventh Line of Defense: If a claim is filed, applicable liability insurance will provide a defense to the claim. In addition, if a facility is found liable for negligence, liability insurance will pay for the resultant damages up to the amount of coverage allowed in the policy, thus protecting the financial assets of the facility. Both general and professional liability insurance should be considered to provide this protection.

FIGURE 14-1 *(Continued)*

The first three lines of defense provide the foundation of a comprehensive risk management plan. The first line of defense—provide a professional environment—is inferred throughout this entire book, as are the second and third lines of defense. There is no doubt that the development and implementation of the risk management strategies described in this book will create a professional environment and enhance the reputation of the health/fitness profession. Knowledge about the law and published standards of practice—reflected in the second line of defense—is necessary to fully understand and appreciate the importance of risk management. The third line of defense—hiring and contracting with only "qualified" and "competent" personnel who are well trained—is essential so that the risk management plan will be carried out properly and professionally.

The fourth line of defense reflects the topics presented in Chapters 5 through 10. Compliance with the law and published standards of practice related to pre-activity health screening (Chapter 6), health/fitness assessments and prescription (Chapter 7), instruction and supervision (Chapter 8), exercise equipment (Chapter 9), and facility risks (Chapter 10) will not only help prevent medical emergencies from occurring in the first place, but also will help defend health/fitness professionals and facilities if a medical emergency does occur and a claim is later asserted. If defendants can prove they met the standard of care (i.e., did not breach any legal duties they owed to a plaintiff), even if the plaintiff is seriously injured or dies, it is likely the defendants will not be liable for negligence.

A written and practiced emergency action plan serves as the fifth line of defense for health/fitness professionals and facilities. If a participant is injured or has some other medical emergency (e.g., cardiac arrest), it is critical that the participant receives proper care. It appears quite conclusively through case law and published standards of practice that health/fitness facilities have a legal duty to provide appropriate first aid, CPR, and in many situations to have and use an AED if needed. The failure to do so can create a substantial liability exposure, as demonstrated through the many case law examples in this book. Some states have even passed legislation requiring health/fitness facilities to have an AED and appropriately credentialed staff members to use one in these settings. It is likely more states will continue with this trend. Chapter 11 presented risk management strategies that address this fifth line of defense.

The sixth line of defense involves the use of various protective legal documents (e.g., waivers, assumption of risk documents) that health/fitness facilities can have their participants sign "before" participation. These documents secured proactively, before activity commences, can help protect health/fitness professionals and facilities "after" a negligence claim or lawsuit is filed against them. Health/fitness professionals and facilities should never rely on these types of documents as their sole risk management strategy. They do nothing to help ensure a reasonably safe environment; nor do they help prevent medical emergencies. It is also important to realize that in some circumstances and in some states (e.g., Virginia) waivers are against public policy and therefore are not effective in providing this level of defense. Chapter 4 addressed this sixth level of defense.

The seventh line of defense—liability insurance—was covered in Chapter 5. Health/fitness professionals and facilities that have incorporated the many risk management strategies in this book—reflected in the first five lines of defense depicted in the Risk Management Pyramid—should be able to minimize significantly any negligence claims or lawsuits against them. However, if they are found liable for negligence (or if a negligence claim is settled out of court), health/fitness professionals and facilities need to protect their financial assets through liability insurance. The best way to do this is to purchase both general and professional liability insurance and to consult with legal and insurance experts to help ensure that all insurance needs are met through appropriate coverage and policies.

SUMMARY

We hope this book has provided health/fitness students and professionals with (a) the *what* (adequate knowledge about law and published standards of practice applicable to the health/fitness field), (b) the *how* (methods and strategies for properly applying the law and published standards of practice to the daily operations of a health/fitness facility), and (c) the *why* (good understanding and appreciation of the importance of risk management) related to the development and implementation of a comprehensive risk management plan in health/fitness settings. In addition, we hope that health/fitness professionals who take the effort to develop and implement a comprehensive risk management plan will reap its many benefits—minimizing legal liability, enhancing the quality of the programs and services provided to participants, and increasing operational efficiency—which all lead to increased professionalism in the field, proper service delivery to participants, and profits for health/fitness organizations.

Glossary

Administrative law Rules and regulations that have the force and effect of law and resolve disputes, similar to court trials, to determine if rules of administrative agencies have been violated and, if so, what sanctions should be imposed.

Answer Response of a defendant that normally denies some or all of the allegations found in the complaint and sets forth applicable defenses.

Attorney–client privilege Rule in the law of evidence that protects certain, private communications between a lawyer and his or her client.

Attractive nuisance Legal doctrine that states if land owners/occupiers maintain a condition on their land that attracts children and there are children around and the condition poses a possible danger, there is not only a duty to warn but also a duty to take reasonable steps to protect a child's safety who is drawn to the nuisance.

Bloodborne pathogens Infectious materials in blood that can cause disease and death in humans; these include, but are not limited to, hepatitis B virus (HBV) and human immunodeficiency virus (HIV).

Breach of contract Breaking a promise(s) specified in a contract; is not typically a crime or a tort, except in unusual cases; if litigation becomes necessary, the breaching party may be obligated by a court to pay compensatory damages.

Breach of duty Act, error, or omission that harmed the plaintiff.

Business invitees Persons who are explicitly or implicitly invited on health/fitness facility premises for the benefit of the facility. An example of a business invitee would be a dues-paying member or guest; see also **Invitee.**

Case law Court decisions that come from the judicial branch of the U.S., state or local government.

Causation The fact that the breach of duty, the negligent act/omission was what caused the injury; courts often use the "but for" or "substantial-factor" tests to satisfy the causation requirement.

Cease and desist notice Penalty resulting in a fine that can occur when someone has violated a state statute (e.g., practicing medicine or some other allied health profession without a license); fines can be charged for each day after the notice was issued if the practice continues.

Civil law Body of state and federal law that pertains to civil or private rights enforced by civil actions.

Common law A body of law that is created through judicial decisions; derived from judgments and decrees in ancient English courts.

Comparative negligence Negligence that is measured in terms of percentages of the parties; damages are allocated in proportion to the amount of fault (negligence) attributable to the plaintiff and the defendant.

Complaint Formal document that initiates a civil lawsuit; briefly states the facts and law the injured party (plaintiff) believes justifies their claim and requests damages, or other relief, that they are seeking from the defendant.

Comprehensive risk management plan Risk management plan that involves implementing risk management strategies that reflect applicable laws (statutory, administrative, and case law) and standards of practice published by professional and independent organizations.

Consortium Benefits that one person, especially a spouse, is entitled to receive from another by reason of relationship, e.g., husband and wife, see also **Loss of consortium.**

Constructive knowledge Prior knowledge of a fact, deemed by the law to have been reasonably known by an individual; gross negligence can result when a health/fitness professional knows about a problem (e.g., a hazard or risk) that has previously caused an injury but then takes no action to correct it.

Contract Agreement that can be enforceable in court; must meet four essential elements: agreement, consideration, contractual capacity, and legality.

Contractual transfer of risks Risk management strategy that transfers risks to a third party (e.g., a health/fitness participant via a waiver or an insurance company through liability insurance).

Contributory negligence Negligence on the part of the person claiming damages (plaintiff); under contributory negligence, if the plaintiff is even slightly negligent, they are barred from recovering any damages.

Criminal law Body of law that declares what conduct is criminal and dictates penalties for its commission.

Damages A loss; can be a physical and/or emotional injury to a person or property damage; compensatory damages cover economic and noneconomic losses; punitive damages can be awarded in addition to compensatory damages to punish the wrongdoer.

Defendant The person(s) or entity the plaintiff is suing.

Deposition Out-of-court oral examination of a witness taken before a trial; attorneys from all parties are typically present at depositions where the witness answers questions, under oath, which are recorded by a court stenographer; similar to interrogatories, deposition transcripts may also be used as evidence at trial.

Design defect Type of product defect that occurs when a product is not designed in a safe manner or when an alternative design could have been used.

Desirable operating practices Standards of practice (e.g., standards, guidelines, and position statements) published by professional organizations that provide benchmarks of staff functions, such as providing emergency care when an injury occurs, conducting pre-activity health screening, and inspecting equipment, as well as the credentials that staff members should possess.

Discovery phase Time period applicable to litigation from the filing of the complaint to the beginning of the actual trial.

Duplication Provision of a second set of documents (written and/or electronic) stored at another location to serve as a backup procedure in case the primary documents are ever lost or destroyed (e.g., in a fire).

Duty Obligation that arises from a special relationship between a health/fitness professional and a participant that requires the health/fitness professional to protect the participant from exposure to unreasonable risks that may cause harm.

Employee Individual who provides defined services to another party or parties or, on behalf of another (e.g., an employer where the individual as an employee renders services within the scope of the employer's authorization and under the control of the employer).

Engineering controls Controls (e.g., sharps disposal containers, safer medical devices, and self-sheathing needles) that isolate or remove the bloodborne pathogen hazard from the workplace.

Exculpatory clause Clause used in waivers/releases that specifies the exculpation of another; the release of another from liability.

Expert witnesses Individuals who are called to educate the triers of fact by sharing their expertise and knowledge through opinion evidence.

Exposure incident Specific eye, mouth, other mucous membrane, nonintact skin, or parenteral contact with blood or other potentially infectious materials (OPIM) that results from the performance of an employee's duties.

Express assumption of risk Written or contractual assumption of risk; see also **Primary assumption of risk** and **Secondary assumption of risk**.

Fact witnesses Individuals who are called because they have specific information (perhaps something they saw, heard, or felt) regarding the alleged incident in question.

Fiduciary relationship Special type of relationship that is formed between professionals and the persons they serve, such as a lawyer–client, agent–professional athlete, and perhaps personal trainer–client, and requires additional duties on part of the professional (i.e., good faith, trust, special confidence, and candor).

Formative evaluation Type of evaluation that is conducted throughout the year on an ongoing basis and during the development/implementation phases of the facility's risk management plan to identify any adjustments or changes that are needed.

General supervision Type of supervision in which the supervisor has the responsibility for overseeing an activity (e.g., supervising the fitness floor and observing participants as they use the exercise equipment).

Governmental immunity Type of immunity that originally barred liability claims against governmental entities, although not, typically, against their individual employees; however, the federal and state governments have passed varying degrees of tort claims legislation that permit injured parties to sue governmental entities under certain circumstances.

Gross negligence Conscious or other voluntary act or omission that involves a reckless disregard of a legal duty and of the consequences to the plaintiff; also referred to as reckless or willful/wanton conduct by which the plaintiff may recover punitive damages.

Handwashing facilities Facility that provides an adequate supply of running potable water, soap, and single-use towels or hot air drying machine.

Health risks Certain medical conditions and/or medical risk factors that can lead to medical emergencies such as cardiac arrest or stroke.

Indemnify Term used to reflect a promise to protect and hold another harmless from legal action and its attendant costs.

Independent contractor Individual who provides services to or for another pursuant to a contract or an agreement under circumstances where the individual as an independent contractor controls the manner and method of service delivery.

Inherent risks Medical emergencies caused by health or injury risks that are inseparable from physical activity or sport; they just sometimes happen due to participation in the activity and are no one's fault.

Injunction Court order that requires an individual or a property owner to do something or to refrain from doing something.

Injury risks Conditions or situations that can lead to medical emergencies such as back injuries and fractured bones.

Intentional tort Tort that requires intent (or purpose) on behalf of the defendant to injure or cause harm.

Interrogatory Set of written questions sent by an attorney representing one party in the lawsuit to the other party involved in the suit, which must be answered under oath, within a certain time period, and may be used as evidence in trial.

Invitee Person who goes on the premises of a land owner/occupier with the express or implied invitation of the land owner/occupier for their mutual advantage; the land owner/occupier owes a duty to act reasonably toward an invitee regarding the activities/conditions on the land, which involves reasonable inspection of the property for dangers and to reasonably repair and/or warn of dangers; see also **Business invitees.**

Legal liability exposure Any situation that (a) creates the probability of medical emergencies occurring, (b) increases the severity when a medical emergency occurs, or (c) reflects nonadherence to laws and published standards of practice.

Liability losses Type of accidental loss related to liability factors (e.g., legal claims or lawsuits due to the negligence of an organization or its personnel).

Licensee Person who enters the premises of a land owner/occupier with the express or implied permission of the land owner/occupier but only for his or her own purposes; the land owner/occupier owes a duty of warning a licensee of any dangerous conditions that exist on the premises if actually known by the land owner/occupier.

Loss of consortium Cause of action, usually by a spouse, for interference by a third party with the relationship of that person with his or her spouse; see also **Consortium.**

Loss of parental consortium Cause of action, by a child, for interference by a third party with the relationship of that person with his or her parent.

Loss prevention Risk management strategies that eliminate or reduce the frequency of medical emergencies occurring (e.g., conducting pre-activity health screening, providing safe instruction, and inspecting exercise equipment).

Loss reduction Risk management strategies that lower the severity of liability loss when medical emergencies occur such as staff members providing appropriate emergency care.

Manufacturing defect Type of product defect that occurs when a product is not manufactured as it was intended to be.

Marketing defect Type of product defect that occurs because of inadequate instructions or warnings.

Negligence Actionable cause of injury due to the fault of the participant and/or the health/fitness facility and its personnel.

Negligence *per se* Type of ordinary negligence that can result from the violation of a state statute; the plaintiff does not have to prove negligence as he or she would in an ordinary negligence case, but does have to show that the violation of the statute caused the harm the statute was intended to prevent and that the victim was in a class of persons the statute was designed to protect.

Occupational exposure Reasonably anticipated skin, eye, mucous membrane, or parenteral contact with blood or other potentially infectious materials (OPIM) that may result from the performance of an employee's job duties.

Ostensible agents Agents who are legally determined to be acting on behalf of another because of the existence of particular facts that tend to demonstrate that agency; these circumstances arise where it appears that the person providing services is an employee or is otherwise so closely connected with the facility that the entity should be liable for his or her actions.

Other potentially infectious materials (OPIM) Body fluids including semen, vaginal secretions, cerebrospinal fluid, synovial fluid, pleural fluid, peritoneal fluid, pericardial fluid, amniotic fluid, saliva in dental procedures, and any other body fluid that is visibly contaminated with blood; they also include any unfixed tissue or organs (other than intact skin) from a human (living or dead), and HIV-containing cell or tissue cultures, organ cultures, and HIV- or HBV-containing culture medium or other solutions, and blood, organs, or other tissues from experimental animals infected with HIV or HBV.

Personal protective equipment Specialized clothing or equipment worn by an employee for protection against a hazard; general work clothes (e.g., uniform, pants, shirts) not intended to function as protection against a hazard are not considered personal protective equipment.

Plaintiff Party who is bringing the lawsuit.

Pleadings The complaint, answer, and other court-filed documents when taken together.

Pre-Activity Health Screening Process Process that involves three major steps: (a) obtaining health information from a participant using some type of a screening device, (b) determining from the health information obtained whether or not the participant should obtain physician clearance, and (c) informing participants of the inherent risks associated with physical activity prior to participation.

Precedent Term referring to a rule or decision made by a court of law that is then followed by future courts in similar cases.

Primary assumption of risk Asserted defense to a negligence claim or lawsuit that involves the plaintiff assuming well-known inherent risks to participating in the activity; a personal injury action wherein the defendant claims that no duty whatsoever was owed to the injured party.

Primary sources Law created by the executive, judicial, and legislative branches of government.

Procedural law That part of the law that prescribes the steps for having a right or duty judicially enforced.

Product liability Type of liability imposed on a manufacturer of a product (and/or distributor) because the product is negligently manufactured, distributed, or sold; liability imposed on the manufacturer for a defect (design, manufacturing, and/or marketing) in a product that makes it unreasonably dangerous to the user; the manufacturer is liable for injuries as long as the product was being used in a foreseeable manner.

Public policy Court determination about what is in the best interest of society; in the context of the enforceability of prospectively executed waiver/release documents, public policy considerations sometimes are defined and used by courts to determine whether or not such documents should be given judicial sanction or, in other words, whether they should be enforced.

Remand Appellate court's decision to send the case back to a lower court for a new trial in compliance with the appellate court's instructions.

Request to produce evidence Request by one party to another to produce, and allow for the inspection of, any designated physical evidence that they currently control or possess, and that is believed to be relevant to the lawsuit.

Respondeat superior Legal doctrine in which a plaintiff can sue multiple defendants for negligence because of a negligent act of one employee; this doctrine imposes vicarious, indirect liability on employers for the wrongful acts of their employees that occur when the employee is on the job.

Risk Element of danger; two categories of risks exist in the health/fitness field, health risks and injury risks, which can both lead to medical emergencies.

Risk management Proactive administrative process that will help minimize liability losses for health/fitness professionals and the organizations they represent.

Risk Management Advisory Committee Committee made up of experts (e.g., from risk management, legal, insurance, medical, and exercise science professions) who assist health/fitness professionals in the risk management decision-making process.

Risk stratification Process that places a participant into a certain risk category using health history data that can then be used to make decisions regarding the need for physician clearance or medical evaluation, as well as what type of health/fitness facility and/or program(s) would best meet the individual's needs.

Scope of practice Activities in which a professional engages when carrying out his or her practice that are within the boundaries or limitations of that particular profession (e.g., health/fitness professionals should practice within the limitations of their education, training, experience, and certification).

Secondary assumption of risk/implied assumption of risk Asserted defense in which the issue is whether or not a particular risk was assumed in a given activity where the participant knows that another has already acted in a negligent manner or will do so, or where established procedures, protocols, rules, or warnings are not followed.

Secondary sources Legal sources that analyze, inform, or summarize various legal topics and issues that are not binding upon courts as precedent or as statutes or regulations.

Specific supervision Type of supervision in which the supervisor is "directly" with an individual or small group and most often involves an "instructional" format.

Standard of care Duty (or degree of care) that is required of a reasonably prudent person acting in the same or similar circumstances.

Stare decisis Legal doctrine that means "it stands decided" and is another term for precedent, which states that if a particular factual dispute has been decided in court and if the same factual dispute arises again, it must be resolved the same way as it was earlier.

Statute of frauds Provision that requires certain types of contracts be written in order to be enforceable.

Statutes of limitations Period of time within which a lawsuit must be filed; usually set by state statutes for personal injury/wrongful death actions, sometimes set at one year or more years, but varies by state; also applies in federal lawsuits and is then set by federal statute.

Statutory law Body of law that has been enacted through our legislative process and is often termed the written law.

Strict liability Type of liability that is not based on fault but instead on public policy; in certain situations, the injured plaintiff does not need to prove intent or negligence; the defendant is liable even if not at fault.

Substantive law Part of the law that establishes the rights and duties of parties.

Sudden cardiac arrest (SCA) Condition when a person's heart stops beating and no longer circulates blood.

Summary judgment Procedural device in which the moving party, the one that requests summary judgment, argues there are not any significant questions of fact and the applicable case law requires that they be awarded judgment; this motion may be made when a party believes discovery has shown there are no real disputes as to the facts; if the motion is granted, a trial will not occur.

Summative evaluation Type of formal evaluation that is conducted annually to address any changes in the laws or published standards of practice and to measure how effective the risk management plan has been in achieving its goals.

Summons Notice commonly delivered by a court officer that informs the defendant a lawsuit has been filed against them and gives them a prescribed amount of time to respond to the complaint.

Technical physical specifications Standards of practice published by independent agencies such as CPSC (Consumer Product Safety Commission) and ASTM (American Society for Testing and Materials) that provide specifications on equipment and facilities.

Tort Conduct that amounts to a legal wrong that also causes harm on which the courts will impose civil liability.

Transitional supervision Type of supervision that involves changing from specific to general and back, perhaps several times during any supervisory session.

Trespasser Person who enters the premises of a land owner/occupier without the permission of the land owner/occupier or without a legal right to do so; the land owner/occupier has no duty in most cases except to refrain from intentionally or willfully injuring the trespasser.

Triers of fact The jury and/or court (judge) whose purpose is to declare the truth based on evidence presented to them.

Unenforceable contract Type of contract that violates a statute or is contrary to public policy.

Universal precautions Approach to infection control whereby all human blood and certain human body fluids are treated as if known to be infectious for HIV, HBV, and other bloodborne pathogens.

Vicarious liability Indirect liability of an employer for the wrongful acts of their employees that occur when the employee is on the job.

Voidable contract Type of contract when an essential element is missing; the contract is said to be voidable, e.g., made by one who lacks legal capacity, for example, a minor, and either party may withdraw without liability.

Work practice controls Controls that reduce the likelihood of exposure by altering the manner in which a task is performed (e.g., prohibiting recapping of needles by using a two-handed technique).

Workers' compensation Type of strict liability in which the employer is liable for injuries sustained by an employee that arise out of or are in the course of employment; no negligence is assumed on part of the employer or employee and state laws establish fixed damages awarded to employees or their dependents.

Case Index

Case Law by Chapter

The following cases, listed by chapter, are found in the text. Those in **boldface** are described in more than one chapter. The page number where they appear is provided in parentheses.

Index

Page numbers followed by *f* denote figures; those followed by *t* denote tables.